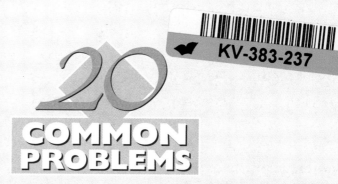

KV-383-237

20 COMMON PROBLEMS

Surgical Problems and Procedures in Primary Care

EDITORS

DANA CHRISTIAN LYNGE, M.D.

Staff Surgeon
VA Puget Sound Health Care System
Assistant Professor, Department of Surgery
University of Washington School of Medicine
Seattle, Washington

BARRY D. WEISS, M.D.

Professor of Clinical Family and Community Medicine
University of Arizona College of Medicine
Tucson, Arizona

SERIES EDITOR

BARRY D. WEISS, M.D.

McGraw-Hill
Medical Publishing Division

New York   St. Louis   San Francisco   Auckland   Bogotá   Caracas   Lisbon   London   Madrid
Mexico City   Milan   Montreal   New Delhi   San Juan   Singapore   Sydney   Tokyo   Toronto

McGraw-Hill

A Division of The **McGraw·Hill** Companies

**20 COMMON PROBLEMS: SURGICAL PROBLEMS AND
PROCEDURES IN PRIMARY CARE**

1 2 3 4 5 6 7 8 9 0 DOC/DOC 0 9 8 7 6 5 4 3 2 1 0

ISBN 0-07-136002-6

This book was set in Garamond by V&M Graphics, Inc.
The editors were Andrea Seils and Susan R. Noujaim.
The production supervisor was Phil Galea.
Project management was provided by Andover Publishing Services.
The cover designer was Marsha Cohen/Parallelogram.
R. R. Donnelley and Sons Company was printer and binder.

This book is printed on acid-free paper.

Library of Congress Cataloging-in-Publication Data

20 common problems: surgical problems and procedures in primary care /
[edited by] Dana Christian Lynge, Barry D. Weiss.
    p.   ;   cm.
Includes bibliographical references and index.
ISBN 0-07-136002-6
        1. Surgery—Complications. 2. Therapeutics, Surgical. 3. Primary care
    (Medical care). I. Title: Twenty common problems in surgery for primary care
    clinicians. II. Lynge, Dana Christian. III. Weiss, Barry D.
        [DNLM: 1. Surgical Procedures, Operative. WO 500 Z999 2001]
RD31.5.A14 2001
617'.9—dc21   00–032922

To our patients
from whom we have learned so much

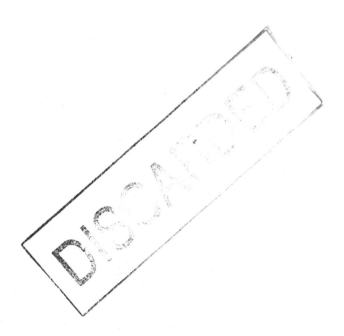

Contents

A color insert falls between pages 304 and 305.

Contributors

Benjamin O. Anderson, M.D.
Medical Director
BioClinical Breast Care Program
Associate Professor of Surgical Oncology
Department of Surgery
University of Washington School of Medicine
Seattle, Washington

Thomas J. Burke, M.D.
Southcentral Foundation Women's Health Service
Alaska Native Medical Center
Anchorage, Alaska

Wallace H.J. Chang, M.D.
Clinical Professor of Plastic Surgery
University of Washington School of Medicine
Seattle, Washington

Jimmy Y. Chung, M.D.
Chief Resident in Surgery
Department of Surgery
University of Washington School of Medicine
Seattle, Washington

John M. Corman, M.D.
Assistant Professor
Department of Urology
University of Washington School of Medicine
Seattle, Washington

Todd G. Dray, M.D.
Assistant Chief
Otolaryngology–Head and Neck Surgery
Kaiser Permanente
Santa Clara, California

Benjamin A. Garnett, M.D.
Southcentral Foundation Women's Health Service
Alaska Native Medical Center
Anchorage, Alaska

David M. Heimbach, M.D.
Professor of Surgery
Director, University of Washington Burn Center
Harborview Medical Center
Seattle, Washington

Robert L. Hogue, M.D.
Assistant Clinical Professor
Texas Tech University Health Science Center
Lubbock, Texas
Active Staff
Brownwood Regional Medical Center
Brownwood, Texas

F. Frank Isik, M.D.
Associate Professor
Department of Surgery
Division of Plastic Surgery
VA Puget Sound Health Care System and
University of Washington
Seattle, Washington

Mary Laya, M.D., M.P.H.
Assistant Professor of Medicine
Division of General Medicine
Department of Medicine
University of Washington School of Medicine
Seattle, Washington

Sarvesh Logsetty, M.D.
Assistant Professor
Associate Director
Firefighter's Burn Treatment Unit
University of Alberta
Edmonton, Alberta, Canada

Dana Christian Lynge, M.D.
Staff Surgeon
VA Puget Sound Health Care System
Assistant Professor
Department of Surgery
University of Washington School of Medicine
Seattle, Washington

Ronald V. Maier, M.D.
Surgeon-in-Chief
Harborview Medical Center
Professor and Vice Chairman
Department of Surgery
University of Washington School of Medicine
Seattle, Washington

Ravi Moonka, M.D.
Staff Surgeon
Virginia Mason Medical Center
Clinical Assistant Professor
University of Washington School of Medicine
Seattle, Washington

Neil J. Murphy, M.D.
Chief Clinical Consultant–Obstetrics and Gynecology
Indian Health Service
Southcentral Foundation Women's Health Service
Alaska Native Medical Center
Anchorage, Alaska

Jeffrey Randall Murray, M.D.
Anesthesiologist
Northern Anesthesia Division
Spectrum Medical Group
Eastern Maine Medical Center and St. Joseph Hospital
Bangor, Maine

John W. O'Kane, M.D.
Assistant Professor of Orthopedics
Adjunct Assistant Professor of Family Medicine
University of Washington School of Medicine
Seattle, Washington

Vanessa B. Peyton, M.D.
Assistant Professor
Department of Family Practice
University of Texas Health Sciences Center
San Antonio, Texas

Susan Reed, M.D.
Assistant Professor
Department of Obstetrics and Gynecology
University of Washington
Seattle, Washington

Peter T. Simonian, M.D.
Associate Professor of Orthopedics
Chief, Sports Medicine Clinic
Department of Orthopaedic Surgery
University of Washington School of Medicine
Seattle, Washington

Matthias Stelzner, M.D.
Staff Surgeon
VA Puget Sound Healthcare System
Assistant Professor
Department of Surgery
University of Washington School of Medicine
Seattle, Washington

T. Al West, M.D., M.P.H.
Assistant Professor
Department of Surgery
University of Texas Southwestern Medical Center
San Antonio, Texas

Introduction

The book you hold in your hands is unique—both in its content and in its preparation. It is also unique among surgical texts in that it was conceived for two very special types of audiences by two very different kinds of physicians.

The first audience is primary care and emergency room clinicians who work in rural areas. These clinicians deal with a variety of acute surgical problems and often do so without the benefit of immediate surgical backup. Presently available books—ranging from simplistic procedure manuals on one hand to all-inclusive texts of academic surgery on the other—do not answer the needs of these practitioners. This book bridges the gap between these extremes and provides clinicians with meaningful and useful information they can immediately put to use.

The second audience is medical students and primary care residents participating in surgical rotations. While most surgical texts cover all surgical conditions and procedures in encyclopedic detail, this book provides information about the 20 most common surgical problems and procedures that primary care clinicians encounter in practice. The book is about what every clinician, regardless of specialty, needs to know about surgery. Thus the information to be gained from reading this book will be of value to clinicians in a variety of specialties, including and especially those who will not be surgeons.

The editors of this book are in a unique position to provide a useful textbook for those two audiences. Each has had a very different, and yet very similar, professional career, and both have had considerable front-line experience handling serious surgical problems in a primary care setting.

One of the editors of this book is Dana Christian Lynge, M.D., who started his career as a general practitioner working in a remote area of northern Canada. In the small Inuit town of Kuujjuaq (pop. 1,000), he provided medical, surgical, and emergency care to a sparsely populated area of arctic Quebec. In that setting it was necessary to deal with surgical emergencies and procedures for which many current primary care physicians feel unprepared, including the treatment of fractures, placement of chest-tubes, endotracheal intubation, and repair of obstetrical tears. It was also necessary to administer anesthesia, to stabilize critically ill and trauma patients, and to transport them from remote villages and camps to the regional hospital and on to urban medical centers—often in small planes in adverse weather conditions.

Following his years in the arctic, Dr. Lynge entered a surgical residency and is now Assistant Professor of Surgery at the University of Washington School of Medicine. In this role, he teaches and supervises surgical residents and students, and also works with family medicine trainees. He receives patients in transport from the remote areas of rural Washington State—sent to him by physicians working in similar settings to those in which he once worked in rural Canada.

Barry D. Weiss, M.D., is the other editor of the book. Dr. Weiss began his career as a solo family physician in the US–Mexico border town of Nogales, Arizona (pop. 15,000). There he staffed an emergency room where he faced surgical problems ranging from traumatic amputations to pericardial lacerations, plus virtually all of the conditions and procedures discussed in this book.

Since his years on the border, Dr. Weiss has worked as an academic family physician, medical journal editor, department chairman, and researcher. He is currently Professor of Clinical Family and Community Medicine at the University of Arizona. Most importantly, he has continued to work as a teacher and supervisor of medical students and family medicine residents at multiple institutions—always focusing on what primary care clinicians need to know to function independently in rural areas where sophisticated technological support may not be readily available.

The authors of the individual chapters of this book bring a wide variety of skills and experiences to the clinical problems they discuss. These authors include surgeons and family physicians from across the US and Canada, all with practice experience in sites ranging from major academic medical centers to small Alaskan villages. We are grateful to each of the chapter authors for their excellent and thoughtful contributions to the book, and for their willingness to share their knowledge and skills with the primary care clinicians.

As mentioned earlier, this book is specifically designed for primary care clinicians and emergency room clinicians—both those working in rural areas and those training in primary care. It is intended for any primary care clinicians wanting to enhance their mastery of the 20 most common surgical problems they see in practice and to perform the procedures necessary to treat those problems. The book is intended to serve them not only as a reference book but also, perhaps more importantly, as a book that can be used on the spot when information is needed about how to perform a specific surgical procedure or evaluate a specific surgical problem.

With advances in telemedicine, biotechnology, and surgery, many changes will occur in rural surgical practice over the next several years. While we have gone to great efforts to assure that this book provides clinicians with practical information to use in their day-to-day practice, it is inevitable that the management of some clinical problems will change. With those changes in management, it is also inevitable that some topics will need to be approached differently than they are in this edition of the book. As you use this book, if you find a need for the book to cover topics in more detail, to cover them differently, or to cover topics not included in the current edition of the book, write to us and let us know. We will be pleased to consider your comments.

Acknowledgments

Finally, we need to say thank you to several individuals without whose help this book would never have been completed.

First, we thank David Ehlert, of *Redehlert* Illustrations and the University of Washington Graphics & Illustration Department, who created all of the original artwork for the book. Surgery is a visual specialty, and David Ehlert's high quality illustrations are central to the success and usefulness of the book.

Second, we thank Susan Noujaim, Development Editor at McGraw-Hill. Ms. Noujaim's hard work and attention to the success of this book—and indeed, to the success of all the books in this series—are very much appreciated.

Finally, we thank our spouses for letting us spend so much time preparing this book. Time devoted to professional projects is time away from the family, and without the support of our families, we would not have been able to develop and edit the book. Thanks to all of you.

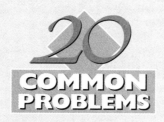

Surgical Problems and Procedures in Primary Care

Basic Problems
and Procedures

Jeffrey Randall Murray

Anesthesia

Introduction

Anesthesia, or the absence of sensation, is critical to the successful management of all of the surgical problems in this book. The skill of the clinician in relieving a patient's pain and anxiety and in understanding how to choose and use the appropriate anesthetic technique will go a long way toward solving many of the problems involved in treating surgical patients.

The purpose of this chapter is to provide basic guidance in the use of local and field anesthesia, regional anesthesia, and conscious sedation. Commonly used drugs and techniques will be described. Emphasis will be placed on anesthetic techniques to use with each of the surgical problems presented in this book.

Principles of Anesthesia

Elements of Anesthesia

The operational definition of anesthesia involves four elements: (1) analgesia, (2) amnesia, (3) skeletal and smooth muscle relaxation, and (4) control of autonomic responses. Depending on the clinical situation, any or all of these elements can be addressed using various combinations of drugs and techniques.

Effective general anesthetics address all four elements, but not all drugs used during a surgical procedure address all four of them. For example, opiates such as morphine provide excellent analgesia but unreliable amnesia, poor relaxation (sometimes rigidity), and moderate blunting of autonomic or reflex responses. Thus, they do not, by themselves, provide complete anesthesia. Barbiturates such as thiopental, on the other hand, provide excellent amnesia but poor analgesia, relaxation, and control of autonomic responses. Some other agents, for example, modern inhaled anesthetics such as sevoflurane, handle all four elements in moderate fashion. Such drugs, however, are so potent at blunting protective reflexes that special considerations such as a separate skilled individual with a specialized delivery system (vaporizer and anesthesia circuit) and special monitoring equipment are required for their safe use.

Phases of Anesthesia

Anesthesiologists speak of an anesthetic as having three phases over time. The first phase, induction, brings a patient from baseline to surgical anesthesia (i.e., no apparent movement or response during surgery). Maintenance of anesthesia is the second phase, which persists until the third phase, emergence. Emergence is reversal, either complete or partial, of the anesthetic agent until the patient achieves an acceptable and safe state of consciousness.

Anesthetic regimens often use multiple agents to achieve induction and maintenance. For example, thiopental causes a rapid loss of consciousness and can be used for induction of anesthesia—but rarely for much else. Then, a slower-acting agent can be used for maintenance, in combination with an opiate for pain and a skeletal muscle relaxant to facilitate intubation.

In many cases the surgical procedure can be performed with a local anesthetic and conscious sedation, with careful attention to the patient's condition and response to drugs. In remote areas where the skills of an anesthesiologist or anesthetist and specialized equipment are not available, local anesthesia and conscious sedation can be used to provide adequate if not excellent anesthesia, but only if the clinician is meticulous and alert for problems associated with these techniques.

Physiology of Pain

ANATOMY OF PAIN PATHWAYS

Nociceptive receptors of the peripheral nervous system are highly organized by type of sensation and type of axonal fibers used to transmit impulses. The sensory impulses follow discrete pathways from peripheral tissues to the central nervous system. Dermatomal, sclerotomal, and myotomal maps allow one to think of these pathways when using field blocks, nerve blocks, and neuraxial blocks, yet the practitioner must also understand that a more detailed understanding is necessary.

Peripheral nerves are divided into somatic and visceral (autonomic) axons having afferent (sensory) or efferent (motor) functions. Somatic afferent axons have specialized sensing organs located in the periphery that respond to pressure, heat, cold, touch, and pain. These axons project back to the dorsal root ganglion and into the dorsal horn and spinothalamic tracts, following both a discrete pathway projected onto the cerebral cortex and a more diffuse pathway with complex connections at many levels above and below within the spinal cord. Especially high densities of peripheral nociceptors and pain fibers are located in fingertips, genitalia, mouth, and bone (periostium). Visceral afferent nerves lack the discrete nature of somatic afferents, as they have many diffuse dendritic projections at multiple levels within the spinal cord and no direct projection to the cerebral cortex. This difference between somatic and visceral nerves explains, at least in part, why local anesthesia and field and nerve blocks can be used to anesthetize somatic afferent nerves but not visceral afferent nerves.

Modulation of nociception occurs both in the periphery and at synapses within the spinal cord and thalamus. Peripherally, mediators of inflammation such as prostaglandins and histamines sensitize nociceptors. Within the spinal cord, neurotransmitter substances both excite and inhibit the nociceptive input and provide reflexive efferent responses, which result in skeletal muscle spasms within the same region of the periphery.

Important adjuncts to modify nociception and reduce efferent reflex responses include aspirin and other nonsteroidal antiinflammatory agents, antihistamines, benzodiazepines, acetaminophen, and opiates. The observation that opiates administered into the spinal canal can provide profound analgesia has caused an explosive growth in the use of neuraxial techniques that combine local anesthetics and opiates.

PREEMPTIVE ANALGESIA

Since the turn of the century it has been theorized that nociceptive input causes excitatory changes in the central nervous system, and that these excitatory changes are a part of the surgical stress response that contributes to increasing postoperative pain. Based on this theoretic construct, if these excitatory changes can be blocked by anesthesia prior to nociceptive input (i.e., prior to pain), the enhancement of postoperative pain can be diminished. Thus, preemptive prevention of this enhancing neuromodulation by the aggressive, early use of local anesthetics and regional techniques has become an increasingly popular anesthetic practice.

Recently, this preemptive use of regional anesthesia has been shown to significantly reduce postoperative pain in humans. Based on experimental data and extrapolated to general use, many anesthesiologist now use infiltration, field blocks, and/or regional blocks in advance of surgery whenever possible, even if general anesthesia is to be used.

Protective Reflexes and Conscious Sedation

PROTECTIVE REFLEXES

Protective reflexes are designed to maintain homeostasis and are divided somewhat arbitrarily into the three categories of airway, respiration, and circulation. The airway, or laryngeal, reflexes (swallowing, coughing, and gagging) prevent the aspiration of foreign material into the lung and the obstruction of the airways. The respiratory reflexes include hyperventilation in response to hypoxemia and hypercarbia and hypoventilation in response to hypocarbia. Circulatory reflexes include bradycardia in response to hypertension and tachycardia in response to hypotension and hypovolemia.

To the anesthesiologist, the most important reflexes are those that protect the airway and prevent hypoxemia and hypercarbia. Normal airway function is related to level of consciousness, tone in the tongue and pharynx, ability to cough and prevent foreign-body aspiration, and integrity of esophageal sphincters and motility.

Protective reflexes are significantly altered—almost always depressed or eliminated—by anesthetic drugs, though the specific effect depends on the type of drug, the dose, the interaction of the drug with other agents, and the route and location of administration. It is easy to demonstrate the effectiveness of sedatives and analgesics in blunting of coughing and swallowing reflexes. For example, the administration of small doses of intravenous fentanyl and midazolam, combined with topical lidocaine spray in the hypopharynx, is usually sufficient to diminish these reflexes to the degree that endoscopic instruments can be passed through the pharynx and larynx without difficulty. Because the reflexes are diminished, however, the practitioner must be always vigilant for airway compromise that may occur and be prepared to assist and, if needed, to secure a patient's airway with tracheal intubation.

Many drugs will not only contribute directly or indirectly to airway compromise, but they also cause respiratory depression. The reflex response to hypoxemia and hypercarbia is very sensitive to systemic anesthetic drugs and can lead to apnea caused by rapid peak effects on the brain-stem regulatory centers. Hypotension from blunting of the circulatory reflexes can also occur, especially in the presence of hypovolemia.

CONSCIOUS SEDATION

The goal of conscious sedation is to relieve pain and anxiety without losing verbal and nonverbal communication with the patient. In general, this assures that protective airway reflexes are not blunted to a critical extent.

The general approach to conscious sedation should consist of setting up monitoring of vital functions, supplemental oxygen (almost never contraindicated), and gradual incremental titration of selected drugs, allowing for the peak effect of each dose to occur before a subsequent dose is given. A common regimen is the combination of midazolam in 0.5-mg doses, alternating with fentanyl in 25-μg doses or propofol in 10- to 20-mg doses (or by infusion at 20 μg/kg/min) and increasing according to the patient's response. Repeated questioning of the patient and engaging the patient in conversation, forewarning of unpleasant events, are very important to successful use of conscious sedation.

Key History

In preparation for adminstration of anesthesia, it is important to obtain information about the patient's general medical history. This will permit identification of contraindications to the use of certain medications and will alert the clinician to specific concerns or cautions that must be exercised in the selection and use of anesthetic agents.

Medications and Allergies

Patients should be questioned about the current use of any medications, the reason for using the medication, and when the last dose was taken. Both prescription and nonprescription medications should be considered.

A history of adverse reactions to medications should also be solicited. In particular, it is important to identify a history of acute hypersensitivity or anaphylaxis in response to the use of any medications or anesthetic agents.

Medical Conditions

Cardiopulmonary and neurologic problems may place the patient at increased risk for complications of surgery and anesthesia, and a history of such problems should be sought. Specifically, it should be determined if the patient has or has had problems with angina, myocardial infarction, congestive heart failure, valvular heart disease, cough, smoking, respiratory infection, asthma, orthopnea, dyspnea, syncope, arrhythmia, stroke, seizures, claudication, weakness, numbness, or activity limitations.

Other systemic diseases that may require special consideration during anesthesia and the perioperative period should also be identified. These include diabetes mellitus, kidney problems (single kidney, stones, renal failure, dialysis), thyroid disease, liver disease, bleeding problems, prior blood transfusions, cancer, pregnancy or possibility of pregnancy, connective tissue diseases (rheumatoid, ankylosing spondylitis, systemic lupus), and substance abuse.

It is also useful to specifically ask about past surgical procedures, the types of anesthesia used, and any problems that occurred with anesthesia. Specific problems about which inquiry should be made include airway problems (e.g., difficulties with intubation), the need for mechanical ventilation or intensive care after surgery, or an unusually prolonged recovery. The clinician should also ask about personal or family history of anesthesia-related problems such as prolonged muscle relaxation (suggesting a cholinesterase deficiency or myasthenia gravis), hyperthermia (suggesting malignant hyperthermia or neuroleptic malignant syndrome), and other disorders that might influence anesthetic management (i.e., acute intermittent porphyria, porphyria variegata, and muscular dystrophy).

Conditions Predisposing to Aspiration of Gastric Contents

GASTROESOPHAGEAL DYSFUNCTION

It is essential to identify conditions that predispose to reflux and aspiration of gastric contents into the respiratory tract, so that the risk of aspiration during sedation and/or intubation can be minimized. Efforts should be made to identify symptoms of esophageal dysfunction such as gastroesophageal reflux disease, heartburn, hiatal hernia, esophageal cancer, prior esophageal, and gastric surgery.

Some patients have reflux symptoms whenever they lie flat and regardless of whether they are fasting. Such manifestations of reflux cause concern about the safety of sedation in these patients, and many anesthesiologists will pretreat such individuals with metoclopramide (10 mg orally or intravenously), an H_2 blocker, and 30 mL orally of a clear nonparticulate antacid such as sodium citrate or modified Shohl's solution (Bictra). If feasible during the surgical procedure, it is also useful to elevate the back of the operating table or place the patient in reverse Trendelenberg's position.

RECENT INGESTION OF FOOD

Recent ingestion of food also may predispose to reflux and aspiration of gastric contents. Thus, it is essential to inquire about the patient's last intake of solids and liquids. The most conservative approach, assuming a surgical procedure it not urgent, is to have the patient take nothing by mouth for at least 8 hours before anesthesia. This approach may be overly restrictive, however, based on several considerations. First, consuming nonfatty and nonalcohol-containing foods actually stimulates gastric emptying, in which case the stomach will be empty before 8 hours have elapsed. Second, liquids, especially clear liquids, are emptied from the stomach in only a few hours. Third, children (especially infants) can safely consume formula 6 hours in advance and pedialyte up to 2 hours in advance of anesthesia without risk of reflux.

Thus, in the absence of the esophageal-dysfunction problems mentioned above, and if the surgical procedure is not urgent, a reasonable approach is to insist on fasting 8 hours for adults for solid food, 6 hours for liquids, and 2 hours for clear liquids. A "clear" liquid includes black coffee, tea, apple juice, and many carbonated beverages.

It is important to remember that gastric motility is altered by trauma and pain, and therefore the risk of aspiration is increased in patients with these conditions. Due to this fact, patients with traumatic injuries and pain should be pretreated as described above.

Key Physical Examination

The patient's height and weight should be determined, as these may influence dosing of anesthetic agents. If direct measurements cannot be obtained, the patient can provide an approximate height and weight, or, if necessary in an emergency situation, they may be estimated by the clinician. The presence of abundant facial hair should be noted, as this often makes an anesthesia mask fit poorly.

While a complete physical examination is appropriate for all patients about to undergo surgery, certain aspects of the examination are particularly pertinent to the adminstration of anesthesia. An anesthesia-focused examination concentrates on issues related to airway management, the cardiopulmonary system, and establishment of intravenous access.

Airway

The airway portion of the physical examination deals with identification of problems that might make it difficult to initiate an airway or maintain good gas exchange. The examination starts by having a patient extend the neck, open the mouth, protrude the tongue, and say "Ah!" During this examination, the clinician should look at the condition of teeth and ask about loose teeth, dentures, and caps or crowns in front; removing dentures may improve the fit of an anesthesia mask. Look at the size of the tongue and how it fills the mouth and at how much of the posterior pharynx is visible beyond. If you can clearly see the tip of the epiglottis and tonsils, that is excellent, and it

portends a relatively easy intubation. On the other hand, if a large tongue-size prohibits visualization of the uvula, it is possible that establishment of an airway will be difficult. In addition, patients with a large tongue may also have obstructive sleep apnea, which is even more common among individuals who are also obese. Patients with sleep apnea can be more sensitive to anesthetics, can obstruct their airway easily, and can readily become hypoxic and hypercarbic.

Check development of the mandible. Micrognathia usually means difficulty in establishing an endotracheal airway. Limitation of mandibular opening, such as occurs in temporomandibular joint syndrome, may also portend a difficult intubation.

The examination should also include an assessment of neck mobility, including flexion, extension, and rotation. If the patient cannot demonstrate good mobility of the neck, it is important to determine if the patient's limitations are the result of pain, lack of cooperation, etc. Limitation of neck motion that occurs with connective-tissue disorders may make intubation difficult. Finally, check the distance between the thyroid cartilage and the chin; short distances can mean difficulty visualizing the larynx if intubation is anticipated.

Cardiopulmonary System

Cardiac auscultation is performed, seeking evidence of murmurs that might indicate the need for endocarditis prophylaxis or arrhythmias that might complicate anesthetic management or postoperative care. The radial pulse is palpated during cardiac auscultation to identify the pulse lag that occurs with atrial fibrillation/flutter and to determine the ease with which the pulse can be identified for insertion of an arterial catheter, if needed.

The next step is to auscultate the posterior lung fields to identify rales that might be caused by congestive heart failure. In addition, auscultation should take place while the patient performs several, forced, expiratory maneuvers. Identification of rhonchi, wheezing, or prolonged expiratory phase usually indicates distal airway obstruction caused by asthma or chronic obstructive pulmonary disease.

IV Access and Position

The final step in an anesthesia-focused examination is to assess the availability of intravenous access sites and the position in which the patient should be placed for the surgical procedure. Depending on the surgical site and procedure, special considerations may be necessary regarding the position of the clinician responsible for anesthetic management and the extent to which topical and regional anesthesia might be used.

Ancillary Tests

The nature of ancillary tests is determined by the specific medical problems presented by the patient, the type of anesthesia to be used, and the nature of the surgical problem. For minor procedures involving local anesthesia with conscious sedation, no ancillary tests are needed unless specifically suggested by evaluation of the patient.

For more significant surgical problems, especially for patients with cardiopulmonary or other chronic medical problems, a variety of laboratory tests can be useful in assessing the patient's operative risk. Such tests include a hemoglobin level to assess oxygen-carrying capacity, creatinine level to determine renal function, electrocardiography to identify ischemia and arrhythmia, a blood glucose if diabetic, coagulation parameters if bleeding risk needs to be assessed, and a chest x-ray if cardiopulmonary pathology needs evaluation.

The use of additional tests must be determined according to what is most likely to alter the care of the patient or reduce risk. Much time and resources can be wasted by excessive use of routine preoperative tests.

Algorithm

An approach for deciding whether local, regional, conscious sedation, or general anesthesia should be used is described in the algorithm (Fig. 1-1). The use of specific drugs and anesthetic techniques is described in the subsequent sections of this chapter. Regardless of the type of anesthesia or route of adminstration, it is essential to keep in mind the primary importance of airway management.

Drugs Used in Anesthesia

Local Anesthetics

The various local anesthetics, along with information about metabolism, allergy, and duration of action, are shown in Table 1-1. Lidocaine is the most commonly used local anesthetic in the United States.

In addition to using the local anesthetics individually, they can also be combined into topical solutions or ointments. One such preparation is a eutectic mixture of local anesthetics (EMLA), which is a mixture of lidocaine (2.5%) and prilocaine (2.5%). EMLA is applied as a topical ointment under an occlusive dressing for 45 to 60 minutes, during which time it will produce an area of dermal anesthesia and cutaneous vasodilation. EMLA is commonly used to anesthetize areas to start intravenous infusion in children and adolescents and can be used when removing small superficial lesions from the skin.

Local anesthetics are also commonly mixed with vasoconstrictors such as epinephrine and then injected or applied topically. The presence of epinephrine prolongs the action of the anesthetic, but it is also associated with certain toxicity, as described below.

Figure 1-1

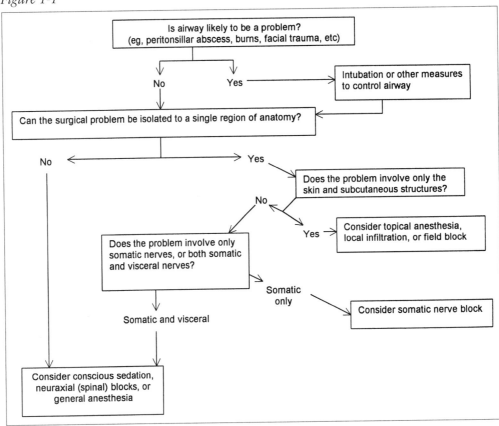

Algorithm for selecting the appropriate anesthetic technique.

TOXICITY OF LOCAL ANESTHETICS

The use of local anesthetics can be associated with toxicity, which can be life threatening. Toxicity can be systemic or local.

SYSTEMIC TOXICITY Systemic toxicity of local anesthetics results from absorption of the drug. Toxicity is typically manifested as nervous system excitation and/or cardiovascular depression. Methemoglobinemia can occur with certain local anesthetics.

Generally, toxicity from systemic absorption of lidocaine begins with subtle signs of central nervous system excitation such as lingual tingling and circumoral numbness. With continued absorption, these symptoms may progress to tinnitus; lightheadedness; sleepiness; and sometimes visual disturbances, myoclonus, and dysphoria. Ultimately, generalized seizures will occur. Unconsciousness, coma, respiratory arrest, and, finally, cardiac arrest rapidly follow seizures if systemic lidocaine levels are high enough.

Systemic toxicity is dose and drug dependent. Local infiltration of the skin and subcutaneous tissues rarely results in toxicity unless intravascular injection occurs. Systemic absorption is higher with some major nerve blocks such as intercostal nerve blocks and brachial plexus blocks and with topical instillation into the tracheobronchial tree.

Facilities for resuscitation and emergency airway management must be immediately available when local anesthetics are used.

Cardiovascular collapse from bupivicaine occurs at lower doses than with lidocaine, and when it does occur, it results in a poor prognosis in part because of high levels of bupivicaine protein binding within the myocardium. Bupivicaine toxicity is associated with ventricular arrhythmias, including fatal ventricular fibrillation, which is not characteristic of lidocaine even when given intravenously. Pregnancy, acidosis, and hypoxemia enhance the cardiovascular toxicity of bupivicaine.

Methemoglobinemia is produced by the systemic absorption of some topical anesthetics, notably prilocaine (and consequently EMLA, of which prilocaine is a major constituent) and benzocaine. Methemoglobin is oxidized (Fe^{+2} to Fe^{+3}) hemoglobin. Normal methemoglobin concentrations are less than 1% of total hemoglobin. Repeated use of 20% benzocaine (Hurricaine) in the oropharyngeal and tracheobronchial tree can produce methemoglobin concentrations greater than 15%. Clinical cyanosis occurs at 10%, symptoms of dyspnea and lethargy at greater than 30%, and pulse oximeter readings do not reflect the degree of tissue hypoxia that occurs (pulse oximeter reading of 85% oxygen saturation can occur in the presence of profound tissue hypoxia). EMLA cream used in infants has resulted in the same problem as oropharyngeal and tracheobronchial benzocaine. Some indigenous peoples (Inuit) have a genetic predisposition toward methemoglobinemia. Treatment is methylene blue, 1 to 2 mg/kg, administered slowly IV.

LOCAL TOXICITY   Vasoconstrictors reduce the risk of systemic toxicity by reducing systemic absorption from surrounding tissues. They also significantly prolong the duration of local action of both lidocaine and bupivicaine. The most commonly used vasoconstrictors are epinephrine and phenylephrine, but epinephrine is the most widely used, and only it will be discussed here. Concentrations vary from 1:100,000 (10 µg/mL) to 1:200,000 (5 µg/mL), and both are equally effective. Vasoconstrictors should not be used in end-arteriolar circulations where ischemia and necrosis might result. These areas include fingers, toes, and tip of nose, ears, and penis.

Local anesthetics can also cause nerve damage, but this is rare. The mechanism of nerve damage is placement of high concentrations of anesthetic directly into or around nerve tissue. Recent reports of cauda equina syndrome resulting from use of spinal catheters through which 5% lidocaine was administered point to the possibility of

Table 1-1

Characteristics of Common Local Anesthetics

ANESTHETIC AND BRAND NAME	STABILITY	METABOLISM	ALLERGY	DURATION OF ACTION
Esters:	Unstable in solution	In plasma by cholinesterase	Para-aminobenzoic acid metabolite causes allergy in some patients	
Procaine (Novocaine)				Short
Chloroprocaine (Nesacaine)				Short
Tetracaine (Pontocaine)				Long
Dibucaine (Nupercainal)				Topical — short
Benzocaine (Hurricaine, Americaine)				Topical — short
Amides:	Stable in solution	In liver by microsomal enzymes	Extremely rare	
Lidocaine (Xylocaine, Lignocaine)				Intermediate
Bupivicaine (Marcaine, Sensorcaine)				Long
Prilocaine (Citanest)				Long

injury if dilution by surrounding tissues does not occur. In the case of spinal anesthesia with 5% lidocaine, dilution by cerebrospinal fluid during injection is considered important to reduce the risk of toxicity. It is wise to remember that many local anesthetics are supplied in concentrations that are much higher than their effective concentrations in tissues.

Benzodiazepines

The term benzodiazepine refers to the benzene and diazepine rings common to all drugs in this class. All have similar pharmacologic effects, causing sedation, hypnosis, anxiolysis, amnesia, anticonvulsant activity, and, in high doses, muscle relaxation. They all exhibit pronounced synergism with opiates, other sedative-hypnotics, and general anesthetics, thus requiring great caution with used in combination with these other drugs. Their most useful properties are anxiolysis and amnesia.

Benzodiazepines are classified as long-, intermediate-, and short-acting agents. Diazepam (Valium), one of the oldest and most widely used benzodiazepines, is a long-acting agent. Doses from 2.5 to 5 mg intravenously and up to 10 mg orally are common for sedation. Diazepam has a slow onset and active metabolites with a half-life of 30 to 60 hours; the half-life is even longer in elderly patients. Lorazepam (Ativan) in doses from 0.5 to 2 mg IV and 2 to 4 mg orally is an intermediate-acting benzodiazepine with a 10- to 20-hour half-life.

Both diazepam and lorazepam have been largely replaced in the practice of anesthesiology by the short-acting benzodiazepine, midazolam

(Versed). Midazolam has a half-life of 1.7 to 2.6 hours and no active metabolites. Because of its water solubility, the commercial preparation of midazolam lacks the burning discomfort sometimes associated with diazepam. Midazolam is suitable for use in continuous infusions. Usual doses are 0.5 to 1-mg IV and 0.2 to 0.5 mg/kg orally. Apnea can occur after IV boluses of midazolam, and is especially likely when used in combination with opiates.

Flumazenil is a specific benzodiazepine-receptor antagonist that can be used to treat benzodiazepine overdose. Flumazenil is administered in small incremental doses of 0.1 to 0.5 mg intravenously, repeated up to a total of 5 mg if necessary.

Opiates

Many opiates are used in the practice of anesthesiology, primarily for their ability to cause effective analgesia. Doses of commonly used opiates are shown in Table 1-2.

Opiates can depress respirations and must be administered cautiously when used in combination with other medications that depress respiratory drive. A typical patient who has received a large dose of an opiate alone may be apneic, but will readily breathe when asked to do so; patients medicated only with opiates may "forget" to breathe despite hypoxemia and hypercarbia.

Opiates exhibit only minor effects on the cardiovascular system, usually bradycardia. One exception is meperidine, which usually causes tachycardia.

Table 1-2
Equivalent Doses of Commonly Used Opiates

DRUG	EQUIVALENT DOSE	ONSET OF ACTION	DURATION OF ACTION
Morphine	10 mg IV	5–10 min	2–4 hours
Meperidine	75–100 mg IV	5–10 min	2–4 hours
Fentanyl	50 μg IV	1–2 min	2–3 hours
Oxycodone	10 mg PO	30–60 min	3–6 hours

Abbreviations: IV, intravenously; PO, orally.

Other prominent opiate side effects include constipation, urinary retention, nausea, vomiting, and pruritis. All opiate effects can be reversed by a specific antagonist, naloxone, which is discussed below.

MORPHINE

Morphine is naturally occurring and derived from the milky extract of the seed pod of the oriental poppy *Papaver somniferum*. Morphine is the prototypical opiate and exhibits a wide range of effects, the most useful of which are analgesia and euphoria. Given intravenously, 10 mg of morphine has a peak effect in 15 minutes, and its effect can last up to 4 hours. Respiratory depression with apnea can occur in higher doses; bradypnea and hypoventilation are common. Respiratory depression outlasts analgesia and is greatly increased by the simultaneous use of propofol, benzodiazepines, and other drugs. Neither amnesia nor unconsciousness occurs unreliably with morphine.

MEPERIDINE

Meperidine (Demerol) was one of the first synthetic opiates, and it remains in widespread use. Meperidine is less potent than morphine, but has a more rapid onset and shorter duration of action. Meperidine has an atropine-like effect, causing tachycardia on administration. It also has important drug interactions. In particular, meperidine can cause a hypertensive crisis if a patient is also taking a monoamine-oxidase (MAO) inhibitor.

FENTANYL

Fentanyl (Sublimaze) has largely replaced meperidine and morphine in anesthesia practice. Like meperidine, it is a synthetic compound, but it is far more potent and specific in its opioid effect (i.e., no atropine-like effect).

Fentanyl is lipid soluble and has an onset of 1 to 2 minutes with a duration 2 to 3 hours. Fentanyl must be administered cautiously, because 1 mL of commercially available solution contains 50 μg of fentanyl, which is the analgesic equivalent of 5 to 10 mg of morphine. A morphine-equivalent dose of fentanyl causes an equal amount and duration of respiratory depression to that of morphine.

In the past, fentanyl was used in a fixed combination with droperidol (Inapsine), called Innovar, for neuroleptanalgesia. Neuroleptanalgesia is a state of stupor in which there is little movement or response on the patient's part. In contrast to a similar state induced by ketamine, hallucinations did not occur with Innovar. Innovar is rarely used today, however, because patients recover from the drug very slowly as a result of the prolonged and intense psychomotor retardation caused by the droperidol, an analog of haloperidol.

OXYCODONE

Oxycodone is an analog of codeine, another naturally occurring compound in *Papaver somniferum*. It is available only in an oral form and is commonly used as a treatment for postoperative pain. Onset of analgesia requires at least 1 hour, and long-acting formulations (Oxycontin) last up to 12 hours.

NALOXONE

Naloxone (Narcan) is the specific antagonist of opiates. One ampule contains 0.4 mg and is diluted 1:10 or 1:20 and given slowly intravenously in 1-mL increments. Onset is very rapid, but may not outlast the effects of all opiates, so one must be vigilant for reoccurrence of an opiate effect and the need for repetitive administration of naloxone. Naloxone is suitable for use as an infusion in cases of severe overdose or methadone poisoning.

Nonstesal Antiinflammatory Drugs (NSAIDs)

Ketorolac (Toradol) is the only NSAID available for intramuscular and intravenous use. It has become very popular in emergency departments and ambulatory surgical areas. A dose of 30 mg of ketorolac is as effective as 10 mg of morphine for treatment of acute pain. Normal-sized patients can receive a single, initial intramuscular dose of up to 60 mg. If repetitive dosing is to be used, the recommended dose is 30 mg, intravenously or intramuscularly, at 6-hour intervals up to a maximum of 120 mg.

Ketorolac shares all the common side effects of NSAIDs, including gastrointestinal side effects, renal dysfunction, and fluid retention with increased blood pressure. It should be used cautiously, if at all, for patients with congestive heart failure and/or renal impairment. If used for patients over 65 years of age or weighing less than 100 pounds, the dose should be reduced to 15 mg every 6 hours.

Nitrous Oxide

Nitrous oxide (N_2O) is an odorless, colorless gas possessing potent analgesic and mild amnestic and hypnotic effects. Commonly called "laughing gas," it is available preblended with oxygen in a fixed ratio of 50%:50% (Nitronox). A 50% mixture of nitrous oxide provides analgesia and amnesia sufficient for minor procedures, but often requires supplementation with other agents such as opiates, benzodiazepines, and propofol.

Nitrous oxide is safe, has a rapid onset and recovery, and has few side effects when used properly. As a gas that displaces oxygen, care must be taken to avoid administering a hypoxic mixture, and facilities must be available to monitor inspired-gas concentration and pulse oximetry. Some patients become agitated and disinhibited, negating any advantage sought by using N_2O.

Chronic exposure to nitrous oxide can cause abnormalities of vitamin B_{12} metabolism and may be associated with an increased rate of first-trimester spontaneous abortions among health-care workers. Therefore, facilities for scavenging of waste gases should be available and used when nitrous oxide is administered.

Ketamine

Ketamine (Ketalar) is a close analog of phencyclidine (PCP), an illicit hallucinogenic drug. Ketamine not only shares the psychomimetic properties (hallucinations and delirium) of PCP but also its relative absence of cardiorespiratory depression. Ketamine is unique among nonopiate anesthetic agents because of its potent analgesic effects and lack of cardiorespiratory depression.

Ketamine causes a unique dissociative state unlike what is commonly observed during general anesthesia. Eyes remain open, pupils dilate, and nystagmus is common. Lacrimation and salivation occur, and it is necessary to administer antisialagogues such as glycopyrrolate if ketamine is to be used repetitively or for a prolonged procedure. Vocalization and spontaneous but purposeless movements may also occur.

Ketamine stimulates respiration and circulation, rather than depressing these functions as many other agents do. In fact, tachycardia and hypertension are common. It is uncertain if protective reflexes are intact, as this has not been well studied.

The dose of ketamine required to cause analgesia is much lower than the dose that causes unconsciousness, and the analgesia lasts much longer than the duration of unconsciousness. This property, combined with lack of cardiorespiratory depression, results in ketamine's popularity for brief but painful procedures such as managing burns and wounds or reducing fractures. A single dose (2 mg/kg IV) causes general anesthesia in 1 minute for 10 to 15 minutes, with complete recovery in 30 minutes.

Ketamine's well-documented ability to cause nightmares and other unpleasant psychologic side effects has resulted in its combination with benzodiazepines. Midazolam given in advance of (and intermittently during) ketamine administration appears to reduce the incidence of these disturbing side effects, but can also markedly prolong the time to recovery. Because of ketamine's unique psychologic side effects, informed consent prior to the use of ketamine is especially important.

Ketamine is useful for patients with asthma because it causes bronchial smooth-muscle relaxation. Because it causes tachycardia, ketamine is relatively contraindicated for patients with unstable coronary disease, uncontrolled hypertension, and cardiac arrhythmias. Because of its psychologic side effects, it generally should not be used for patients with a serious psychologic disorder. It should not be used for patients with head injury when the possibility of increased intracranial pressure exists, because ketamine can elevate blood pressure.

Propofol

Propofol (Diprivan) is the newest IV anesthetic agent and one of the most important. It is a polysubstituted phenol and therefore lipid soluble. Propofol is suitable for general anesthesia, continuous infusions, and conscious sedation. It exhibits no appreciable analgesic effects.

A bolus of 2 mg/kg causes rapid unconsciousness, recovery in 10 minutes, and less depression of mood afterward as compared with thiopental. Propofol lowers blood pressure by 25 to 40%, reduces cardiac output by 10% to 15%, but has little effect on heart rate. Propofol is more likely to cause prolonged apnea than other IV induction agents, and this effect is increased by concomitant use of opiates. A desirable effect is that propofol exhibits minor antiemetic activity, even in subanesthetic doses.

Sedation with propofol (30% to 60% μg/kg/min) produces reliable amnesia and more rapid recovery than midazolam. As with all drugs, elderly and sick patients may require a substantially lower dose; titration to effect is the rule. Side effects include pain on injection, especially in small veins, which can be reduced or eliminated by giving lidocaine IV 50–200 mg slowly prior to propofol. Myoclonus may occur, but is less common than with methohexital and more common than with thiopental. Cardiorespiratory depression is more common and hypotension can be severe in the hypovolemic patient.

Propofol is prepared as an emulsion with egg lecithin, soybean oil, and glycerol at a concentration of 1% (10 mg/mL). The emulsion readily supports bacterial growth, so once exposed to air unused drug should be discarded within 6 hours.

Barbiturates

Until the 1990s thiopental (Pentothal) was the most common induction agent used for general anesthesia. Thiopental is an ultrashort-acting barbiturate whose onset is less than 1 minute, and its duration of action is short because of rapid redistribution from the vessel-rich organs (brain, heart, lungs, muscles, gut) to the vessel-poor organs (skin, fat, connective tissue, bone). Elimination of thiopental is much slower than distribution and depends on saturable hepatic mechanisms, leaving patients with a sometimes not-so-subtle depressed feeling for hours after a single dose. Thiopental and other barbiturates exhibit dose-dependent cardiorespiratory depression that can include apnea, hypotension, and tachycardia.

Methohexital (Brevital) is another ultrashort-acting barbiturate that is more potent than thiopental and more likely to cause myoclonus. Methohexital is frequently used for short procedures such as electroconvulsive therapy and cardioversions, but propofol appears to be equally or better suited for this task.

It is of note that barbiturates exhibit a unique antianalgesic effect that is clinically important. Sedating a patient for a painful procedure with a barbiturate alone results in the patient perceiving increased, rather than decreased, pain.

Useful Adjuncts to Anesthetic Agents

NONPHARMACOLOGIC ADJUNCTS

Distraction is one of the most useful nonpharmacologic adjuncts. Used successfully, distraction can significantly reduce anxiety and the need for repeated doses of medications. The more adept one is at communication and reassurance, and at distracting the patient during painful procedures, the better the outcome is likely to be. Some patient's personalities respond more readily than others.

In addition to verbal communication, several other techniques can be used. For example, sometimes listening to music through headphones can bring a patient through a long procedure with less pain and anxiety. Similarly, mild hypnosis and meditation will often help. For some patients, even something as innocuous as talking about significant life events and asking for a patient's opinions can be a successful distracting technique.

MUSCLE RELAXANTS

Skeletal muscle relaxants are useful for securing an emergent airway by facilitating intubation. It is important, however, to induce unconsciousness first with an agent such as propofol.

Succinylcholine (Anectine) is the muscle relaxant of choice for most patients because of its rapid onset and rapid elimination. The dose of succinylcholine is 1 mg/kg IV or 3 mg/kg IM. The intubation procedure should begin as soon as vis-

ible muscle fasciculations occur. It is important to note that occasional patients have low levels of cholinesterase enzymes and will have a prolonged drug effect caused by inability to metabolize the succinylcholine.

Succinylcholine causes pronounced skeletal muscle contractions (fasiculations) during which K^+ is released extracellularly. As a result, serum K^+ rises 0.5 to 1.0 mEq/L, and the response is exaggerated in the presence of recent denervation injuries (such as from burns and from brain and spinal-cord injuries). It can also complicate preexisting hyperkalemia, resulting in cardiac arrest. Succinylcholine is also a well-known trigger for malignant hyperthermia.

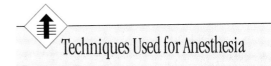

Techniques Used for Anesthesia

This section of the chapter describes a number of techniques for administering the various medications described in the previous section. Table 1-3

Table 1-3
Anesthetic Techniques for the Surgical Problems Discussed in This Book

SURGICAL PROBLEM	USUAL ANESTHETIC TECHNIQUE	ALTERNATE TECHNIQUES
Acute abdomen	General	Saddle block, w/neuraxial opiates
Anorectal disorders	Epidural	Saddle block
Abscesses	Infiltration or field block	
Breast lesions	Infiltration, field (breast) block	
Burns (dressing change)	Sedation	
Epistaxis	Local (topical)	
Peritonsillar abscess	Infiltration, topical, field block, sedation	
Lacerations	Infiltration, field and/or nerve blocks	
Skin lesions	Infiltration, field and/or nerve blocks	
Fractures	Infiltration, sedation, hematoma or nerve blocks	
Dislocations	Infiltration, sedation, hematoma or nerve blocks	
Spontaneous abortion	Sedation, paracervical block	
Episiotomy	Infiltration	
Cesarean delivery	General, epidural	Saddle block

lists many of the surgical procedures discussed in this book, along with the usual and alternate anesthetic technique for each of those procedures. In remote areas in which regular anesthesia services are not readily available, the alternate anesthetic techniques listed in the table are effective and acceptable methods.

Infiltration of Local Anesthetics

A simple and widely used technique for administering local anesthetics is by injecting into the skin and subcutaneous tissues where a surgical incision is to be made. The choice and dose of anesthetic agent is based on the desired duration of action (short-, intermediate-, or long-acting), on whether epinephrine is appropriate (1:200,000/5 µg per mL or 1:100,000/10 µg per mL), and on the safe maximum dose. The dosing characteristics of lidocaine and bupivicaine, the most commonly used local anesthetics, are shown in Table 1-4.

Small-diameter (25 to 30 gauge) needles should be used for injection whenever possible. Begin with an intradermal wheal and through this wheal slowly expand and enter the subdermal tissue, spreading the agent deliberately around the area to be incised. If injections occur in the vicinity of blood vessels, it is essential to aspirate periodically to identify and avoid intravascular injection. Allow a few minutes for the agent to reach surrounding nerves and penetrate axonal sheaths to effect a blockade.

Field Blocks

Several field blocks can be achieved with injections of local anesthetic—usually bupivicaine. Field blocks involve infiltrating tissue surrounding a specific area of the body, thus providing anesthesia without infiltration into the actual site in which the surgical procedure is to be performed. An advantage of this technique is that it avoids distortion of the skin from the edema caused by direct infiltration of anesthesia into the surgical site.

Although many different areas can be anesthetized with these techniques, the discussion here will focus on ear blocks, which are useful for repairing ear lacerations, and breast blocks, which are useful for breast biopsies. Paracervical blocks are another type of field block that are useful during dilation of the uterine cervix or treating cervical dysplasia with cryotherapy or loop electrosurgical excision. The technique for paracervical block is described in Chapter 18.

EAR BLOCK

Because the tissues of the ear are thin and closely associated with cartilage, it is often difficult to inject directly into the pinna or other parts of the ear. However, reasonable anesthesia for laceration repair can often be achieved by injecting local anesthetic completely around the base of the ear. In performing an ear block, local anesthetic is infiltrated not into the base of the ear itself but rather into the adjacent skin of the scalp and preauricular area (Fig. 1-2).

Table 1-4
Dose and Duration of Action of Lidocaine and Bupivicaine

ANESTHETIC	CONCENTRATION	MAXIMUM DOSE WITHOUT EPINEPHRINE	DURATION	MAXIMUM DOSE WITH EPINEPHRINE	DURATION
Lidocaine	1.0%	30 mL (4.5 mg/kg)	1 hr	50 mL (6–7 mg/kg)	2–3 hrs
Bupivicaine	0.25%	70 mL (2.5 mg/kg)	2–3 hrs	90 mL (3.3 mg/kg)	3–6 hrs
	0.5%	35 mL (2.5 mg/kg)	>3 hrs	45 mL (3.3 mg/kg)	>5 hrs

Figure 1-2

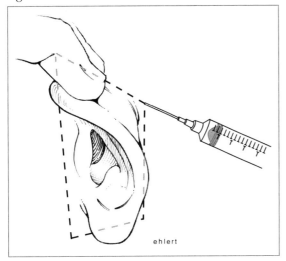

Ear block. To anesthetize the ear for laceration repair, local anesthetic is injected completely around the base of the ear, rather than into the ear itself.

BREAST BLOCK

To perform a breast block, the patient is placed in a supine position with the arm abducted and behind the head. Up to 60 mL of 0.25 to 0.375% bupivicaine with 1:200,000 epinephrine can be injected. It is imperative to stay superficial and parallel to the ribs, thereby avoiding the possibility of pneumothorax caused by intrapleural injection. It is also important to aspirate to detect and avoid intravascular injection.

By injection around the breast, four nerve groups entering the breast are anesthetized. The first is the anterior and lateral cutaneous branches of the T2-T5 intercostal nerves in the retromammary space superficial to the pectoralis muscle. The second is the descending branches of the supraclavicular nerve from the superficial cervical plexus inferior to the clavicle and from the sternum toward the axilla. The third group is the medial anterior cutaneous branches of intercostal nerves along the medial border of the sternum. The fourth injection is into the medial and lateral pectoralis nerves from the brachial plexus at the midpoint of the clavicle, inferiorly within the body of the pectoralis muscle. The location of these nerves can be found in any standard anatomy text.

Nerve Blocks

Specific peripheral nerves can be anesthetized using injections of local anesthesia. Primary-care clinicians can use many of these blocks to anesthetize a particular area of the body prior to laceration repair or skin excision. Nerve block offers the advantage of permitting skin excision or laceration repair without the need to inject directly into the surgical site.

To be successful at peripheral nerve blocks, it is necessary to have an understanding of the location of the pertinent peripheral nerves. It is also essential to avoid injecting directly into a nerve. Instead, the injection should be made near and around the nerve sheath. Finally, because most nerves are situated in conjunction with arteries and veins, it is important to aspirate before infiltrating local anesthetic to avoid intravascular injection.

MENTAL NERVE BLOCK

Anesthesia of the mental nerve, which innervates the lower lip and a portion of the chin, can permit repair of lip lacerations without the deforming edema caused by infiltration of local anesthetic directly into the lip. The bilateral mental nerves exit from the mandible through small bilateral depressions in the mandible that are palpable about 1 cm below the mandibular bicuspid teeth. While some clinicians inject anesthetic directly through the skin of the chin, a preferable way to inject anesthetic is through the gingival-buccal sulcus overlying the mandibular exit of the mental nerve. Lidocaine with epinephrine can be used.

DIGITAL NERVE BLOCK

The nerves that innervate the fingers and toes can be anesthetized using a digital nerve block (Fig. 1-3). This technique involves injection of lidocaine into the distal webbed space on both sides of the digit to be anesthetized and then across the dorsal and ventral aspect of the digit. The total injected solution is about 6 cc (2 cc on either side of the digit and 1 cc on the dorsal and ventral surface) for the toes and about 4 cc (1 cc on each side and 1 cc dorsally and ventrally) for the fingers. All authorities recommend using lidocaine without epinephrine. The technique for digital nerve block is also discussed in Chapter 12.

POSTERIOR TIBIAL NERVE BLOCK

Injections into the sole of the foot are extraordinarily painful. Posterior tibial nerve blocks are useful for anesthetizing the medial sole of the foot because they achieve anesthesia without injections into the sole itself.

The posterior tibial nerve is found posterior to the medial malleolus, anterior to the Achilles tendon, and just posterior to the palpable posterior tibial pulse (Fig. 1-4). About 5 cc of local anesthetic can be infiltrated into the area. It is essential to avoid injection directly into the posterior tibial

Figure 1-4

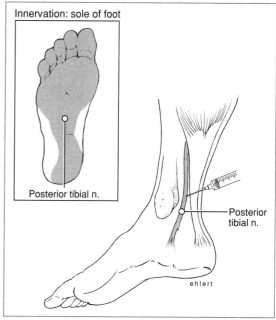

Posterior tibial nerve block. The medial aspect of the sole of the foot *(inset)* can be anesthetized with a posterior tibial nerve block. About 5 cc of local anesthetic is injected in the vicinity of the posterior tibial nerve, which is found just posterior to the posterior tibial pulse.

Figure 1-3

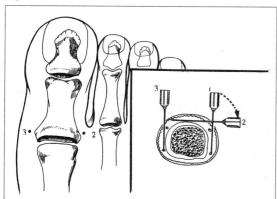

Digital nerve block. Local anesthetic is injected into the webbed space on both sides of the digit to be anesthetized and on the dorsal and ventral aspect of the digit. The same technique can be used for fingers or toes. *(Reproduced with permission from Arpey CJ, Whitaker DC, O'Donnell MJ: Cutaneous Surgery: Illustrated and Practical Approach. New York, McGraw-Hill, 1997.)*

vessels, so the syringe should be aspirated before injection takes place.

SURAL NERVE BLOCK

The lateral aspect of the sole of the foot can be anesthetized with a sural nerve block. The sural nerve passes anterior to the Achilles tendon and posterior to the lateral malleolus of the ankle; it is often ramified into multiple branches. To achieve a sural nerve block, the needle should be inserted just anteriorly to the Achilles tendon and advanced anteriorly toward the lateral malleolus (Fig. 1-5). Anesthetic should be injected in a fan-shaped distribution to ensure that the nerve's multiple branches have been anesthetized.

Figure 1-5

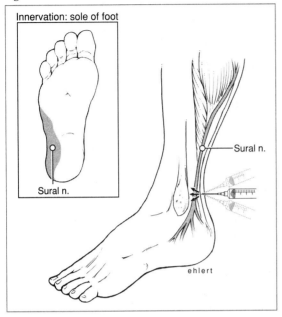

Sural nerve block. A sural nerve block can be used to anesthetize the lateral aspect of the sole of the foot *(inset)*. Local anesthetic is injected in a fan-shaped distribution anterior to the Achilles tendon in the direction of the lateral malleolus.

Hematoma Block

Hematoma blocks are often the anesthetic of choice for pain relief during closed reduction of a Colle's fracture. If necessary, a hematoma block can be supplemented with any form of conscious sedation and/or opiates.

In this simple technique, 10 mL of 1% lidocaine is injected through a 22-gauge needle, directly into the hematoma. With the needle positioned so that the tip is angled slightly toward the radial head, the examiner "walks" the needle tip toward the fracture line, ideally until a step-off is identified through which the needle can enter the fracture site. Blood is aspirated from the hematoma, and lidocaine is injected slowly, observing for signs of toxicity that might indicate intravascular injection.

Intravenous Regional (Bier) Block

Although Bier blocks are most often applied during surgery on the hand or forearm, they can also be used on the foot and leg. The technique involves the injection of a large volume of dilute local anesthetic, usually 40 mL 0.5% lidocaine, into the vein of an exsanguinated upper extremity kept pulseless by a proximal tourniquet maintained much above systolic blood pressure. Bier blocks are tolerated well for up to an hour, at which point limb ischemia and tourniquet pain require that the technique be stopped. A step-by-step approach to this technique is shown in Table 1-5, and the setup for the procedure is illustrated in Figure 1-6.

Table 1-5

Step-by-Step Instructions for a Bier Block

1. Start a small (20- or 22-gauge) IV in the surgical hand; flush and cap.
2. Prepare 0.5% lidocaine 40–50 mL solution in a syringe.
3. Apply proximal and distal cuffs over cast padding on the upper arm, making sure they fit well, do not leak, and can be inflated to 250 mm/Hg (or 50% above measured systolic blood pressure). Leave deflated for now.
4. Apply routine monitors, and establish IV access in the other extremity.
5. Elevate surgical arm, and tightly apply eschmarch bandage, wrapping from the hand to the upper arm, to exsanguinate limb for at least 1 minute.
6. Inflate proximal cuff to preset pressure.
7. Remove eschmarch bandage.
8. Radial pulse should now be absent.

Table 1-5

Continued

9. Attach lidocaine syringe, and slowly inject contents, observing patient for signs of toxicity. Veins in hand and forearm should be prominent. Patient should experience warmth and tingling followed by numbness of entire arm and hand within a few minutes. Patient will not have substantial motor weakness and will be able to move arm.
10. Wait 2–3 minutes, and then inflate distal cuff to preset pressure.
11. Deflate proximal cuff pressure, observing for signs of systemic toxicity. Now lidocaine will decrease sensation under the distal cuff.
12. Remove IV in surgical hand, prep, and proceed with procedure.
13. After about 30 minutes the proximal cuff can be inflated, and then the distal cuff can be deflated. This should provide 15–30 minutes more of tolerable anesthesia to extremity.
14. If procedure is finished before 30 minutes after the lidocaine was injected, slowly deflate the cuff, watching for signs of toxicity.
15. Local anesthesia can be added directly at the surgical site as needed.

Figure 1-6

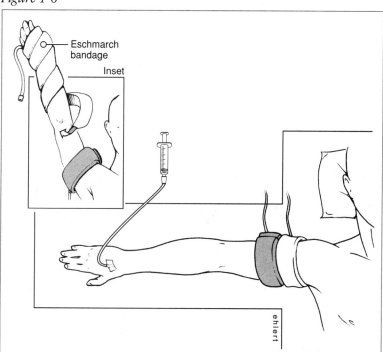

Bier block. The Bier block is used to anesthetize an extremity after "exanguinating" the extremity by the use of an eschmarch bandage *(inset)*. Local anesthetic is administered via intravenous infusion and retained in the extremity by the use of blood pressure cuffs that serve as tourniquets.

Neuraxial Block

Of the several forms of neuraxial blocks, a simple spinal anesthetic ("saddle block") is easiest to administer. It can sometimes be used when general anesthesia or more-sophisticated, neuraxial blocks are unavailable. Procedures for which saddle blocks are well suited include cesarean delivery, laparotomy for acute abdomen, and treatment of lower-extremity fractures and dislocations.

Saddle block involves the administration of a hyperbaric local anesthetic solution into the sub-arachnoid space while the patient is in the sitting position. A saddle block provides reliable dense anesthesia to the perineum, pelvis, both lower extremities, inguinal region, lower peritoneum, and genitourinary/gastrointestinal tract. It does not provide reliable anesthesia for upper abdominal procedures.

A saddle block of lidocaine without epinephrine will last from 45 minutes to 1.5 hours. The technique for administering a saddle block, which is similar to that involved in performing a lumbar puncture, is outlined in Table 1-6.

Table 1-6
Step-By-Step Instructions for Administering a Saddle Block

1.   Place patient in sitting position, leaning forward on an assistant.
2.   Attach monitors, start IV, and administer 500–1000 mL fluid.
3.   Have emergency airway equipment, ephedrine, and phenylephrine available.
4.   Sedate patient if desired, and administer oxygen.
5.   Widely prep and drape the lumbar spine midline and 4 inches laterally in both directions.
6.   With sterile gloves palpate the lateral pelvic brim on both sides, and visualize a straight line between both sides. They cross the lumbar spine at approximately the L_{4-5} interspace.
7.   With your fingertips palpate the spinous processes above and below, determining relative size of space and curvature.
8.   Reposition patient in flexion, and straighten shoulders if needed, paying special attention to flexion of the lumbar spine.
9.   Administer 1 mL of 1% lidocaine intradermally over the interspace and 1–2 mL deeper in the midline between spinous processes, angling slightly cephalad toward the umbilicus.
10. With spinal needle and stylette fully inserted advance into the same interspace by passing through interspinous ligament. Stabilize spinal needle using one hand against patient's back and the other hand around the hub of the needle to avoid sudden uncontrolled advancement. If bone is encountered, redirect without bending the spinal needle.
11. On advancing halfway up the shaft of the needle, remove the stylette and observe fluid return. CSF is clear and colorless; blood should rapidly clear.
12. Advance slowly and stop if patient notices paresthesias. If yes, ask where felt and in what location; this is very helpful as it can signal wandering from midline. It is OK to advance as long as paresthesias are no longer present; if so, then redirect slightly.
13. Usually a slight change in resistance is felt as the subarachnoid space is entered.
14. Remove stylette and observe continuous dripping of CSF.
15. Attach syringe containing 1.0 mL of 5% lidocaine (50 mg) and 7.5% dextrose.
16. Aspirate gently and observe CSF slowly whisping and mixing with lidocaine; withdraw at least 0.25 mL CSF.
17. Slowly begin injection. It should be easy to inject.
18. Stop halfway, repeat #16–17.

Table 1-6

Continued

19.	Before removing syringe repeat #16–17 a final time, and then remove needle and syringe entirely in one move.
20.	Keep talking to the patient throughout the procedure, explaining what you are doing and forewarning of pain.
21.	Ask about warmth in feet, tingling in toes. Spinal onset is 1–3 minutes and should be very obvious to patient within 5 minutes.
22.	After 5 minutes assist patient in assuming supine position (they will be weak!)
23.	Spend the next few minutes assessing the extent of spread of the spinal, taking frequent blood pressures. The cephalad spread of a spinal can be influenced greatly by the position of the patient during the first few minutes after injection. Thereafter, changing position of the table becomes less and less effective.

Abbreviations: CSF, cerebrospinal fluid; IV, intravenous.

Conscious Sedation and Other Brief Anesthetic Techniques

Conscious sedation is an anesthetic regimen in which patients remain communicative and generally able to cooperate with clinicians. The medication most often used for conscious sedation is midazolam, frequently in combination with a narcotic analgesic (fentanyl) or sometimes with propofol. Patients undergoing conscious sedation with midazolam experience amnesia for the procedure they have undergone. The most important adverse effect from administration of midazolam is apnea.

The usual dose of midazolam for conscious sedation is an initial 0.5 to 1.0 mg intravenous bolus. This is followed by an intravenous infusion at a rate of 0.5 to 1.0 μg/kg/min.

Several of the other medications discussed earlier can also be used for brief intravenous or inhalation anesthesia. Propofol is perhaps the most common agent used for this purpose, but inhalation of nitrous oxide may sometimes be appropriate. Opiates are frequently combined with these agents to ensure an adequate analgesic effect.

Every patient that undergoes conscious sedation or other brief anesthesia regimens should be monitored by someone who is capable of making an accurate assessment of cardiopulmonary and neurologic status and of intervening if the patient becomes unstable. The minimum monitoring routine for conscious sedation, or for any of the regional anesthetic techniques (i.e., neuraxial or Bier blocks) described in this chapter, is shown in Table 1-7.

General Anesthesia

General anesthesia involves endotracheal intubation, administration of anesthetic and analgesic medications, and sophisticated monitoring of vital functions. Clinicians who administer general anesthesia must have mastered skills of airway management and should be familiar with the use of agents such as succinylcholine, propofol, opiates, and other agents discussed earlier in this chapter.

A detailed discussion of how to administer general anesthesia is beyond the scope of this chapter. However, for clinicians practicing in remote areas where general anesthesia services are not readily available, many of the anesthetic techniques outlined above can be used as alternatives to general anesthesia when patients cannot be safely transported to other facilities. As seen in the anesthetic techniques recommended in Table 1-3, clinicians who develop skills at

Table 1-7

Basic Requirements for Monitoring Patients During Conscious Sedation

1. Intravenous access
2. Pulse oximeter
3. Blood pressure cuff with measurement of blood pressure every 5 minutes
4. Three-lead electrocardiography
5. Direct observation of breathing frequency, depth, and pattern
6. Supplemental oxygen (minimum 2 L by nasal prongs)
7. Repeated verbal communication with patient, especially after repeated doses

regional blocks, neuraxial blocks, and conscious sedation will be able to manage many cases for which general anesthesia might otherwise be used in larger centers. These skills, combined with an understanding of the information outlined in Chapter 4 about how to appropriately stabilize and transport patients, will permit clinicians to effectively handle most surgical problems.

References

Bergman SA: Ketamine: review of its pharmacology and its use in pediatric anesthesia. *Anesth Prog* 46:10, 1999.

Bhatt-Mehta V, Rosen DA: Sedation in children: current concepts. *Pharmacotherapy* 18:790, 1998.

Bissonnette B, Swan H, Ravussin P, et al: Neurolept-anesthesia: current status. *Can J Anaesth* 46:154, 1999.

Brown DL (ed): *Regional Anesthesia and Analgesia*. Philadelphia, WB Saunders, 1996.

Dahl JB, Jeppesen IS, Jorgensen H, et al: Intraoperative and postoperative analgesic efficacy and adverse effects of intrathecal opioids in patients undergoing cesarean section with spinal anesthesia: a qualitative and quantitative systematic review of randomized controlled trials. *Anesthesiology* 91:1919, 1999.

Goodman AG, Rall TW, Nies AS, et al (eds): *Goodman and Gilman's The Pharmacological Basis of Therapeutics*, 8th ed. New York, Pergamon, 1990.

Goodwin SA: A review of preemptive analgesia. *J Perianesth Nurs* 13:109, 1998.

Harris LG: Spinal and combined spinal epidural techniques for labor analgesia: clinical application in a small hospital. *AANA J* 66:587, 1998.

Lazarov SJ: Office-based surgery and anesthesia: where are we now? *World J Urol* 16:384, 1998.

Lowson SM, Sawh S: Adjuncts to analgesia. Sedation and neuromuscular blockade. *Crit Care Clin* 15:119, 1999.

McCarty EC, Mencio GA, Green NE: Anesthesia and analgesia for the ambulatory management of fractures in children. *J Am Acad Orthop Surg* 7:81–91, 1999.

Miller RD (ed): *Anesthesia*, 4th ed. New York, Churchill Livingstone, 1994.

Mirakhur RK, Morgan M: Intravenous anaesthesia: a step forward. *Anaesthesia* 53:(suppl 1):1, 1998.

Mulroy MF: Extending indications for spinal anesthesia. *Reg Anesth Pain Med* 23:380, 1998.

Pfenninger JL, Fowler GC: *Procedures for Primary Care Physicians*. St Louis, MO, Mosby–Year Book, 1994.

Shelly MP, Nightingale P: ABC of intensive care: respiratory support. *BMJ* 318:1674, 1999.

Smith DW, Peterson MR, DeBerard SC: Local anesthesia. Topical application, local infiltration, and field block. *Postgrad Med* 106:57, 1999.

Smith DW, Peterson MR, DeBerard SC: Regional anesthesia. Nerve blocks of the extremities and face. *Postgrad Med* 106:69, 1999.

Spencer HC: Postdural puncture headache: what matters in technique. *Reg Anesth Pain Med* 23:374, 1998.

Stewart GM, Simpson P, Rosenberg NM: Use of topical lidocaine in pediatric laceration repair: a review of topical anesthetics. *Pediatr Emerg Care* 14:419, 1998.

Wilhelmi BJ, Blackwell SJ, Miller J: Epinephrine in digital blocks: revisited. *Ann Plast Surg* 41:410, 1998.

Wallace H.J. Chang

Suturing Techniques and Materials

Introduction

The basic biologic reaction to injury initiates a process that ultimately leads to healing in all tissues, including skin. The healing process initially involves an inflammatory response, and the degree of inflammation is proportional to the degree of tissue destruction caused by the injury. In skin, the presence of a gap between the margins of the wound prolongs the inflammatory process and can result in excess scar formation with various consequences, including hypertrophic (keloid) scars, contractures of adjacent tissues and structures, restriction of motion, and gross physiologic dysfunction. Approximation of the wound edges decreases the degree of inflammation, leads to healing by primary intention, and thereby reduces the likelihood of these untoward consequences.

The act of approximating wounds is probably as old as the human species. The natural reflex of grasping a wound and holding it together with whatever means available must have been the first and simplest maneuver in wound repair. In modern times we have a variety of techniques available to close wounds, resulting in potentially excellent cosmetic and functional results.

The purpose of this chapter is to discuss the various aspects of wound repair, including selec-

Figure 2-1

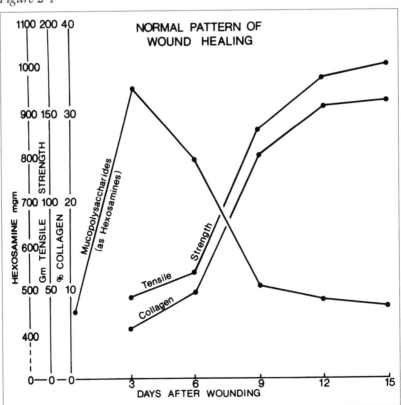

Tensile strength of healing wounds. Note that at 7 days after injury, the usual time of suture removal, tensile strength of wounds is still relatively low. (*Reproduced with permission from Chang W: Fundamentals of Plastic and Reconstructive Surgery. Philadelphia: Lippincott Williams & Wilkins, 1980.*)

tion of sutures and instruments, suturing techniques, and wound care after suturing, including timing of suture removal. While a considerable portion of the chapter is devoted to descriptions of sutures and instruments, it is important for the reader to keep in mind that technical finesse—through proper wound preparation, reduction of tension, and atraumatic approximation of wound edges—is far more important than the choice of suture materials and instruments for obtaining a superior result.

Chapter 2

Pathophysiology

It is beyond the scope of this chapter to include a detailed discussion of wound physiology. In brief, wound healing involves an initial inflammatory phase, followed by synthesis of collagen to close and provide tensile strength for the wound. It is important to note that the tensile strength of wounds (Fig. 2-1) is still quite low at 7 days following wound repair (a popular time for suture removal), and does not achieve 75% of its normal strength until about 42 days after injury. The obvious implication of this fact is that, if sutures are removed at 7 days after wound repair and no subcutaneous sutures were used to provide strength to the wound, the scar needs to be splinted to avoid spreading of the scar.

Instruments and Supplies

Suturing is broadly conceptualized as the use of any material or device to approximate the edges of a wound. Therefore, surgical staples can also be considered a form of "suture," as can tissue glue or tape. Stapled methods of wound closure will not be discussed in this chapter, except to briefly discuss here when surgical staples should and should not be used. If speed of wound clo-

sure is more important than the appearance of the final scar, stainless staples do a fine job of holding the wound edges. Staples can also be used for temporary wound approximation when dealing with large wounds as "trial" sutures to identify appropriate points of wound approximation; they are then removed during surgery when conventional suturing is performed. It should be emphasized that staples leave permanent marks on the skin, and, therefore, they have no place in wound repair about the face and neck.

Instruments

The basic instruments required to suture most wounds in an office or emergency room setting are listed in Table 2-1. Several of the instruments deserve specific comment in this chapter. Photographs of some of these instrument are presented in the next chapter.

SCALPEL

Although #4 flat scalpel handles are the most prevalent and least expensive, round scalpel handles are more maneuverable, especially for

Table 2-1

Instruments for Basic Suture Repair

Quantity	Instrument
1	Scalpel
	#4 handles with
	#15 disposable blades
3	Forceps, Adson type
	1 plain
	1 with teeth
	1 Brown modification
1	Curved iris scissors
1	Straight iris scissors
2	Skin hooks
2	Hemostat clamps
1	Needle holder, Webster type

cutting around curves, for excisional debridement of devitalized tissue, and for converting jagged wound margins to clean, straight edges. Regardless of the type of scalpel handle, the use of a scalpel is less traumatic than scissors.

The #15 disposable blades are adequate for most head, neck, and upper extremity areas. The larger #10 blades will facilitate excisions on the trunk and lower extremities where the skin is generally thicker (Fig. 2-2).

Skin Hook

In most instances a skin hook should be used to hold tissue instead of forceps, to avoid unnecessary crushing of the tissues between the forceps blades. If necessary, two skin hooks are applied at opposite ends of a wound to stablize the wound margins for excision or undermining, as needed

Figure 2-2

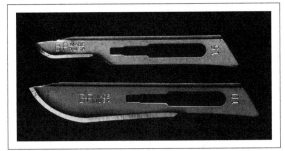

Scalpel blades. The most commonly used scalpel blades are the smaller #15 and the larger #10. The #10 blades are most useful for cutting in thick skin such as on the trunk and lower extremities.

to relieve tension with a minimum of trauma to the new wound edges (Fig. 2-3). Skin hooks can also be used during suture placement for eleva-

Figure 2-3

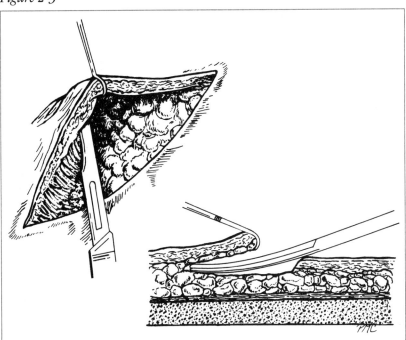

Skin hook. The skin hook is used to elevate skin, to expose the wound, and to stabilize skin during suture placement or tissue undermining, as shown here. (*Reproduced with permission from Chang W:* Fundamentals of Plastic and Reconstructive Surgery. *Philadelphia: Lippincott Williams & Wilkins, 1980.*)

tion of the skin and for retraction of the wound to provide better exposure. In addition, skin hooks can be used to reduce tension across a wound during the tying of the first few sutures.

When skin hooks are unavailable, a makeshift skin hook can be fashioned by bending the tip of a fine hypodermic needle into a hook. Insertion of a dry, cotton Q-tip into the hub of the needle makes a nice handle, and moistening the Q-tip after insertion secures the fit.

FORCEPS

Forceps are used to pick up tissues for excision and for holding the needle during passage of the suture. Unfortunately, forceps are often used instead of a skin hook to handle the wound edges, resulting in undue pressure to the wound margins. Crushing of the tissues with every suture along the wound margin will cause increased inflammation, swelling, delayed wound healing, and an unfavorable scar.

The choice of forceps is largely personal. Of the three types of forceps listed in Table 2-1, two have teeth at the tips for holding tissue (Fig. 2-4). The Brown-Adson (multiple-teeth) forceps distributes the applied force to many fine teeth, whereas the standard, single-tooth forceps has only one point

Figure 2-4

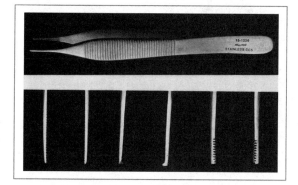

Forceps. The Brown-Adson forceps, commonly used for wound repair, are shown on the top. Forceps are available with multiple small teeth *(bottom left)*, single teeth *(bottom center)*, and larger teeth *(bottom right)*.

of contact. Both forceps can be abused if too much force is applied. The plain Adson forceps (without teeth, but has fine serrations) is better for picking up small tags of tissue during debridement.

HEMOSTATIC CLAMPS

Hemostats are used for clamping bleeding vessels. Remember that only the cut ends of the vessels are bleeding, and therefore only the ends of the vessels need to be clamped and ligated. One must avoid clamping blindly in a bleeding area, as this results in the unnecessary incorporation of excess tissue in the clamp and in the ligature. This is undesirable, because all clamped and ligated tissues become necrotic and add to the inflammatory phase of healing. If the end of the bleeding vessels is not readily visible because of the bleeding, digital pressure on the adjacent skin surface usually stops or slows the bleeding enough to allow identification of the source.

NEEDLE HOLDERS

Needle holders are specialized types of clamps, modified by heavier jaws with reinforced surfaces of more dense metal plates, and designed to grip and hold a needle firmly in all positions and angles. This capability allows the clinician to pass the needle in various directions simply by changing the position of the needle in the needle holder, thereby avoiding the awkwardness of needing to twist the wrist.

The proper placement of the needle in the needle holder is to grasp the needle at a point on the curve of the needle, approximatuely one-half to two-thirds the distance from the needle tip and one-half to one-third the distance from the threaded end (Fig. 2-5). Placement of the needle holder any closer to the threaded end increases the torque force on the the distal portion of the needle and may cause the needle to bend. Placement of the needleholder any closer to the tip makes it more difficult to pass enough needle through the tissue so it can be grasped as it emerges on the other side.

Figure 2-5

Selection and Use of Needleholders

1. The needleholder must be an appropriate size instrument for the size needle selected.

2. It must be made from good quality steel with a secure jaw design.

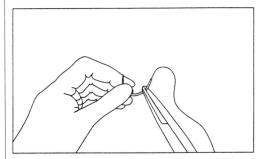

3. Needles should be grasped in an area about ⅓ to ½ of the distance from the swaged area to the point. Avoid placement on or near the swaged area.

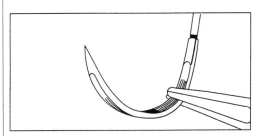

4. The needle should be placed securely in the tip of the needleholder jaws.

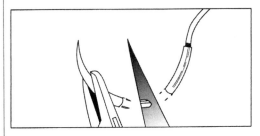

5. Do not damage taper points or cutting edges when using the needleholder to pull the needle out through the tissue. Grasp as far back as possible.

6. When placing the needle in tissue, any force applied should be in the direction following the curve of the needle.

7. Do not take excessively large bites of tissue with small needles.

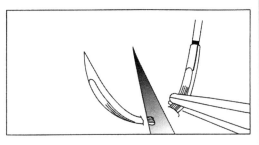

8. Do not force or twist the needle in an effort to bring the point out through the tissue—withdraw the needle and replace in tissue.

9. Do not force a dull needle through tissue—obtain a new one.

10. Avoid using the needle to bridge or approximate tissues for suturing.

11. If the needle is held too tightly in a sharp or hard jawed or defective needleholder, the needle may be damaged or notched in such a manner that it will have more of a tendency to bend or break on successive passes through tissue.

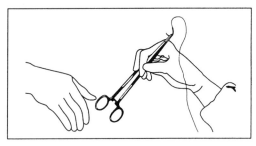

12. When the needleholder with needle is passed to the surgeon, the needle should be pointing in the direction in which it will start to be used without need for readjustment.

13. In some patients, the tissues may be tougher or fibrosed more than normal and require the use of a heavier gauge needle.

14. In a deep confined area, ideal positioning of the needle may not be possible. The surgeon should proceed with caution or use a heavier gauge needle.

An ATRALOC needle is an instrument that complements the surgeon's skills. The variety of ETHICON needles offers the surgeon a choice of needles which are dependable for consistent quality and for practically all surgical applications.

Needle holder. Note proper location of needle in the needle holder. (*Courtesy of Ethicon.*)

Supplies

SUTURE

An ideal suture not only closes the wound effectively with minimal tension on the wound edges, but also glides through tissue with the minimum amount of resistance. It should also be easy to tie with a needle holder, incite the least amount of inflammatory reaction, and when appropriate, be absorbed completely.

There are four basic considerations in the selection of suture—the type of suture material, the caliber of the suture, its filamentous structure, and the type of needle that is attached to the suture.

SUTURE MATERIALS Suture materials can be divided into two categories: nonabsorbable and absorbable. Nonabsorbable suture includes suture made from materials like silk, steel, and nylon. Common types of absorbable suture are shown in Table 2-2. The absorbability of the suture depends on the type of material used and the mass of the suture—a larger size of the same type of suture material will take longer to completely dissolve.

Plain catgut suture will disolve and lose much of its tensile strength within 7 to 10 days, whereas chromic (treated with tannic acid) catgut will last perhaps two to three times as long. There are

Table 2-2

Absorption Time of Common Absorbable Suture Material

TYPE OF SUTURE MATIERAL	TIME TO DISSOLUTION (DAYS)
Synthetic suture	
Polyglactin 910 (Vicryl)	55–70
Poliglecaprone 25	
(Monocryl)	90–120
Polydioxanone (PDS)	120–180
Natural suture	
Fast-absorbing catgut	< 7
Plain catgut	7–10
Chromic catgut	15–30

also fast-absorbing catgut sutures whose strength wanes in less time than plain catgut.

Synthetic absorbable sutures such as Vicryl (polyglactin 910), Monocryl (Poliglecaprone 25), and PDS (Polydioxanone) last longer and are totally absorbed in 55 to 70 days, 90 to 120 days, and 4 to 6 months, respectively.

SUTURE CALIBER The caliber of the suture is usually expressed by a number followed by a hyphen and a zero, such as 3-0 nylon or 4-0 catgut. The caliber of the sutures increase as the number designation decreases (i.e., 4-0 is thinner than 3-0).

One must keep in mind that using a fine-caliber suture does not guarantee a fine, hairline scar. In fact, a very fine caliber suture, especially when tied too tightly or in the presence of postoperative swelling, will actually cut into the epidermis and the superficial dermis, giving rise to tissue damage and the classic "railroad track" scar marks on the skin.

FILAMENTOUS STRUCTURE Suture material is made as a single strand (monofilament), as with nylon or stainless steel wire, or it can be braided, as with silk, catgut, and other synthetic materials. Monofilament sutures glides through tissue easier, but have an intrinsic spring quality that makes instrument–knot-tying more difficult for the novice. Braided sutures are easier to tie, but glide through tissue with more resistance and are more difficult to remove than the monofilament sutures that glide with equal ease when removed.

Type of Needle

In general, the size and caliber of the needle is proportional to the caliber of the suture. However, they vary in their type and curvature.

There are generally two types of needles—taper and cutting. The taper needle is round and smooth throughout. A cutting needle, in contrast, is usually triangular in cross section at the tip. All three corners of the triangle are honed to fine-cutting edges. When the apex of the triangle is on the inside of the curved needle, it is called simply "cutting." When the apex of the triangle is on the outside of the curve, it is referred to as "reverse-cutting." These and other types of needles are shown in Figure 2-6.

Cutting needles pass through tissue with less resistance and are particularly useful for suturing dense and fibrous tissue such as the normal skin, dermis, tendons, ligaments, and fascia. Taper needles, in contrast, are more useful for approximating tissues such as muscle, mucosa, serosa, vessels, and nerves, when it is particularly desirable not to introduce a tear in the tissue being approximated.

Needles are also available in a variety of curves, expressed in terms of full curve to straight (Fig. 2-7). The half-curve needle represents one complete half of a circle. The selection of the appropriate curvature of the needle depends somewhat on the type and thickness of the tissue being approximated and the space available around the tissues in which to maneuver.

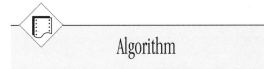

Algorithm

In the selection of the appropriate suture material, one must first decide what one is asking the suture to do. The type of tissue being approximated; the tension, if any, across the wound; and the general thickness and density of the tissue are some of the factors in the selection of the type and caliber of the suture material and the size and shape of the needle. For example, while an absorbable suture is suitable for dermal approximation, it is not as reliable as a nonabsorbable nylon suture in a vascular anastomosis. Figure 2-8 is an algorithm that correlates suture type and size with the type of tissue. As noted earlier, the number of days before all the absorbable suture material is gone is related to the size of the suture; that is, a heavier suture of the same type of suture material will last longer than a finer one.

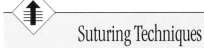

Suturing Techniques

Wounds heal better when the edges are approximated with the proper amount of tension and when the wound gap is eliminated. Thus, the purpose of suturing is to eliminate the gap by appoximating and immobilizing the wound until the tensile strength of the healing wound is sufficient to prevent dehiscence, at the minimum, and, ideally, sufficient to oppose any external spreading forces that tend to attenuate the scar. In addition, although clinicians cannot influence the wounding event, they can improve outcomes by avoiding further tissue damage with proper wound preparation (debridement), handling of tissue, and suture techniques.

Wound Preparation—Debridement

Improper or inadequate wound preparation prior to suturing may prolong healing and result in inadequate tensile strength of the wound. Most open wounds are contaminated by bacteria introduced during penetration of the skin. In addition, many wounds contain devitalized tissue.

A common cause of inadequate wound preparation is failure to remove devitalized tissue from within the wound. Devitalized tissue increases the likelihood that infection will be established within the wound, and the approximation of devitalized tissue prolongs the inflammatory phase of wound healing and decreases tensile strength of the wound.

Whenever possible, therefore, the wound margins should be sharply debrided by excision with the scalpel, that is, removal of contaminated wound edges, thereby exposing fresh, healthy tissue. Debridement is particularly important in dealing with wounds that are grossly contaminated or that are treated several hours after wounding. Excision of the wound edges in these cases converts a contaminated wound into a surgically clean wound by

Figure 2-6

ATRALOC Stainless Steel Needles

Types

Taper Point
For soft, easily penetrated tissues.

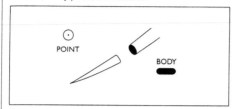

ETHIGUARD* Blunt Point Needle
Taper body. For blunt dissection and suturing friable tissue.

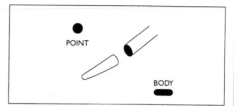

Conventional Cutting
Two opposing cutting edges, with a third on inside curve. Change in cross-section from a triangular cutting tip to a flattened body.

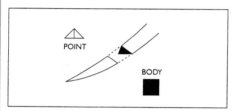

Reverse Cutting
Cutting edge on outer curve. For tough, difficult-to-penetrate tissues.

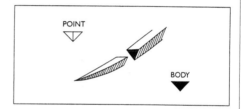

TAPERCUT* Needle
Cutting tip, taper body. For tough tissue, like two needles in one.

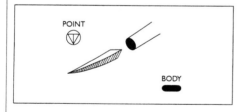

Precision Point
For delicate plastic or cosmetic surgery. Cutting tip electropolished for added sharpness.

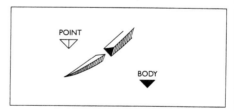

Precision Cosmetic—Conventional Cutting PRIME
For delicate plastic or cosmetic surgery. Conventional cutting tip and PRIME geometry for increased sharpness.

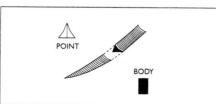

*Trademark

Types of needles. This figure illustrates a variety of types of needles, but note that all fall into one of two basic categories: (a) taper, which is rounded in cross section through its shaft, and (b) cutting, which has sharp edges and is usually triangular in cross section. (*Courtesy of Ethicon.*)

Figure 2-7

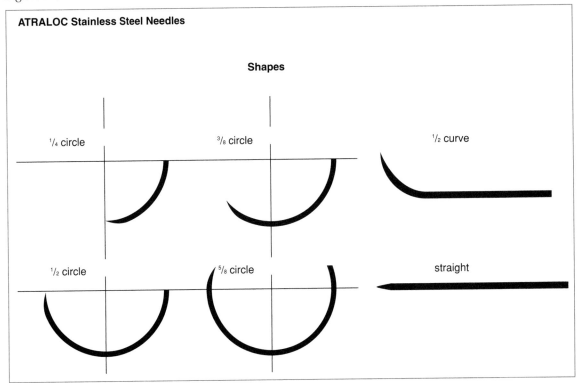

Needle curves. The curvature of needles is expressed in relation to the curve of a full circle. (*Courtesy of Ethicon.*)

removing devitalized tissue and reducing tissue bacterial count.

The ability to successfully debride a wound will depend on the availability of adjacent tissue and/or absence of adjacent vital anatomic structure. In certain anatomic regions or, specifically, if the laceration transects normal anatomic structures, excisional debridement must be tempered to avoid distortion of the normal anatomy. In eyebrow and hair-bearing scalp areas, the plane of excision must recognize the normal obliquity of the hair shafts as they emerge from the skin surface; otherwise, there will be a scarred area that is devoid of hair.

Handling Tissue

In handling wound edges during debridement and suturing, the use of a skin hook or the tip of an opened forceps avoids crushing the wound edges further. Using the scalpel blade for debridement is probably less traumatic than doing the same with a scissor.

With practice, tissues can be stabilized and needles passed without undue handling or crushing of tissues. However, in situations where the placement or passing of the needle is difficult, the reflex is to exert more pressure by the forceps on the tissue. If forceps are used to

Figure 2-8

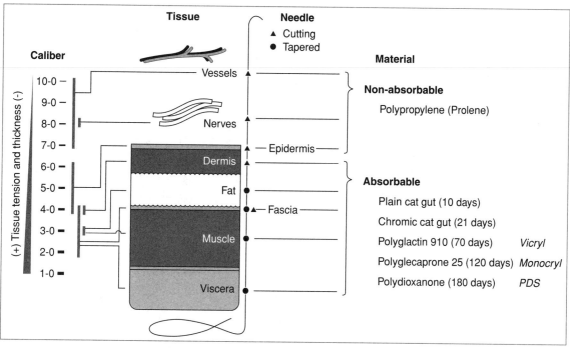

Algorithm for selection of needle(s) and caliber and type of suture(s). One can select the proper suture and needle by first identifying the tissue to be sutured in the center of the diagram. The diagram is then followed to the left to determine the appropriate caliber of suture. The diagram is followed to the right to identify the correct type of needle and suture. (*Reproduced with permission from Chang W:* Fundamentals of Plastic and Reconstructive Surgery. *Philadelphia: Lippincott Williams & Wilkins, 1980.*)

handle the wound margin, grasping the subdermal layers as much as possible spares trauma to the epidermis.

Techniques of Closure and Positioning of Sutures

There are a variety of suture techniques that can be used in different situations. It is helpful to become familiar with several of them as different wounds may require different techniques for optimal closure.

When possible, one should close wounds with subcuticular sutures because scar results are superior. Monocryl and PDS meet all the desirable suture characteristics for such closures. Either paper tape or very fine (6-0), fast-absorbing, plain catgut sutures can then be used for the fine approximation of the epidermis and superficial dermis and for leveling of the epidermal surface to avoid uneven edge levels.

SINGLE-LAYER CLOSURES

Single-layer closures are appropriate only when the depth of the laceration extends incompletely through the dermal layer. In this situation, the remaining dermal integrity prevents distraction of the wound, and all that is required is fine approximation of the epidermal and superficial dermal edges.

Either interrupted, running, interrupted horizontal mattress, or running horizontal mattress

Figure 2-9

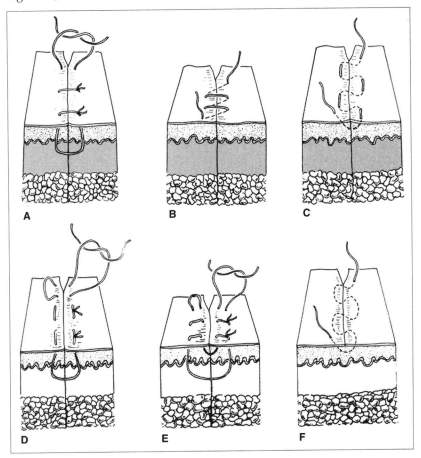

Types of suturing. **A.** Simple interrupted. **B.** Simple running. **C.** Horizontal running mattress. **D.** Horizontal mattress.**E.** Vertical mattress. **F.** Running subcuticular. (*Reproduced with permission from Chang W:* Fundamentals of Plastic and Reconstructive Surgery. *Philadelphia: Lippincott Williams & Wilkins, 1980.*)

sutures can be used (Fig. 2-9). For very superficial wounds, paper-tape strips can be just as effective as sutures.

Single-layer closures are also appropriate in certain specific locations, even if the wound is completely through the dermis. Specifically, single-layer closure is indicated for repairing wounds in the eyebrows and hair-bearing scalp areas, as too much handling and/or dermal/subdermal sutures may interfere with hair growth and create conspicuous, hairless scars.

MULTILAYER CLOSURES

Multilayer closures are necessary when the wound is deep and when multiple layers of tissue are involved. Obviously, a knowledge of the associated anatomy is mandatory for a successful repair.

By convention, nonabsorbable sutures are used for repair of tendons, fascia, blood vessels, and nerves, while fat, muscle, and dermis are approximated with absorbable sutures. However, there is no scientific reason for not using an

Figure 2-10

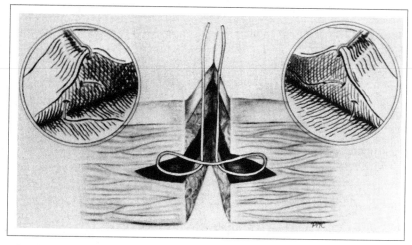

Subcuticular sutures. Placement of subcuticular sutures under the dermis and lateral to the cut edges, rather than through the opposing wound surfaces, will evert the approximated wound margins. (*Reproduced with permission from Chang W: Fundamentals of Plastic and Reconstructive Surgery. Philadelphia: Lippincott Williams & Wilkins, 1980.*)

absorbable suture in a tendon repair, as long as the suture does not dissolve before the tendon has regained its normal breaking strength. Likewise, a nonabsorbable nylon suture can be used in the dermis, placed very close to the epidermis for a long-lasting effect against attenuation. A colorless, 4-0, clear nylon is selected to avoid the visibility of the suture through lightly pigmented skin.

POSITION AND NUMBER OF SUTURES

The position and number of sutures cannot be arbitrarily decided, as they are often dictated by the condition of the wound and the types of tissue being approximated. In general, more sutures are not better. In fact, experienced surgeons strive to achieve ideal wound approximation with the least number of sutures. Too many sutures can potentially compromise the local circulation especially if tied too tightly, and they serve as foreign material that may increase the risk of infection.

At times, if a wound is very contaminated, no sutures should be used and the wound should be left open for delayed primary repair. If drainage

(e.g., bleeding) from the wound is anticipated, more space should be left between sutures or a drain should be used.

To avoid the suture marks that are often seen flanking a linear scar, it is often desirable that all sutures be placed at the subcuticular level (Fig. 2-10). The final epidermal approximation can then be acheived with paper tape (SteriStrips). As noted earlier, use of fine sutures is contraindicated when postoperative swelling is anticipated, as thin suture material can cut into the skin as swelling develops, leaving scars and increasing tissue damage. Tying the knots properly, selecting a larger-caliber suture, and removing sutures earlier are preferred when swelling is anticipated.

Tying Sutures

Sutures can be tied manually or by instrument. Manual ties can be performed one-handed or two-handed. In an instrument tie, a needle holder takes the place of one of the clinician's hands. Some practice is mandatory with all of these techniques; otherwise, one will spend an inordinate amount of time closing a wound.

MANUAL TIES

Manual tying may be done two-handed or one-handed (Figs. 2-11 and 2-12), and the result should be a square knot. The technique for tying a square knot involves crossing the hands to opposite sides with each half of the tie (the right strand of the suture over and then under the left strand of the suture, followed by the left strand of the suture over and then under the right strand of the suture, or vice versa). Note the importance of achieving a square knot, which does not slip and holds well. Failure to alternate the direction of the two halves of the knot results in a "granny" knot, which is actually the wrapping of one strand of

Figure 2-11

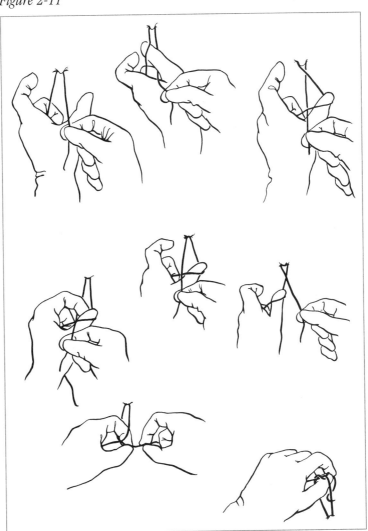

Two-handed knot tying. Follow the diagram from left to right. (*Reproduced with permission from Chang W:* Fundamentals of Plastic and Reconstructive Surgery. *Philadelphia: Lippincott Williams & Wilkins, 1980.*)

Figure 2-11 (continued)

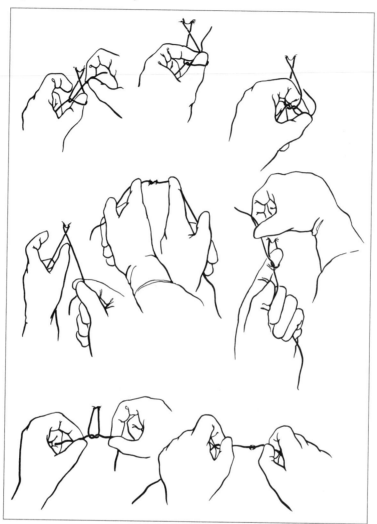

the suture around the other. Granny knots slip and untie.

Manual ties are usually used only in areas where maneuvering a needleholder is hampered by the size and location of the wound, or when controlling the position of the first half of the knot is desirable. Two-handed manual knots are essential for approximating subcutaneous tissues such as fascia that may be under tension across the wound. Sometimes, this tension is such that the first half of the knot is not sufficient to hold the first tie. In such instances two-handed control

(i.e., maintenance of tension on both ends of the suture) while tying the second half of the knot will effectively maintain wound approximation. A third square tie will ensure security of the knot.

INSTRUMENT TIES

Instrument tying (Fig. 2-13) requires a good deal of practice, but, once learned, is easier and quicker, and uses less suture than manually tied knots. In an instrument tie, the needle holder takes the place of one of the clincian's hands. One

Figure 2-12

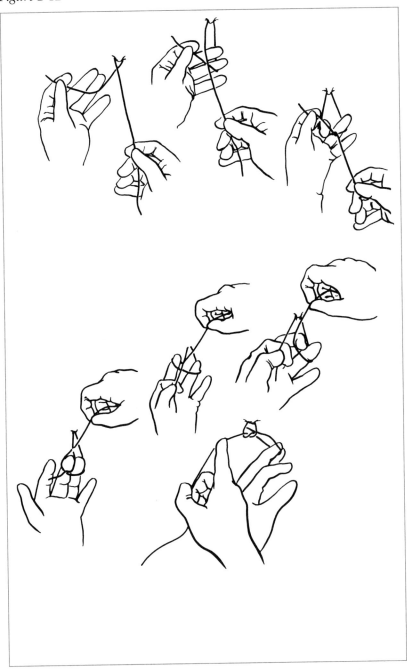

One-handed knot tying. Follow the diagram from left to right. (*Reproduced with permission from Chang W:* Fundamentals of Plastic and Reconstructive Surgery. *Philadelphia: Lippincott Williams & Wilkins, 1980.*)

Figure 2-12 (continued)

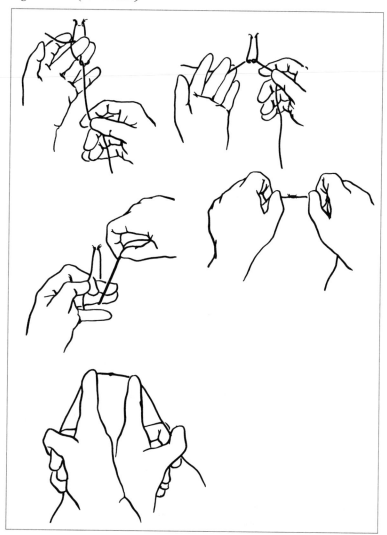

must be careful to alternate the direction of the suture loop around the needle holder to ensure a square knot. This can be done by wrapping the long end of the suture, alternately, clockwise and counterclockwise around the end of the needle-holder with each throw of the knot. If the long end of the suture is wrapped around the needle-holder in the same direction for both halves of the knot, a "granny" knot will result.

Special Considerations

SUBCUTANEOUS SUTURES

In the sequential placement and tying of sub-cutaneous sutures, the exposure progressively diminishes, making each successive suture—especially the last suture—more difficult to place. It is helpful to hold the next-to-the-last suture untied and not tie it until the last suture is placed.

Figure 2-13

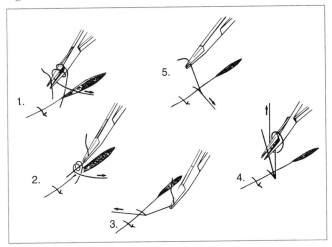

Instrument knot. Instrument-tied knots are easier, quicker, and use less suture material than manually tied knots. (*Reproduced with permission from Chang W: Fundamentals of Plastic and Reconstructive Surgery. Philadelphia: Lippincott Williams & Wilkins, 1980.*)

SURGEON'S KNOT

Most monofilament nylon sutures have some internal springiness, which makes them somewhat difficult to tie, especially when performing an instrument tie, and especially when tying tissues under tension. As one tries to set the second half of the knot, the spring effect causes the first half to slide and loosen. This can usually be prevented by tying a "surgeon's knot." A surgeon's knot is tied by wrapping the long end of the suture around the end of the needleholder twice when tying the first half of the knot, before grasping the short end. This will result in a knot that will not slip in most circumstances.

If this surgeon's knot is still inadequate to overcome the tension across a wound and maintain approximation for placement of the second half of the square knot, simply lock the first knot. Locking the first knot is accomplished as follows: First, set the first surgeon's knot down (the hand holding one end of the suture and the needleholder are pulling in opposite directions at this point). Then, while maintaining the tension on the ends of the suture, bring both ends of the suture to the

same side of the wound (it is not important which side). Finally, with the first knot now locked, set the second half of the square knot.

If the above maneuver is still not adequate to maintain approximation in tying the square knot, a two-handed tie can be performed. A little practice with the two-handed approach will permit tying the second half of the square knot, while maintaining tension on the first. If the two-handed method is still inadequate to allow tying, the clinician should reexamine the wound and seek other solutions to reduce the tension (e.g., undermining the wound, as shown in Fig. 2-3) or use alternative methods of wound closure.

SPECIAL TISSUES

FAT   Fatty tissues do not hold sutures well. However, there are superficial fascial layers throughout the body that do hold sutures and can be used to approximate the adjacent fat. In most instances, it is not necessary to suture the fat that is passively approximated when adjacent fascial and dermal layers are sutured.

FASCIA   Fascial tissues hold sutures very well, but the type of suture material selected should have a longevity that exceeds the time necessary for the fascia to attain sufficient tensile strength (Fig. 2-8). Permanent suture material like nylon or long-lasting absorbable suture materials like Monocryl should be used.

MUSCLE   Muscle can hold sutures fairly well, as long as the sutures are not tied too tightly and not placed parallel to the direction of the muscle fibers. If the suture is placed parallel to the direction of the muscle fibers and tied tightly, the suture will tear through the muscle tissue.

However, most muscles are surrounded by a fascial layer that can be used to approximate the muscle tissue passively. In this situation, the needle is passed through both the fascia and the muscle. The fascia will hold the suture and allow approximation of the muscle without tearing.

TENDONS   Tendons are usually sutured with non-absorbable, monofilament sutures because of the longevity and tensile strength of such suture material. Successful healing of a tendon repair, however, is measured beyond the mere joining of cut ends. It is ultimately judged on restoration of the preoperative functional range of motion of the injured tendon.

Lacerations involving more than 50% of the cross-sectional area of a given tendon must be repaired, as not repairing such injuries is associated with a high incidence of subsequent tendon rupture. Lesser degrees of partial tendon laceration require individual considerations, including, but not limited to, the condition of the wound, the location of the injury, the function of the involved tendon, and associated injuries. Therefore, the clinician performing the repair must have an intimate knowledge of the anatomy and physiology of the injured part. If the clinician does not possess knowledge and experience in tendon repair, the case should be referred to or discussed with a clinician with the requisite knowledge and experience.

NERVES   Nerves are specialized tissue consisting of nerve fascicles, each of which is surrounded by epineureum. All the epineureum-enclosed fasicles are, in turn, enclosed in a layer of perineureum to form a nerve. Each nerve fascicle can be repaired individually, with the aid of magnification, by suturing the epineureum. Or, more commonly, only the perineureum is approximated, in which case joining of fascicles occurs passively and at random. Statistically, there is little difference in the outcome when these two methods are compared. Nerve repair should be undertaken only by those with adequate training and/or clinical experience in the repair technique.

BLOOD VESSELS   The success of vascular repair is determined not only by proper approximation of vascular tissue but also by the restoration of blood flow through a patent anastomosis. Like nerve repairs, vascular repairs should only be attempted by those with specialized training and/or experience.

When a clinician who does not have the requisite training encounters a wound with major arterial bleeding, it is essential to avoid unnecessary trauma and attempt to control the bleeding by manual pressure. Thus, one must avoid the temptation to blindly clamp bleeding vessels, as this may injure the ends of the vessels and preclude a successful subsequent anastomosis.

Suture Removal

As noted earlier, the tensile strength of skin wounds is low at 7 to 10 days following repair, the precise time when sutures are usually removed. However, sutures should nonetheless be removed at this point to avoid the development of cosmetically undesirable suture marks.

There are two types of suture marks. One is a dotlike scar at the sites of entry and exit of the sutures material. These suture marks may be impossible to avoid, but timely removal of suture minimizes the likelihood that they will develop. The other type of suture mark is the so-called "railroad-track" mark, which is created by "cutting" of the skin by the suture itself. The risk of developing railroad-track suture marks can be minimized by ensuring that surface sutures are not tied too tightly, especially when swelling is anticipated.

In removing a suture (Fig. 2-14), the suture loop is cut at the skin surface. The knot or the

other end of the loop is grasped with forceps and pulled toward, rather than away from, the midline of the wound to avoid distracting the healing wound.

Because surface sutures are removed when tensile strength of the wound is low, it is mandatory that wound strength be preserved by one of two measures. One measure is the use of subcutaneous sutures. The second measure, which is especially important in the absence of subcutaneous sutures, is splinting the wound with skin tape (Fig. 2-15).

Figure 2-14

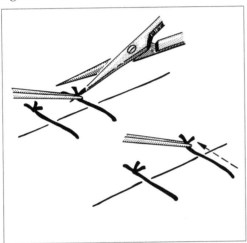

Suture removal. Note that when applying traction on the suture during removal, the direction of traction is toward the midline of the wound instead of applying traction that might result in opening the wound. (*Reproduced with permission from Chang W:* Fundamentals of Plastic and Reconstructive Surgery. *Philadelphia: Lippincott Williams & Wilkins, 1980.*)

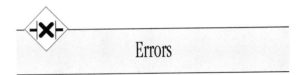

Errors

The most common errors in wound closure are errors of technique relating to approximation of the wound edges. Other errors relate to selection of suture material.

Errors of Technique

There are three common errors in approximation of the wound. The most common error is inversion of the epidermal edges caused by improper

Figure 2-15

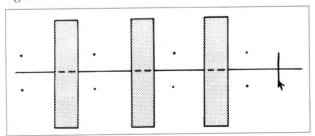

Adhesive skin tapes. Adhesive skin tapes are used to maintain strength of the wound after suture removal. (*Reproduced with permission from Chang W:* Fundamentals of Plastic and Reconstructive Surgery. *Philadelphia: Lippincott Williams & Wilkins, 1980.*)

placement of the suture. The second most common error is telescoping (sliding of one epidermal edge under the opposite edge). Other errors include a discrepancy in the levels of the approximated wound edges caused by improper placement of the sutures, creation of "dog ears," and errors in management of bevelled and triangular wounds.

INVERSION OR TELESCOPING OF THE EPIDERMAL EDGES

The inversion and telescoping are most likely to occur when the skin being approximated is thin and when the suture is placed too far from the edge of the wound. In this situation, when the suture loop is tightened or closed, the two skin edges within the loop come together at random by inverting or by one sliding under the other. The solution to these errors in thin skin is to use a horizontal mattress suture (Fig. 2-9), which will evert the edges of the wound. In using horizontal mattress sutures, it is important to tie the suture with just enough tension to approximate the edges. Tying the suture too tightly will exaggerate the eversion of the wound edges, make suture removal difficult, and may leave a prominent suture mark. Used properly, the horizontal mattress suture will give the most consistent, fine, and level approximation of wounds.

In thicker skin, inversion of the edges is caused by improper passage of the needle through the skin, thereby incorporating more epidermis than dermal and subdermal tissues. The solution is to pass the needle obliquely away from the edge of the wound, thus incorporating less epidermal and more dermal and subdermal tissue. On cross section the path of the suture should be an equilateral trapezoid with the longer base in the subdermal level (Fig. 2-16).

DISCREPANCY IN THE LEVELS OF THE WOUND EDGES

Discrepancy in the levels of the approximated wound edges is caused by placement of the suture at different levels. Often, after placement of the dermal sutures, the clinician is presented with uneven epidermal levels. To correct this discrepancy with the skin suture, it is necessary to place the suture more superficially on the "high" side and more deeply on the "low" side (Fig. 2-17). When the suture is tied, the lower side is lifted by the suture loop. The same principle can be applied to both interrupted and running sutures and is effective in both cutaneous and dermal suturing.

Figure 2-16

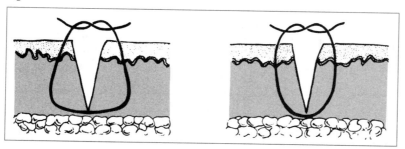

Proper placement of sutures in thick skin. Inversion of the wound edges can be avoided in thick skin by placing sutures in the shape of an equilateral trapezoid, with the longer base of the trapezoid in the subdermal level. The correct placement of the suture is shown on the left, while a common error in suture placement is shown on the right. (*Reproduced with permission from Chang W:* Fundamentals of Plastic and Reconstructive Surgery. *Philadelphia: Lippincott Williams & Wilkins, 1980.*)

Figure 2-17

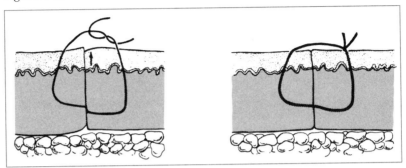

Technique in leveling wound margins. Note on the left that the suture is placed more superficially on the "high" side and more deeply on the "low" side. This results in correct leveling of the wound margins (*right*). (*Reproduced with permission from Chang W:* Fundamentals of Plastic and Reconstructive Surgery. *Philadelphia: Lippincott Williams & Wilkins, 1980.*)

DOG EARS

Dog ears result when approximating wounds with edges of unequal lengths. If the discrepancy is minor, the difference in lengths can be corrected by spacing sutures differently on each side of the wound. If a more substantial discrepancy exists, or if a dog ear occurs, it can be corrected by a triangular excision of excess tissue (Fig. 2-18).

Figure 2-18

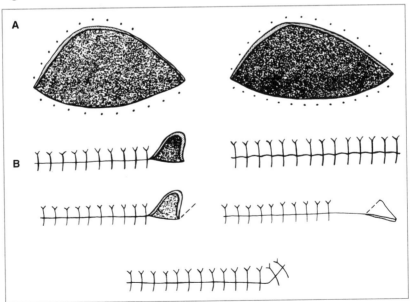

Dealing with "dog ears." Dog ears occur when the two sides of the wound are of unequal length. They can be removed or prevented by a triangular excision of excess tissue. (*Reproduced with permission from Chang W:* Fundamentals of Plastic and Reconstructive Surgery. *Philadelphia: Lippincott Williams & Wilkins, 1980.*)

BEVELLED AND TRIANGULAR WOUNDS

Bevelled lacerations should be corrected by creating new wound edges before suturing; otherwise, the edges with the acute angle will be advanced over the opposite edge during suture tying (Fig 2-19). When repairing a triangular laceration, the tip of the triangular laceration should be approximated with a buried, horizontal mattress suture to avoid the placement of too many sutures at the tip of the triangular flap, where the vascularity is often most vulnerable (Fig. 2-20).

Errors in Suture Selection

Perhaps the most widely held misconception is that fine scars are the result of using fine sutures. As discussed earlier, sometimes fine sutures can produce adverse results by cutting through the epidermal layer to leave "railroad track" marks. Actually, all other factors being equal, the selection of suture size makes no difference in the final outcome of the scar, provided that the sutures are removed early and the wound properly protected with external splinting (Steri-Strips).

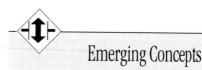

Emerging Concepts

Important emerging concepts and trends in wound closure include the use of tissue adhesives and developments in our understanding of the biochemical basis of wound healing.

Tissue Adhesives

Topical skin adhesives such as 2-octyl cyanoacrylate (Dermabond, Ethicon) show some efficacy in the closure of traumatic lacerations. General use of adhesives to close wounds will follow more clinical experience. If further research can resolve concerns about tissue toxicity and hypersensitivity, tissue adhesive will have a place in general

Figure 2-19

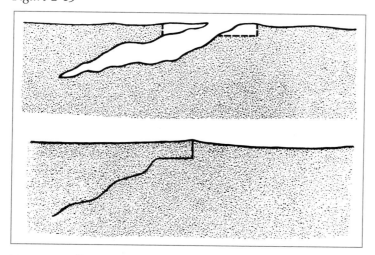

Management of bevelled wounds. Prior to closure, perpendicular edges are created for the wound by partial excision of the wound margins. (*Reproduced with permission from Chang W: Fundamentals of Plastic and Reconstructive Surgery. Philadelphia: Lippincott Williams & Wilkins, 1980.*)

Figure 2-20

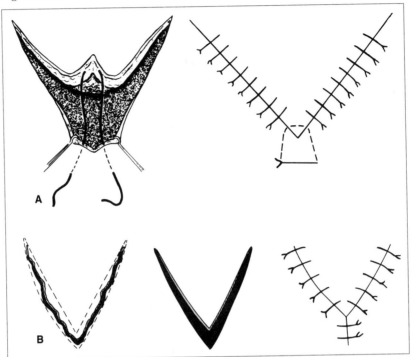

Management of triangular wounds In repairing a triangular laceration, the first step is to place a suture at the apex of the triangle. (*Reproduced with permission from Chang W:* Fundamentals of Plastic and Reconstructive Surgery. *Philadelphia: Lippincott Williams & Wilkins, 1980.*)

wound repairs, although use of adhesives around the face may be limited. Tissue adhesives are discussed in more detail in Chapter 10, which reviews repair of lacerations.

Biochemical Basis of Wound Healing

With the rapid strides in research into growth hormones and other tissue factors, it is conceivable that these substances will have a role in altering the rate of wound healing. Similarly, as we gain a better understanding of the process of tissue regeneration (as observed in lower species), it may someday be possible to induce wound healing by regeneration of the injured tissue instead of by the formation of scar. Such advances will potentially eliminate the need for suturing and will achieve the ultimate in wound repair.

References

Burke M: Scars. Can they be minimised? *Aust Fam Physician* 27:275, 1998.

Castille K: Suturing. *Nurs Stand* 12:41, 1998.

Kanegaye JT: A rational approach to the outpatient management of lacerations in pediatric patients. *Curr Probl Pediatr* 28:205, 1998.

Niessen FB, Spauwen PH, Kon M: The role of suture material in hypertrophic scar formation: Monocryl vs. Vicryl-rapide. *Ann Plast Surg* 39:254, 1997.

Orozco-Covarrubias ML, Ruiz-Maldonado, R: Surgical facial wounds: simple interrupted percutaneous suture versus running intradermal suture. *Dermatol Surg* 1999 25:109, 1999.

Penoff J: Skin closures using cyanoacrylate tissue adhesives. Plastic Surgery Educational Foundation DATA Committee. Device and Technique Assessment. *Plast Reconstr Surg* 103:730, 1999.

Romfh RF, Cramer FS: *Technique in the Use of Surgical Tools*. Norwalk, CT, Appleton & Lange, 1992.

Saxena AK, Willital GH: Octylcyanoacrylate tissue adhesive in the repair of pediatric extremity lacerations. *Am Surg* 65:470, 1999.

Smoot EC: Method for securing a subcuticular suture with minimal buried knot. *Plast Reconstr Surg* 102: 2447, 1998.

Toriumi DM, O'Grady K, Desai D, Bagal A: Use of octyl-2-cyanoacrylate for skin closure in facial plastic surgery. *Plast Reconstr Surg* 102:2209, 1998.

Robert L. Hogue

First-Assisting in Surgery

Introduction

Most primary-care clinicians seek to provide continuity of care for their patients, and many believe they must participate in all phases of their patients' medical care. Family physicians, in particular, are trained to deal with some 90% of the conditions for which their patients seek medical attention, and they see continuity of care as a central dogma of their specialty. Increasingly, however, primary-care training and practice do not include the experience and competencies necessary to assist in the operating room, making true continuity of care difficult to achieve.

Benefits of Surgical Assisting

There are a number of benefits to having primary-care physicians assist at surgery. First, in remote and rural areas, and even in some urban underserved areas, the limitations of the health-workforce supply often mandate that primary-care clinicians serve as surgical assistants. In such situations, if the primary-care clinician is not capable of serving as an able surgical assistant, there may be no one else available to fill that role.

Second, patients frequently request and desire that their primary-care clinician participate in surgery. Such patients often report less anxiety when they know that their personal physician will "be there" and is assisting in the operating room.

Third, primary-care clinicians are often in an excellent position or serve as the patient's advocate in communicating with the surgeon, as patients or their families may look to the primary-care clinician for explanations of diagnosis, prognosis, and surgical procedures. This communication can strengthen bonds between primary-care clinicians and their patients and can enhance the patient's confidence in the surgeon. To be effective in this role, however, primary-care clinicians must enter the operat-

ing room to see what the surgeon does. With this firsthand knowledge, a clinician can be more effective at counseling patients about what to expect from an operative procedure.

Finally, when primary-care clinicians participate in surgical care on a regular basis, they are better able to evaluate patients with surgical problems. They have a better understanding of diagnosis, prognosis, and surgical considerations for treatment and will be able to request earlier and more appropriate surgical consultation.

Disadvantages of Surgical Assisting

Despite the benefits outlined above, there are potential disadvantages for primary-care clinicians that choose to serve as surgical assistants. For one thing, time spent in the operating room may not justify, from an economic point of view, the time spent outside the office practice. Typically, Medicare and commercial insurance companies pay the surgical assistant between 20% to 30% of what they pay the surgeon. Depending on the specific surgical procedure, these payments may be less than the income that could be earned during a similar period in office practice.

Another consideration is that primary-care clinicians who assist as surgery incur a higher risk of malpractice litigation and, therefore, in many parts of the country must pay higher malpractice-insurance premiums. This adds to the economic cost of assisting in surgery. The risk of malpractice litigation may be even higher when assisting on cases involving patients known only to the surgeon. Some primary-care clinicians will, therefore, choose only to operate on patients with whom they have a preexisting relationship.

Only individual clinicians can balance the pros and cons of assisting in the operating room and decide if assisting in major surgical procedures will fit into their daily practice routines. Such considerations may not, of course, apply in remote isolated areas in which the exigencies of practice require the primary-care clinician to assist the surgeon.

Epidemiology

According to a 1998 survey by the Association of Operating Room Nurses, the most common general and gynecologic surgical procedures for which an assistant is used are total abdominal hysterectomy, cesarean delivery, laparoscope-assisted vaginal hysterectomy, and laparoscopic cholecystectomy. However, there are no universal rules about which surgical procedures require an assistant and which do not. In fact, many hospitals have no list of procedures or criteria that identify which operations require an assistant. Furthermore, even when such a list exists, the type of assistant (i.e., physician, physician assistant, or registered nurse) is often not delineated, and even a surgical scrub technician may serve as assistant for selected surgical procedures.

There is, however, a source that indicates which surgical procedures might warrant a physician as assistant at surgery. This is a booklet, published by the American College of Surgeons, entitled *Physicians as Assistants at Surgery*. This reference, which is updated periodically, is the result of a collaboration of surgical specialists who review the procedures applicable to their specialties and determine which operations require the use of a physician as an assistant at surgery. The results are given in a table rating the need as "(1) almost always; (2) almost never; or (3) some of the time." This booklet can be obtained by contacting the American College of Surgeons at 1640 Wisconsin Avenue NW, Washington, DC 20007. The phone number is 202-337-2701, and the fax number is 202-337-4271.

The Royal College of Surgeons in the United Kingdom is currently preparing a similar document. It will include guidelines on what surgical procedures require an assistant, who should assist at surgery, and training standards and certification for those who do.

Finally, the American Academy of Family Physicians maintains a database that gives some information regarding the hospital activities of its members. While this will not exactly translate into numbers of surgical cases assisted by family practitioners, it does indicate to some extent the relative prevalence of this type of work in different geographic regions. These data are summarized in Table 3-1 and demonstrate that there is wide variation in the level of family physicians' surgical practices, ranging from performance of major surgery to assisting at surgery to no surgical practice at all.

Instruments

To be proficient in any type of surgery, one must have a working knowledge of the instruments designed for general surgical use and of some instruments designed for use in special situations. It would be impossible to discuss all surgical instruments in this brief chapter. In addition, the instruments that surgeons use vary widely according to their training and personal preferences. Therefore, this chapter will focus on the most commonly used surgical instruments, about which all surgical assistants should have some working knowledge.

Many instruments are named after the surgeon who designed or popularized them. In many cases there are only subtle differences between various types of very similar instruments, yet each has its own specific name. These variations in names may cause confusion when different surgeons refer to very similar looking instruments by different names. For example, there may be several names for hemostats or needle holders, depending on size, shape, and whether their grasping surface is smooth or serrated, even though these instruments might look similar or identical to an inexperienced surgical assistant. Paying attention during the surgical procedure to what instruments the surgeon uses and what they are called will be especially helpful in developing skills as a surgical assistant.

Table 3-1

Surgical Care Provided by Family Physicians in Regions of the United States

GEOGRAPHIC REGION	RESPONDENTS	PERFORM MAJOR SURGERY PERCENT	ASSIST IN MAJOR SURGERY PERCENT	PERFORM MINOR SURGERY PERCENT
All Regions	1909	4.5	35.7	47.5
New England	180	1.2	23.6	42.4
Middle Atlantic	210	.5	9.4	33.5
East North Central	212	3.5	30.7	46.1
West North Central	249	6.2	57.0	61.6
South Atlantic	223	1.6	13.8	30.4
East South Central	195	6.3	17.2	40.6
West South Central	193	9.0	39.7	49.4
Mountain	221	4.3	60.5	58.3
Pacific	226	8.2	66.3	66.2

Data excerpted from a 1998 survey of active members of the American Academy of Family Physicians. Data were adjusted by the sampling fraction and the response percentage for each geographic region.
SOURCE: American Academy of Family Physicians Practice Profile Survey, Kansas City, MO, 1998.

DEFINITIONS OF GEOGRAPHIC AREAS:
New England—Connecticut, Maine, Massachusetts, New Hampshire, Rhode Island, Vermont
Middle Atlantic—New Jersey, New York, Pennsylvania
East North Central—Illinois, Indiana, Michigan, Ohio, Wisconsin
West North Central—Iowa, Kansas, Minnesota, Missouri, Nebraska, North Dakota, South Dakota
South Atlantic—Delaware, District of Columbia, Florida, Georgia, Maryland, North Carolina, South Carolina, Virginia, West Virginia
East South Central—Alabama, Kentucky, Mississippi, Tennessee
West South Central—Arkansas, Louisiana, Oklahoma, Texas
Mountain—Arizona, Colorado, Idaho, Montana, Nevada, New Mexico, Utah, Wyoming
Pacific—Alaska, California, Hawaii, Oregon, Washington

The assistant's dexterity and smoothness of handling instruments often determines the degree to which the surgeon will allow the assistant to perform many tasks such as grasping tissue, cutting tissue, and tying suture. One technique that is often used in medical school surgical clerkships and which remains helpful to developing instrument-handling skills is to practice opening and closing a clamp (hemostat) or similar instrument without putting one's fingers into the holes on the instrument's handles. By using the thenar eminence or proximal interphalangeal joint of the thumb, along with the hypothenar eminence, to open and close the instrument, efficiency is greatly improved. The ability to use these instruments without fingers in the holes also makes it less likely to get caught with the thumb and finger stuck in the holes. There are times when, for the sake of accuracy, one must put fingers into the holes (e.g., cutting with scissors), but insertion of fingers into the holes should be done sparingly and then only with the fingertips.

Table 3-2 lists and Figure 3-1 displays the instruments in a general surgical set at one hospital. Additional instruments with which assistants should become familiar include Lahey tenaculum forceps, Brown-Adson forceps, Russian forceps (short and long), Ferris Smith forceps, and Bonney forceps. Each of these instruments is discussed below.

Clamps

CRILE HEMOSTAT

Crile hemostats (Fig. 3-2) are the most familiar type of clamp. They are used in numerous situa-

Table 3-2

Components of the General Surgical Set at One Hospital[a]

Oschner clamps	Sponge (ring) forceps
Kelly clamps	Thumb forceps (with and without
Crile hemostats (variable lengths,	teeth)
delicate and regular serration)	Adson forceps (with and without
Needle holders (standard and small)	teeth)
Towel clips	Richardson retractors (small, large,
Allis forceps	and appendectomy type)
Babcock forceps	Malleable retractors
Mayo scissors (straight and curved)	Bard Parker retractors
Metzenbaum scissors	Knife handles
(straight and curved)	

[a]Brownwood Regional Medical Center, Brownwood, TX.

tions and are the clamps most often used for grasping bleeding vessels and small portions of tissue. Small-tipped Crile clamps are often called "mosquitoes."

OSCHNER CLAMP

Oschner clamps, also called Kocher clamps (Fig. 3-3), are straight clamps with teeth at the very end. They are used to clamp across tissue,

Figure 3-1

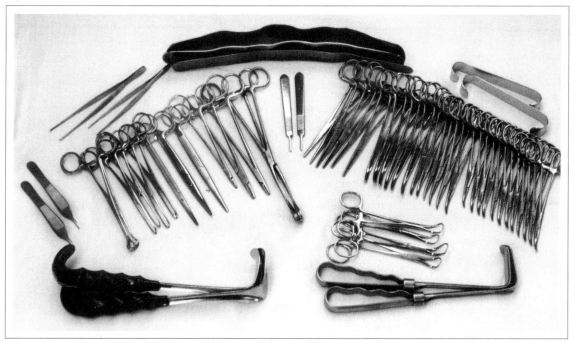

General surgical set. The photograph shows the general surgical instrument set used at the author's institution.

Figure 3-2

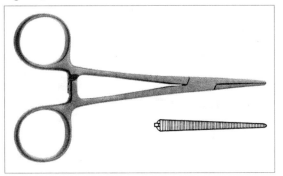

Crile hemostat.

Figure 3-3

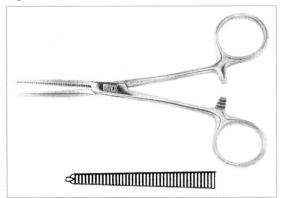

Oschner (Kocher) clamp.

Figure 3-4

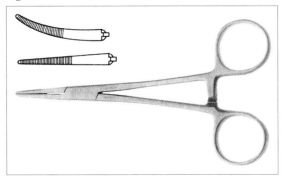

Kelly clamp.

Figure 3-5

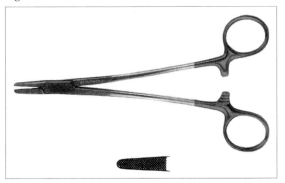

Needle holder.

particularly when it is essential that no tissue slip out of the clamp. The teeth can act as an outside border or may bite into the tissue for security. They are often used to hold fascia during closing.

KELLY CLAMP

Kelly clamps (Fig. 3-4) are used when the curve of the clamp helps with grasping of certain tissue. They are less traumatic than Oschner clamps, but they give good length and can hold larger portions of tissue.

Needle Holders

Needle holders (Fig. 3-5) can be large or small, depending on the size of needle and suture to be used. They can also be straight or curved, the latter design facilitating use in difficult-to-reach areas. The Haney needle holder is most often used in gynecologic surgeries.

Figure 3-6

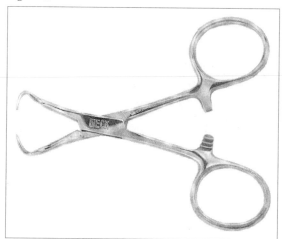

Towel clip.

Figure 3-7

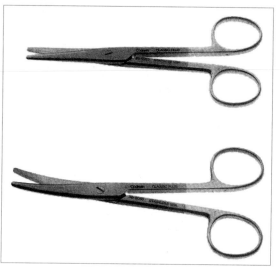

Mayo scissors. The straight-tipped variety are shown at top and the curved variety at bottom.

Towel Clips

Towel clips (Fig. 3-6) can be used not only for securing towels, but also for holding tissue. They are particularly good to isolate a piece of tissue when a larger instrument would traumatize it too much or be too large to grasp it without being in the way.

Scissors

MAYO SCISSORS

Mayo scissors come in straight and curved varieties (Fig. 3-7). The curved Mayo scissors are typically used to cut tissue and are most often used for larger and tougher tissue. The straight type is most commonly used to cut suture and is often referred to as "suture scissors."

METZENBAUM SCISSORS

Metzenbaum scissors are used to cut smaller and more delicate tissue. These can be straight, as shown in Figure 3-8, or curved. They are used frequently for dissecting.

Forceps

SPONGE (RING) FORCEPS

Sponge forceps (Fig. 3-9), also known as ring forceps, are most commonly used to hold a 4 × 4 gauze sponge to wipe tissue, absorb fluid, or retract structures. They can also be used to grasp tissue such as the uterus during a cesarean delivery or the products of conception in a spontaneous abortion. Ring forceps are also very good for holding omentum.

Figure 3-8

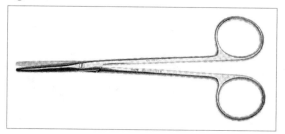

Metzenbaum scissors.

Figure 3-9

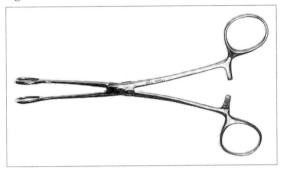

Sponge (Ring) forceps.

Figure 3-11

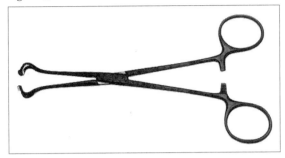

Babcock forceps.

ALLIS FORCEPS

Allis forceps (Fig. 3-10) are fairly atraumatic, but have small teeth that can easily hold tissue for retraction. They are often used for vaginal retraction during anterior or posterior repair.

BABCOCK FORCEPS

Babcock forceps (Fig. 3-11) have curved tips that are good for holding tubular structures such as the fallopian tubes or appendix. They can also hold any tissue when the surgeon must exercise care not to tear the tissue (e.g., bowel).

THUMB FORCEPS

Thumb forceps (Fig. 3-12) are used to grasp tissue for retracting. They come in various sizes and

are available with and without teeth. The ones without teeth can have serration or be smooth, and the choice of which to use depends on what type of tissue is being handled.

ADSON FORCEPS

Adson forceps are small forceps with fine teeth (Fig. 3-13). They are used for less traumatic grasping and are particularly useful for skin.

LAHEY FORCEPS

Lahey forceps (Fig. 3-14) are doubled-toothed, short forceps that are good for grasping larger and bulkier tissue. They are often used for grasping thyroid and uterus.

Figure 3-10

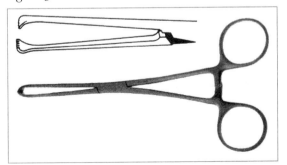

Allis forceps.

Figure 3-12

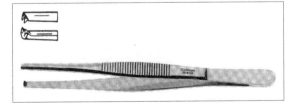

Thumb forceps.

Figure 3-13

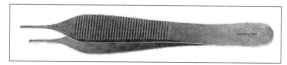

Adson forceps.

BROWN-ADSON FORCEPS

Brown-Adson forceps (Fig. 3-15) are very atraumatic and, therefore, excellent for use during skin closure. Skin margins should be handled gently to minimize necrosis that may promote infection and delay healing. Skin hooks, not shown, are also excellent for pulling back skin borders (see Chapter 2).

RUSSIAN FORCEPS

Russian forceps (Fig. 3-16) are versatile forceps that can be used to handle tissue of all types. They provide a wider grasping surface than most other types of forceps.

FERRIS-SMITH AND BONNEY FORCEPS

Ferris-Smith forceps and Bonney forceps are used for sturdier tissue such as fascia. The Ferris-Smith forceps have a very wide belly (Fig. 3-17), which helps with control. Bonney forceps (Fig. 3-18) are much narrower so that they can be used in tighter locations.

Figure 3-14

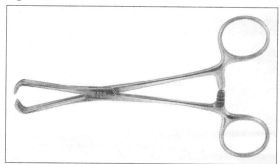

Lahey forceps.

Figure 3-15

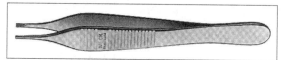

Brown-Adson forceps.

Figure 3-16

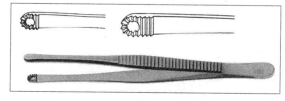

Russian forceps. The inset above shows the appearance of the grasping surface.

Figure 3-17

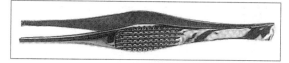

Ferris-Smith forceps.

Figure 3-18

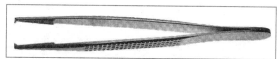

Bonney forceps.

Retractors

There are assortments of retractors (Fig. 3-19). The Richardson retractors are used to retract the abdominal wall. Depending on the required depth and width of retraction, a small- or large-sized Richardson retractor can be used. The appendiceal type is especially helpful in small incisions needing

Figure 3-19

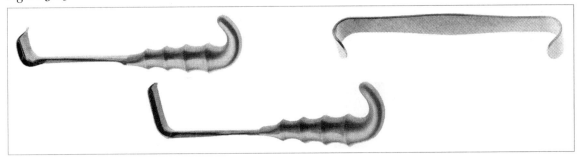

Retractors. The figure shows the Richardson *(left)*, appendiceal *(center)*, and Parker *(right)* retractors.

longer or deeper reach. The Parker retractors are for more shallow areas such as skin or fascia.

First Assisting Technique

Preliminary Considerations

Perhaps the most important role of the surgical assistant is to pay attention—even through long and laborious operations. One cannot anticipate what is needed to assist the surgeon if the mind is wandering. One step of preparation that can help maintain alertness is to become familiar with the procedure to be performed. The more the assistant knows about the procedure, the easier it will be to understand what the surgeon is trying to accomplish. This knowledge will then lead to the ability to anticipate the next step and what instruments will be needed.

Before entering the operating room, therefore, it is essential that the assistant be as familiar as possible with anatomy and the techniques used for the operation. For most primary-care clinicians, medical school anatomy class and surgical clerkships are years in the past, and it is usually necessary to consult an operative atlas (e.g., Zollinger and Zollinger, see reference list). Such reference texts should be available in all hospitals in which nonsurgeons serve as surgical assistants. For physicians

located in remote areas, such resources are increasingly available through the Internet (e.g., www.texmed.org) or through central book repositories such as the Huffington Memorial Library at the American Academy of Family Physicians.

General Considerations in the Operating Room

The environment in the operation room should be as free of bacterial contamination as possible, and much of what is done in the operating room and perioperative period aims at diminishing the likelihood of infection. While the patient is probably the most common source of infection, the personnel in the operating room are the secondary sources. Therefore, solutions containing iodophors and hexachlorophene are frequently used to wash the patient and scrub the hands and arms to the elbows of the operative team. Caps, gowns, shoe covers, and masks all compose the equipment that protects both the patient and members of the surgical team.

Gloves should be comfortable, yet snug enough to give good tactile capabilities. Double gloving should be considered mandatory. There is now abundant literature proving that double gloving reduces exposure to blood (caused by rips or leaks in gloves and from suture or needle punctures) when compared with single gloving. The relative size of the two pairs of gloves is a matter of personal preference, but it often works best to wear a half-size larger glove under one's regular-sized glove.

Sterile drapes are used to define and preserve the sterile field during the operation. They should not be moved or lifted once they are in place. All persons in the room should watch for potential or actual compromise of the sterile field. When moving within or around a sterile area, do so in a manner that will maintain its integrity. Keep all sterile items, including hands, above waist level. If personnel positions must be changed, do so back to back or face to face, maintaining sufficient distance to avoid contact.

The Surgeon's Expectations

What the operating surgeon expects from a first assistant is help in completing the operation more quickly and safely. Everything the assistant does should be aimed at making the job of the surgeon easier and more efficient. There are many components involved in this process.

COMMUNICATION

Communication with the surgeon is paramount in developing a good working relationship. It helps to have a clear understanding of what the surgeon expects of the assistant. Some surgeons will want to do everything themselves, with the assistant only providing exposure by holding retractors. Others will want the assistant to tie knots, and still others may want the assistant to cut tissue.

Successful assisting, therefore, requires clear expectations. The assistant should never be shy about asking what the surgeon expects or prefers the assistant's role to be. As an assistant works repetitively with the same surgeon and demonstrates skills in handling instruments, tying sutures, and providing exposure, the assistant's participation in the procedure will often increase.

Communication and coordination with the surgeon are particularly important in laparoscopic surgery where the assistant is often the person "driving" the camera. The camera needs to be kept steady and centered on the area where the surgeon is working. It is essential to understand how to focus the camera and, when employing an angled scope, how to use this to advantage. For maximum safety, the camera should always follow the instruments and trocars in and out of the abdominal wall.

EXPOSURE

A primary responsibility, and perhaps the most critical, for any assistant is to provide exposure of the operative area, because surgeons cannot safely operate on what they cannot see. Poor exposure can lead to grasping the wrong tissue or cutting the wrong structure. The key to success in providing exposure is always to be thinking about what the surgeon needs to best visualize the surgical field.

The importance of anticipation cannot be overstated. Thinking ahead to the next step and adjusting the exposure will greatly enhance your value as an assistant. Request a particular instrument if it will be required. Never drop the exposure until the case is completely done.

Maintaining exposure often involves holding of retractors. Retraction can be tiring and often boring in a long surgical case, but it is essential to expediting the work of the surgeon and improving safety for the patient.

Suction is another important adjunct in exposure. A surgical field covered with blood is difficult, if not impossible, to work in. Thus, suction is used to keep the operative area clean and dry; the suction device can also be used to retract structures.

One can also use surgical sponges to blot the field dry and to improve exposure. This can be accomplished with either a piece of 4 × 4 gauze attached to the sponge forceps or by use of a lap sponge, which is much larger. Lap sponges can also be placed in the abdomen to pack off bowel and expose a larger area of the abdominal cavity. Additionally, forceps can be used to move tissue around or hold it out of the way.

While one wants to create the best exposure, one must remember not to be so aggressive in blotting, suctioning, and changing retraction angles that it becomes a nuisance or a hindrance to the surgeon. Similarly, adjustment of the lighting can help with exposure, but the assistant should never adjust the light when the surgeon is cutting or applying suture or cautery.

HEMOSTASIS

Another important responsibility of the assistant is helping with hemostasis. The objectives are to decrease blood loss and prevent hematoma formation.

HEMOSTATS   Maintaining a clean, bloodless field during dissection can be accomplished in several ways. Often, especially with larger blood vessels, one may need to grasp the cut end of the vessel with a hemostat. If possible, grab the vessel with the tip of the hemostat pointed upward. A tie of suture material can then be used to occlude the vessel. When placing the tie around the hemostat, continue to keep the tip up. Often the surgeon will say, "Show me the tip."

It is essential to exercise care when grasping vessels with a hemostat, and assistants should never grasp what they cannot see. A better approach is to apply pressure for a short period, 15 to 20 seconds, to see if natural clotting will stop the bleeding or at least slow it down enough to see the bleeding structure, after which the hemostat can be applied. If essential to grasp with poor visibility, let the surgeon do the grasping. The only exception to this rule might be in the subcutaneous tissue where there is very little to harm from blind clamping.

Often a rhythm can be helpful as the assistant blots the field and the surgeon dissects. It is important, however, to blot, not wipe. Wiping may remove small clots that are aiding in the very hemostasis you are trying to achieve. Packing an area off with lap sponges for a while can often help significantly with hemostasis. In addition, metal clips may be used at times.

ELECTROCAUTERY   Electrical cautery can also be used to stop bleeding. Both unipolar and bipolar electrosurgical units can be used.

Unipolar electrosurgical units are used for dissection and for hemostasis. The grounding plate must be well attached to the patient, and it is important to remember that the cautery will conduct through any metal material. Therefore, one must be especially careful to not allow the cautery tip to touch the retractors or the patient could get a severe burn. Likewise, the cautery spark from a unipolar unit can arc to adjacent metal instruments that, if attached to tissue, can cause a burn. Therefore, the cautery spark should not be permitted to arc to adjacent instruments unless that is the intention of the surgeon. Finally, if there is a hole in the surgeon's or assistant's glove, an electrical shock may occur. Intact gloves and double gloving will minimize this risk.

A bipolar cautery spark, and resulting tissue damage, does not extend as far from the cautery tip as that of unipolar cautery and is more precise than unipolar cautery. It typically confines the damage to the tissues between the tips of the cauterizing forceps.

In summary, while cautery can save time and diminish blood loss, it can create increased tissue damage and can result in susceptibility to infection. Most cauterization injuries occur from the unipolar device.

TENSION

The proper amount of tension on tissue is yet another important aspect to be considered when assisting. Tissues being cut must always be held under tension or countertraction, as this permits cut tissue to come apart more easily, and structures can be more easily seen.

When suturing, on the other hand, the tissue being sutured should be under no tension whatsoever. If under tension, the suture may become loose when it is relaxed, thus allowing bleeding to occur or tissue to come apart. The general rule is summarized by the axiom: "approximate, don't strangulate" the tissue. This is especially true in bowel and skin (though it does not apply to suture applied for the purpose of hemostasis; such sutures should be tied tightly). When tying a knot in a suture, follow the loop of suture all the way down to the knot, and be sure it is secure before the next throw. Holding some mild tension on the suture between throws will ensure that the knot does not loosen.

Finally, when dissecting, it is important to follow natural tissue planes, as this will cause the least amount of tissue trauma. Often, a finger will suffice to dissect, or a sponge forceps with a damp gauze or a Kuttner pledget can be used to separate tissues. When cutting with scissors, it is essential to cut only with the tips of the scissors. If cutting is performed with the body of the scissors, the tip may cut something else unintentionally. Blunt-tipped scissors such as the Metzenbaum type are helpful for dissecting dense tissue and opening tissue planes.

Postoperative Care

Depending on the geographic setting and the relationship between the surgeon and assistant, the management of postoperative care may be the responsibility of either. In remote areas, "visiting" surgeons may perform the operation and then depart, leaving postoperative care to the patient's on-site clinician. In more populated areas, in which both the surgeon and assistant are present daily, it is essential that there be a clear understanding about who will write orders and supervise daily-care instructions. Misunderstandings in this area can be a source of significant conflict if not resolved in advance. Who participates in and supervises postoperative care will depend on the surgeon's routine, whether the patient was self-referred to the surgeon or referred by the primary-care clinician, the surgeon's perceived level of responsibility for the patient, and the level of surgical skill and experience of the primary-care clinician.

When the primary surgeon delegates postoperative care to the primary-care clinician that assisted at surgery, the care will involve several general management issues, including diet, activity, laboratory monitoring, medication, intravenous fluids, drains, wound care, pulmonary toilet, and measures to reduce the risk of thromboembolism.

Diet

In general, the patient should be allowed to eat as soon as safely possible. In almost all operations not involving invasion of the chest, abdomen, or pelvis, the patient should be able to drink, if not eat regular food, as soon as consciousness allows.

If resection and anastomosis of a portion of the gastrointestinal tract has been performed, the need and duration for a nasogastric tube and timing of oral feedings should be specifically discussed with the surgeon. For other procedures in the abdomen or pelvis, one can often begin liquids after 8 to 10 hours, but must always be mindful that bowel function may return slowly after such procedures. A good indicator of readiness to eat is the presence of bowel sounds and the passage of flatus. It is not necessary to have a bowel movement before the patient can have solid food. Indeed, if adequate bowel preparation was performed preoperatively, there may be some delay in the stool. Once the patient is passing flatus, solid food should be no problem.

Activity

The patient should be ambulated as soon as possible. To the extent possible, it is often desirable to at least have the patient sit on the side of the bed with nursing help on the operative day. Obviously, the severity of the patient's condition and the nature of the surgery may have some adverse effect on activity; however, except in certain orthopedic procedures, most patients can be up and out of bed on the first postoperative day. With early activity, the soreness abates more quickly, and the patient has fewer pulmonary problems than with delayed activity.

Laboratory Monitoring

For most uncomplicated surgical procedures, postoperative laboratory monitoring is directed at detection of occult bleeding and abnormalities in serum electrolytes. In addition, individual surgical procedures may have specific needs for postoperative laboratory monitoring, a discussion of which is beyond the scope of this chapter.

Intravenous Fluids

Intravenous fluids should be aimed at replenishing fluid lost through urine, drains, third-spacing, stool (if liquid), and insensible losses. On average, in healthy adults following uncomplicated surgery that required short-term intravenous fluid for short periods, 3 liters in 24 hours is a reasonable target for fluid administration. Care should be taken to closely monitor the intake and output, which should be well documented in the graphic chart or nursing notes. Patients who have had major abdominal surgery often have increased fluid requirements for 24 to 48 hours after surgery because of third-space losses. Enough fluid should be given to keep urine output at a minimum of 20 to 30 cc/hour.

Particular attention should be given to fluid balance in elderly individuals and those with cardiac compromise to avoid fluid overload. Having said that, it is important to note that the most common postoperative error made by nonsurgeons is underadministration of fluids.

Medications

Preoperative and postoperative antibiotics are used in a wide variety of operations. Operations associated with a high risk of infection are candidates for prophylactic administration of antibiotics. These procedures include cesarean deliveries, hysterectomies, bowel procedures, operations associated with implantable devices, and cardiovascular procedures. Recommendations for antibiotic selection and dosage for these procedures are widely available in antibiotic prescribing manuals. First- or second-generation cephalosporins are the most commonly used agents for patients who are not allergic to lactam antibiotics. For most procedures, antibiotics are administered one-half hour before the operation begins (to ensure adequate tissue levels) and are continued for two to three doses afterward.

Pain medicine is required following most surgical procedures and is usually administered intravenously to avoid the discomfort of intramuscular injections. Morphine is the most widely used analgesic for severe pain, but other narcotics agents such as meperidine and butorphanol are also frequently prescribed. Narcotics are often administered using patient-controlled anesthesia devices. For patients with less severe pain, oral narcotics (e.g., codeine or oxycodone) and/or nonsteroidal antiinflammatory drugs (e.g., ketorolac, ibuprofen) or even acetaminophen are appropriate.

Surgical Drains

Surgical drains may be either the passive or active type. The type of drain should be chosen according to the viscosity and volume of anticipated drainage. Drains are frequently used in situations in which there may be an infection draining pus, collections or accumulation of serous fluid, or the possibility of bleeding. Drains are commonly left in place until drainage diminishes to negligible levels, after which they are removed.

In certain instances (e.g., bile leak after cholecystectomy), drains may be required for a substantial length of time, but it is important to remember that while drains provide for the egress of fluid, they are also a potential conduit for infection to enter the body. Accordingly, they should not be left in place any longer than necessary. Primary-care clinicians responsible for postoperative care should always understand the placement and purpose of the drain and should have made a plan with the surgeon for its removal.

Wound Care

Details of wound healing are discussed in Chapter 2. In managing postoperative patients, the wound dressing should protect against bacterial contamination and mechanical trauma. For years, it was thought that covering the incision for many days would help to prevent postoperative infection. The trend now is to remove dressings much earlier—often within 48 hours after surgery. The patients are typically permitted to shower after 48 hours.

Pulmonary Toilet

Routine deep breathing after surgery has been shown to decrease the risk of atelectasis and other pulmonary complications. Incentive spirometry is the most widely used technique, but requires the patient's cooperation and motivation.

Prevention of Thromboembolic Complications

Much is written about avoiding venous thromboembolic complications, which include deep venous thrombosis and pulmonary embolism—a potentially lethal complication most often seen after abdominal, pelvic, and orthopedic surgery.

When possible, early ambulation is perhaps the most effective measure for preventing venous thromboembolic complications, but a variety of other modalities are also important. For example, the current standard of care following intra-abdominal surgery is to use thigh-high antiembolic stockings (e.g., TED hose) and mechanical sequential decompression stockings (SCDs). Postoperative care following orthopedic surgery often involves SCDs along with administration of dextrans and low-molecular-weight heparins.

Thus, the need for and choice of these various modalities depends on the surgical procedure performed, along with a consideration of the patient's risk factors and underlying medical conditions. The clinician responsible for postoperative care should review the antithromboembolic management with the surgeon and should be conversant with current literature regarding optimal interventions for the specific surgical procedure performed.

Controversies and Emerging Concepts

The Decreasing Surgical Role of Primary-Care Clinicians

Of the major primary-care specialties (general medicine, general pediatrics, and family practice), only physicians in family practice have ever been significantly involved in operating-room surgery. From the point of view of family-practice physicians, therefore, an important trend in recent years has been a decrease in the rates with which primary-care clinicians are involved in surgical care. This includes their roles as both primary surgeons and as surgical assistants.

ROLE AS PRIMARY SURGEONS

Prior to the early 1970s, it was not unusual for family-practice physicians to perform and assist at surgery. Even as recently as 1982, family physicians constituted about one-quarter of the surgical work force, with 21% of family physicians performing surgery and 40% assisting as surgery. By 1998, however, these figures had fallen to 5% and 36%, respectively, with almost no family-practice physicians performing surgery in the eastern United States (Table 3-1).

The availability of surgeons in a particular geographic region appears to have a distinct bearing on the attitude of the medical community about what type of physicians can and should perform surgery. Most family physicians who currently perform surgery are either older physicians, whose careers have always involved surgical care, or those working in rural and underserved areas. Many young, family-practice physicians in the United States seek additional surgical training (often an elective surgical rotation during residency) if they expect to work in a remote area in which they will be expected to have surgical skills.

While the limited involvement of primary-care clinicians in surgery and surgical assisting is not unique to the United States, primary-care clinicians in some industrialized nations still perform substantial amounts of surgery. In Canada, for example, a 1995 study involving 101 smaller hospitals showed that 56 (55%) of the hospitals provided surgical services and that, at 45 (80%) of those hospitals, general practitioners provided some surgical services. At 15 (27%) of the 56 hospitals, the only physicians performing surgery were general practitioners—many of whom had limited surgical training. This surgical staffing appeared to be adequate, in that three-quarters of the administrators at those hospitals reported their community's surgical needs to be well met. Similarly, a 1998 survey of 57 rural hospitals in South Australia found that only 39 had active operating facilities. General practitioners performed most of the surgical procedures in 26 of those 39 hospitals.

ROLE AS SURGICAL ASSISTANTS

The issue of who should and can assist in surgery has been under discussion in recent years. As with the role of family physicians as primary surgeons, attitudes about their roles as surgical assistants in a given geographic areas are also related to the availability of surgeons in that area.

Some surgeons recommend, and some medical staffs require, that only surgeons serve as surgical assistants. In many of those same hospitals, family-practice physicians no longer assist in surgery and are unable to obtain hospital privileges to do so. Yet, in other areas of the United States, nonphysicians (physician assistants and, to a lesser extent, advanced-practice nurses) rou-

tinely assist in surgery, with some evidence that involvement of these nonphysician practitioners in operative and postoperative care results in excellent outcomes and decreased lengths of hospitalization. Because of the good outcomes with nonphysician assistants, many question the validity of policies that prohibit primary-care physicians from serving in the same role.

Implications for Training

The changing role of nonsurgeons in surgical care raises interesting questions about the surgical training that should be included in the general education of medical students. That is, what surgical knowledge and skills should all physicians have—even those who will enter primary-care disciplines or specialties that do not involve surgery at all? Current surgical training for medical students often involves a considerable amount of operating-room time, and it is not clear that this is the best approach to educating medical students—most of whom will not become surgeons.

To address this question, one survey research team questioned family-practice residency directors regarding urologic surgery skills and found that cognitive and diagnostic skills were considered more important for primary-care clinicians than were procedural and surgical skills. Similarly, in a recent survey of members of the American Academy of Family Physicians, 90% of respondents reported that emphasis in surgical training should be on diagnosis and management, with an understanding of when to refer to a surgeon. Technical skills, while still felt to be important, were considered less significant than the aforementioned knowledge of diagnosis and management.

Neither of these studies, however, addressed the need of physicians who practice in remote or rural areas, where surgical skills can be particularly valuable. The information contained in this chapter should be of particular assistance to these physicians, providing basic guidelines to enhancing surgical assisting skills.

Acknowledgements

Photographs and drawings of surgical instruments in this chapter are from the *Codman Surgical Products Catalog* and the *Weck Surgical Instrument Catalog*, reproduced with permission by courtesy of Codman & Shirtleff, Inc., and Linvatec, Inc., respectively.

References

American Academy of Family Physicians: *Practice Profile Survey.* Kansas City, MO, American Academy of Family Physicians, May 1998.

American College of Surgeons: *Physicians As Assistants at Surgery.* Washington, DC, American College of Surgeons, 1996.

Bates T, Siller G, Crathern BC, et al: Timing of prophylactic antibiotics in abdominal surgery: trial of a pre-operative versus an intra-operative first dose. *Br J Surg* 76:52, 1989.

Brough SJ, Hunt TM, Barrie WW: Surgical glove perforations. *Br J Surg* 75:317, 1988.

Bruening MH, Maddern GJ: The provision of general surgical services in rural South Australia: a new model for rural surgery. *Aust NZ J Surg* 68:764, 1998.

Cahill H: Role definition: nurse practitioners or clinicians' assistants? *Br J Nurs* 5:382, 1997.

Chiasson PM, Roy PD: Role of the general practitioner in the delivery of surgical and anesthesia services in rural western Canada. *Can Med Assoc J* 153:1447, 1995.

Codman Surgical Product Catalog. Raynham, ME, Johnson & Johnson Professional, 1996.

Cruse PJ, Foord R: The epidemiology of wound infection: a 10-year prospective study of 62,939 wounds. *Surg Clin North Am* 60:27, 1980.

Dayton M: *Manual of Surgical Objectives,* 3rd ed. Springfield, IL, Association for Surgical Education, 1990.

Edwards C, Keeley O: Competency-based learning for the surgical assistant. *Nurs Stand* 12:44, 1998.

Greco RJ, Wheatley M, McKenna M: Risk of blood contact through surgical gloves in aesthetic procedures. *Aesthetic Plast Surg* 17:167, 1993.

Hopkins CC: Antibiotic prophylaxis in clean surgery: peripheral vascular surgery, non-cardiovascular thoracic surgery, herniorrhaphy, and mastectomy. *Rev Infect Dis* 13(suppl 10):869, 1991.

Mainen MW: The surgical role of family physicians. *Am J Public Health* 72:1359, 1982.

Miller W, Riel E, Napier M, et al: Use of physician assistants as surgery/trauma house staff at an American College of Surgeons — verified level II trauma center. *J Trauma* 44:372, 1998.

Nora P (ed): *Operative Surgery: Principles and Techniques.* Philadelphia, WB Saunders, 1990.

Quebbeman EJ, Telfors GL, Hubbard S, et al: In-use evaluation of surgical gowns. *Surg Gynecol Obstet* 174:369, 1992.

Romfh RF, Cramer FS: *Technique in the Use of Surgical Tools.* Norwalk, CT, Appleton & Lange, 1992.

Sabiston DC, Lyerly HK: *Textbook of Surgery: The Biological Basis of Modern Surgical Practice,* 15th ed. Philadelphia, WB Saunders, 1997, pp 105–111.

Sprat JS, Papp KK: Practicing primary care physicians' perspectives on the junior surgical clerkship. *Am J Surg* 173:232, 1997.

Teichman JMH, Weiss BD, Solomon D: Urological needs assessment for primary care practice: implications for undergraduate medical education. *J Urol* 161:1282, 1999.

Tissier J, Rink E: Evaluation of minor surgery courses for general practitioners. *Med Educ* 30:333, 1996.

Weck Surgical Instrument Catalog. Largo, FL, Linvatec, 1992.

Williams JL: Assistants in surgical practice: a discussion document. *Ann R Coll Surg Engl* 81(2 suppl):63, 1999.

Zollinger RM, Zollinger RM: *Atlas of Surgical Operations,* 6th ed. New York, Macmillan, 1998.

Dana Christian Lynge

Chapter 4

Consultation, Stabilization, and Transport

Introduction

A 23 year-old male was driving alone on an icy road in rural eastern Washington State late on a Friday night in midwinter. While crossing a patch of "black ice," the back end of his truck skidded and he lost control of the vehicle, which ran off the road, rolled, and came to rest in a ditch. The accident took place on the outskirts of a small town (population 3000).

A passing motorist witnessed the accident and called 911. The 911 dispatcher passed the information on to the local volunteer emergency medical technicians. They found the driver unrestrained and smelling of alcohol in the cab of his overturned truck.

The victim was initially unresponsive, but he was breathing regularly and had a palpable pulse. Emergency personnel extricated him from the truck—being as careful to protect his spinal column as circumstances allowed—and placed him on a backboard with a cervical restraint collar.

The patient's vital signs at the accident scene included a pulse of 120 beats per minute, blood pressure 110/60 mm Hg, and a respiratory rate of 30 breaths per minute. The patient could be aroused by painful stimuli, but he was confused. Emergency personnel transported the patient to the local emergency room (travel time 10 minutes), where he was seen and examined by the family physician on duty, who was already present in the emergency room.

The family physician in the emergency room found the patient to have a clear airway and to be breathing spontaneously at a rate of 35 breaths per minute. The patient's pulse was 110 beats per minute, and his blood pressure was 120/70 mm Hg. The patient responded incoherently to painful stimuli and was otherwise somnolent. The physician called for administration of 100% oxygen by mask, the intubation kit, and placement of two large-bore intravenous catheters. Blood testing was also requested (complete blood count, standard blood biochemistry tests, liver function tests, type and cross-match for blood, toxicology screen, arterial blood gasses), and x-rays (cervical spine, chest, pelvis) were ordered.

The physician then completed her secondary survey of the patient's injuries. The findings were as follows. There was tenderness over the left frontoparietal area of the skull, but no step-off was palpable. There was no hemotympanum or cerebrospinal fluid rhinorrhea. The pupils were equal in size and reactive to light, extraocular movements were normal, and the midface and dentition were intact. There was no tenderness over the cervical spine. Respiratory examination revealed no tracheal deviation, but there were decreased breath sounds on the left side of the chest with tenderness on the left side of the chest wall. The abdomen was soft and nontender. The pelvis was stable, the limbs were intact, and there were no step-offs over the thoracic and lumbar spine. Genitorectal examination revealed heme-negative stool, no high-riding prostate gland, and no blood at the urethral meatus. The plantar reflexes were downgoing bilaterally.

Initial laboratory and x-ray results came back as follows. Radiographs of the cervical spine and pelvis were normal; chest x-ray showed a small left pneumothorax. The first hematocrit, drawn prior to administration of intravenous fluids, was 42%. Other laboratory studies were normal except for a blood alcohol level of 0.2 mg per deciliter and moderate respiratory alkalosis.

The physician asked for a second hematocrit to be drawn and for a tube thoracostomy (chest tube) kit. She placed a 32-French chest tube at the left fifth intercostal space at the anterior axillary line. There was a rush of air on placement of the tube and good movement of the water column in the Pleurovac when the tube was connected to it. Repeat chest x-ray showed reexpansion of the left lung, but increased opacity in both lung fields (left side greater than right).

It was then decided to intubate the patient because of his fluctuating mental status and increased respiratory rate to 40 breaths per minute.

Arterial blood gas sampled subsequent to intubation revealed a decreased PaO_2.

The family physician contacted a trauma center in Seattle, and the trauma surgeon on duty agreed to accept the patient in transfer for neurosurgical evaluation and treatment, as well as intensive care for probable pulmonary contusions. Arrangements were made for helicopter transport with a flight nurse accompanying the patient. The patient was stable during the 1-hour flight to Seattle. He was hyperventilated during the flight to reduce intracranial pressure. The flight nurse was able to relay data to and consult with the trauma surgeon concerning the patient's status throughout the flight.

On arrival at the trauma center, the patient was seen and evaluated by the trauma team in the emergency department. The patient was already intubated and sedated. Vital signs and hematocrit were stable, but the patient's PaO_2 was lower than before transport. Computerized tomography of the head revealed diffuse cerebral edema, but no intracranial bleeding. Computerized tomography of the abdomen (done because the patient's blood alcohol level and neurological status made his abdominal exam unreliable) was unremarkable. The patient was transferred to the surgical intensive care unit where he underwent placement of an intracranial pressure monitor by the neurosurgical team and was placed on a ventilator with sufficient positive end-expiratory pressure (PEEP) to improve his oxygenation.

The patient's hospital course was complicated by a nosocomial pneumonia that responded to appropriate antibiotic treatment. His chest tube was removed on hospital day 3, with no residual pneumothorax. His intracranial pressure monitor was removed on hospital day 7 when his pressures had decreased and neurologic examination had normalized. His pulmonary contusions resolved with supportive care. He was extubated on hospital day 8 and transferred to a general surgical ward bed on hospital day 9. He was discharged from the hospital 11 days after admission.

This case, a not-unfamiliar scenario for clinicians staffing emergency departments in rural areas, illustrates three salient features of rural surgical problems. The first is the critical importance of local emergency responders and primary-care clinicians in stabilizing patients with an emergent surgical problem. The second is the benefit of well-coordinated emergency transport systems. The third is the role of consultation and the surgical consultant in the management of surgical problems in rural areas where no surgeon is present.

Each of these issues, as well as related topics, will be covered in this chapter. While the emphasis will be on consultation, stabilization, and transport for trauma patients, the points made in this chapter are applicable to many of the other surgical problems covered in the other chapters of this book.

Epidemiology

Shift from Rural to Urban Surgical Care

Approximately 25% of the United States population lives in areas defined as rural by the US Office of Management and Budget. No data are collected about how much surgical care for the rural citizens is performed in rural areas and how much surgery is referred to urban medical centers. Determining how much surgery is referred to urban centers is complicated by the fact that referral patterns for both elective and emergency surgery vary widely depending on availability of local surgical resources, the presence or absence of trauma systems, and managed care networks.

There are, however, data to substantiate an increasing trend in recent years for patients from rural areas to receive their surgical care in urban centers, rather than at their local rural hospitals. For example, a study in the mid 1990s revealed that 60% of surgical charges for services provided to residents of rural Washington were billed by urban hospitals. In some cases, performance of surgery in the urban hospital occurred clearly because the specific surgical service needed (e.g,, neurosurgery) was not available at the rural hospital. However, the same study found that almost one-third of patients undergoing cholecystectomy (a routine general surgery procedure—commonly performed in rural areas) had their surgery at an urban hospital, rather than at their local rural hospital.

This trend probably has its origin in many factors, including the ease of modern transportation, the marketing and practice-purchasing by urban-based managed-care entities, the shifting preferences of patients, the changing referral patterns of primary-care clinicians, the shortage of rural surgeons, and rural hospital closures. This trend is unlikely to reverse. Rural family practitioners will increasingly consult urban surgeons for both elective and emergency problems. Those with emergent problems will be stabilized and transported to urban medical centers for definitive treatment. Given this reality, it is important for the rural primary-care clinician to learn about and develop the best methods for consultation, stabilization, and transport.

Lessons from Trauma Care

While general data on surgical care are somewhat limited, there is an extensive amount of literature on the interaction between rural and urban centers in the management of trauma. A review of this trauma literature reveals important facts about the transfer of injured patients, and the findings suggest several areas of improvement that can be applied to the transfer of all surgical cases from rural to urban settings.

The most striking finding in this literature is that victims of trauma in rural settings are almost twice as likely to die as those whose trauma occurs in an urban setting. There are multiple factors thought to be responsible for the poorer outcome in rural areas. They include immutable factors particular to the rural environment such as prolonged time to the discovery of the accident scene, prolonged transport time to the treating facility because of distance and weather, and

extreme mechanisms of injury (i.e,, agricultural vehicles, outdoor recreational injuries). There are, however, several modifiable factors—mostly in the areas of training of and communication between health-care personnel—in which improvements have been shown to result in less morbidity and mortality for trauma victims in rural areas.

PERSONNEL TRAINING

There is evidence to suggest that outcomes can be improved by increasing training and education for rural emergency medical technicians (EMTs), many of whom serve on a volunteer basis. In particular, certification in Advanced Life Support (ALS) can result in more thorough evaluation and treatment of rural trauma patients by EMTs. There is also evidence that increased training and education for rural physicians—specifically, Advanced Trauma Life Support (ATLS)—can have similar beneficial results.

TRAUMA SYSTEMS

The implementation of a "trauma system" also results in better outcomes, both because it facilitates the aforementioned training for rural health-care personnel and because standardized transfer protocols are often developed that are suitable to the realities of a particular region. In such systems, the local rural hospital is often designated a level III hospital and serves as a stabilization and transfer station, sending more severely injured patients on either to a larger, more resource-rich rural level II center or to an urban level I trauma center. The implementation of such a system at the local rural level usually requires a "dedicated individual" (often a general surgeon or family practitioner). The benefits include not only better care for patients but also an increase in the emergency-care capabilities of rural hospitals.

AIR TRANSPORT

The influence on mortality rates of air (usually helicopter) versus land evacuation of rural trauma patients has been much debated. Helicopter evacuation from the scene of injury was developed by the military during the Korean War and perfected during the Vietnam War, when it led to a marked reduction in death rates resulting from penetrating trauma.

"Medevac" helicopters are now a common feature of trauma centers and systems. Their use has been extended into many rural areas of the United States and other countries, and some studies of their use have been conducted. These studies reveal that the advantage of helicopter evacuation over ground transport is not necessarily because of shortened transportation time. In fact, in some instances transport times by helicopters were longer because of stabilization and resuscitation performed by helicopter crews at the accident scene or rural hospital prior to airlift back to the urban trauma center. Rather, decreased mortality rates associated with air transport appear to be the result of the higher degree of skill (in areas of resuscitation, intubation, chest-tube placement, etc.) of medevac flight crews, and the fact that these crews are in constant communication with receiving physicians at the urban trauma. The flight crews act as a direct extension of the trauma center. In the final analysis, it appears that education (e.g., ALS for rural EMTs, ATLS for rural physicians, and the advanced skills and experience of the medevac flight crews) makes the biggest difference in patient mortality during stabilization and transport from rural areas to urban centers.

TELEMEDICINE

All aspects of rural surgical care are being influenced by telemedicine technology (the use of telecommunications to aid in medical diagnosis and patient management). Telemedicine is rapidly becoming available throughout rural America. This technology will have a profound effect on consultation concerning and the stabilization/transport of the surgical patients in rural areas. Telemedicine has, of course, been practiced in a literal sense ever since the advent of the telephone.

However, with the recent of addition of videoconference capability, store-and-forward techniques, and the digital transfer of images, the technologic capability and practical application of telemedicine have expanded considerably.

Data from the Office of Rural Health Policy indicate that nearly 30% of rural hospitals now have telemedicine programs in place. Given that Congress has recently approved Part B Medicare reimbursement for telemedical consultations to rural, health-personnel-shortage areas, there is likely to be an increase in the use of telemedicine.

Increased use of telemedicine for rural surgical problems has several potential benefits. These include avoiding the costs and logistic problems inherent in transfer/transport when telemedicine consultations permit management of problems in the rural community. The quality of stabilization and transport when it is necessary, after guidance by surgical consultants in urban centers, is also likely to improve. Other potential benefits of telemedicine include increased continuity of care by local clinicians, retention of revenue by rural institutions and clinicians when telemedicine-guided local management is possible, and decreased overall costs by reducing the number of inappropriate transfers.

A review of the telemedicine research literature indicates that the bulk of current telemedicine involves radiology, cardiology, dermatology, and pathology—all areas of medical endeavor that are centered on electronic or pictorial data. Orthopedic cases comprise nearly a quarter of all telemedicine consultations. A study from North Dakota on the use of telemedicine in orthopedic problems revealed high satisfaction on the part of both orthopedic consultants and rural practitioners, and no adverse outcomes in 91 cases handled by telemedicine consultation over a 2-year period.

Additional research is needed to identify the specific surgical disciplines and clinical conditions for which telemedicine will provide the best and most cost-effective outcomes. Until such studies are available, it is likely that telemedicine will remain underused.

Key History, Physical Examination, and Ancillary Tests

Most key points of the medical history, physical examination, and tests that can influence outcomes for surgical patients are discussed in the chapters of this book that deal with specific surgical problems; details specific to trauma patients are reviewed in Chapter 13. However, the trauma literature and the personal experience of many surgeons offer additional insights into aspects of the history, physical, and laboratory testing that influence outcomes during transfer from rural to urban health care facilities—both for patients with traumatic injuries and for those with non–trauma-induced surgical problems. These points deserve emphasis and will be discussed here.

Trauma Patients

HISTORY

It is important to collect information on the mechanism of injury and vital signs/physiologic status at the time the patient was first assessed in the field. Thus, for example, a when transferring an apparently stable patient who was the unrestrained driver of a compact car that collided head on at high velocity with a large truck, the accepting surgeon will have more suspicion of potentially lethal injuries because of the mechanism of injury, even though the patient appears stable. This will lead to a search for injuries such as cardiac contusion and/or tamponade or traumatic disruption of the aorta. Given this example involving a severe mechanism of injury, the accepting surgeon will be more likely to ask for a second chest x-ray just prior to transport to rule out the development of a pneumothorax—a complication that can be difficult to diagnose and treat while in flight.

PHYSICAL EXAMINATION

Physical assessment of trauma patients should follow the ATLS protocol and should be reported to the consulting surgeon in this format. While a reiteration of the ATLS manual is beyond the scope of this chapter, the evaluation of trauma patients must focus on the "ABCs" (airway, breathing, and circulation) and an adequate neurologic examination.

There have been several studies evaluating treatment of trauma patients in emergency departments, each revealing frequent (more than half the time) deviation from the ATLS standard of practice. In these studies, failure to detect problems with airway and breathing and the consequent failure to intubate the patient prior to transfer were common occurrences. Failure to detect problems with circulation (e.g., that the patient was bleeding to death and in need of urgent surgery) was also surprisingly frequent. Lastly, failure to perform and document a thorough neurologic examination on initial assessment was a frequent omission from evaluations of patients.

ANCILLARY TESTS

The key investigations for trauma patients, based on the ATLS protocol, are serial hematocrits and initial radiographs (x-rays of the chest, pelvis, and lateral cervical spine). There is good evidence in the literature that spending time getting extremity films in trauma patients who need to be transferred for definitive treatment of a more serious injury should be avoided, as it prolongs transfer time—resulting in a worse outcome for the patient.

Nontrauma Patients

For evaluating patients being referred from rural areas with non–trauma-induced surgical conditions, the appropriate history, physical, and laboratory assessments vary with the nature of the surgical problem. Recommendations for evaluating most common surgical problems are contained in the various chapters of this book. However, based on my experience both as a primary-care clinician in a remote locale and as a consultant surgeon in an urban, tertiary medical center, two general points deserve emphasis—the importance of succinct case presentations and the need to provide pertinent medical records and laboratory results.

BE SUCCINCT

Be succinct and direct when communicating with the consulting/accepting surgeon. Long, all-inclusive reports of the type demanded for internal medicine grand rounds, in which every possible diagnosis must be considered, are not appropriate for surgical consultation.

In the case where the diagnosis is known (e.g., fracture, epistaxis, etc.), it is essential to collect information that the surgeon will want. This information includes the patient's gender, diagnosis, relevant past surgical/medical history, treatment measures already taken, stability of the patient (if relevant), and why it is necessary to transfer the patient.

In the case where the diagnosis is unclear (e.g., nonspecific abdominal pain with acute abdomen), state the age, gender, and the most probable diagnosis in your opinion, before going on to describe the history, physical examination, and diagnostic workup in appropriate detail. The point of stating your most probable diagnosis at the beginning of your consultation, providing the consulting surgeon with a "headline" as it were, is that it gives the surgeon an idea of the severity of the problem. It also enables the surgeon to more easily rule out or in different diagnoses as the whole story unfolds, and it gives the surgeon an idea of whether it will be necessary to have a fully staffed operating room ready for the patient on arrival.

PROVIDE PERTINENT RECORDS

When sending patients for consultation or referral, whether elective or emergent, it is essential for the referring clinicians to send a brief note stating the highlights of the workup and what treatments, if any, have already been implemented. To avoid needless duplication of studies, make sure that all relevant images go with the patient. Referring clinicians should resist the temptation to photocopy and send comprehensive medical records (e.g., the last 5 years of the patient's chart); such a practice wastes everybody's time.

In return, the referring clinician should expect to receive a telephone call or written communication from the consultant concerning an opinion about the diagnosis and what treatments were administered. This is not only polite and good business practice, it makes for better patient care.

Treatment

To ensure stability and suitability for safe transport, the first step is to address the ABCs (airway, breathing, and circulation) of the patient. These issues are discussed in many of the chapters in this book in relation to specific surgical problems, but they will be reemphasized here. In addition to dealing with the ABCs, other interventions will also enhance the safety of transport. These include cardiac monitoring, spine stabilization for trauma patients, monitoring circulatory status of injured extremities, and a variety of other interventions discussed in the individual chapters in this book.

Airway and Breathing

A secure airway with adequate ventilation and oxygenation is the first priority. If there is any uncertainty about the patient's ability to maintain an airway and ventilate spontaneously during transport, the patient should be intubated prior to leaving the rural facility. Patients with neurotrauma who might lose their ability to maintain an airway or ventilatory drive during transport also should be intubated. A further advantage to intubating such patients is that it enables hyperventilation, which may decrease intracranial pressure. If the patient is unable to be intubated, then crico-thyroidotomy should be performed (Chapter 13).

It is almost always appropriate to administer oxygen (by nasal prongs, mask, or endotracheal tube) with monitoring by pulse oxymetry. Ventilation with PEEP may be necessary in some patients. As discussed in Chapter 13, the nature of some traumatic injuries will require placement of a chest tube(s) prior to transport.

Circulation

If the patient is bleeding heavily—either from a traumatic injury (e.g., a ruptured spleen) or from a nontraumatic cause (e.g., a ruptured abdominal aortic aneurysm)—and no local surgeon is available to deal with the situation, it is important to ensure adequate circulation prior to transport. The first step in doing this is to access to the circulation with short, large-bore intravenous needles. Blood and fluid (warmed Ringer's lactate is best) resuscitation is then administered at a rate and in sufficient quantity to ensure circulatory stability.

Studies from the trauma literature indicate that a common problem among transported patients is insufficient administration of intravenous fluids and blood, that is, underresuscitation. It is likely that this phenomenon results in large part from the nonsurgeon's fear of inducing congestive heart failure. Suffice it to say, it is very difficult to volume overload patients who are bleeding to death or experiencing major third-space losses caused by inflammation (i.e., infection, trauma, burns, etc.).

When in doubt, establish adequate intravenous access, insert a Foley catheter to monitor urine output, and give fluid and blood in large quantities. Monitoring urine output with a Foley catheter is underutilized by nonsurgeons. Having a urinary catheter in place and assessing urine output in relation to the volume of fluid administered is a simple, low-tech way to ensure adequacy of resuscitation and thus end-organ perfusion.

Education

The most common reasons for patient transfers are patient/family request, the need for additional diagnostic technology and/or expertise not available in the local health-care facility, or the need for health-care resources or treatments only available in the referral center. Patients and their families should be fully informed of the reasons for transfer of the patient, its purported benefits, and the possible risks—just as one would obtain informed consent for a procedure. Transport of patients is not risk-free, as unstable medical or surgical problems may develop or become evident during transport when effective assessment and treatment may be difficult in the cramped quarters of the transport vehicle.

While most patients and families will readily accept the need for transport to an urban center when diagnostic and therapeutic expertise is unavailable locally, rural clinicians will occasionally encounter patients who argue against the recommendation for transport. These patients are often elderly individuals with fragile, social support systems, who fear that they will not be able to return home from the urban facility, or who fear loss of control in an out-of-town institution with unfamiliar health-care providers. While it is sometimes tempting to acquiesce to such a patient's request, the temptation should be resisted. In the presence of a life-threatening surgical problem that requires therapy unavailable in the home community, it is rarely appropriate to "negotiate" with patients about suboptimal alternative modes of therapy that might be administered locally. Patients who initially refuse transport should understand the nature of the problem that requires diagnostics and treatments that are unavailable locally and the likely outcome if appropriate care is not provided.

Legal Issues

Antidumping Laws

The "antidumping" provisions in Section 1867 of the Social Security Act and the Emergency Medical Treatment and Active Labor Act apply to all patients in the United States. These laws were enacted to prevent the needless transfer of patients from one institution to another to avoid financial loss. They forbid refusal to treat indigent patients (or, for that matter, *any* patients) for emergency medical conditions. They also prohibit the transfer of patients prior to stabilization. The legislation suggests that clinicians initiating the transfer take responsibility for certifying that the benefits of transfer outweigh the risks.

Liability

Based on the provisions of the aforementioned legislation, physicians have a responsibility to patients seen in rural areas when transport or referral is being considered. They also have potential liability if they do not act appropriately. The basic questions of liability for consultation and transfers are probably the same as for medical practice in general. That is, was there a patient-physician relationship between the consultant and the patient? Was there a breach of the standard of care? Was there an injury to the patient as a consequence of that breach?

There is some controversy, however, about the liability of clinicians participating in a patient's care when the consultant is not physically present. That is, the consultant may have been contacted by phone or other electronic medium and may not have personally seen the patient.

REFERRING CLINICIAN

Clinicians involved in the in-person evaluation and treatment of the patients clearly have liability for the patient's care when consultation occurs and transport is being considered. The main legal and ethical duty for the on-site consulting physician is to provide an accurate history and representation of the patient's condition to the consultant.

CONSULTANT/ACCEPTING CLINICIAN

For the consultant, the main question in terms of telephone and telemedicine consultations usually revolves around whether there was a patient-physician relationship with the remote consultant. Several factors inform this determination. Has the consulting physician met the patient or know the patient's name? Has the consulting physician examined the patient and/or the patient's record? Did the consulting physician charge a fee for services provided? Issues regarding patient-physician relationship are usually decided on a case-by-case basis in the courts, and the laws vary widely from state to state.

In the case of telemedicine consultations, there are a whole host of nascent legal issues that have yet to be worked out. In which jurisdiction should the case be tried—that of the referring physician or the consultant? Do consultants need to have a valid medical license in every state in which they "teleconsult?" It is likely that with increased use of telemedicine, legal interpretations and answers for the questions will evolve.

Errors

Common errors, or rather inefficiencies, in consultation have already been described. These include failure to provide a succinct history, failure to provide a brief summary of the patient's diagnostic workup and treatment prior to transfer, and failure to send relevant records and diagnostic images with the patient. Common errors in stabilization and transfer have also been dis-

Table 4-1

Common Clinical Errors in Stabilization and Transport of Surgical Patients

Delaying transport to obtain unnecessary x-rays
  (e.g., plain films of long bones and skull)
Failure to document neurologic status
Inadequate cervical-spine immobilization when
  indicated
Failure to intubate patient when indicated
Failure to place tubes (chest tubes, nasogastric
  tubes, and Foley catheters) when indicated
Inadequate fluid resuscitation with crystalloid
  and/or blood
Failure to recognize problems that need urgent
  surgical attention

cussed. These errors are emphasized in Table 4-1. They can be avoided, in large part, by adherence to ATLS protocols.

Controversies and Emerging Concepts

Scoop and Run

A long-standing but unresolved controversy in the area of stabilization is the issue of whether to "scoop and run" with a patient directly from the scene of injury to the tertiary trauma center, rather than stopping for stabilization at the accident scene or local health-care facility. Many experts advocate this approach as an alternative to stabilizing the patient (either at the injury scene or in a nearby health-care facility) before transport. Research on this controversial topic suggests that patients who are bleeding to death (i.e., penetrating trauma with vascular injury) are best served by the "scoop and run" approach, as various stabilization measures only serve to delay definitive surgical treatment.

Patients with central nervous system injuries, on the other hand, often profit from stabilization prior to transfer. In particular, endotracheal intubation to secure the airway and provide hyperventilation prior to transport may result in better outcomes for patients than transporting them without instituting such interventions.

IVs in the Field

Recent research suggests that for many trauma patients (up to half) routine placement of intravenous access in the field is unnecessary and leads to delay of transport that may result in unfavorable outcomes for patients. Further investigation is needed to determine the situations in which it is desirable to take the time for establishing intravenous access.

Benefits of Air Evacuation

Despite its widespread use, the merits of routine air evacuation of trauma patients continue to be debated. Studies indicate that it is the most severely injured patients, rather than all trauma patients, who experience the largest decrease in morbidity and mortality rates if evacuated by air. As stated earlier in this chapter, the improved outcomes appear to be as much the result of the skills of the flight crew—acting as a *de facto* extension of the trauma center staff—as from any reduction in transport time. Given the cost and relative danger of air evacuation and a desire to reduce the number of unnecessary air evacuations, more research is needed to determine which patients most benefit from air transport.

Elderly Trauma Victims

Another area of controversy involving stabilization pertains to elderly individuals who are victims of trauma. Several studies from rural hospitals, involving both major and minor trauma, have revealed that the majority of the deaths deemed preventable or unexpected were in elderly patients. The increased death rate among elderly trauma victims in rural areas is higher than one would expect based on the experience in urban trauma centers. The reason for this disproportionately higher death rate among elderly trauma victims is unexplained, but may be the result of more than the decreased "physiologic reserve" that accompanies aging. Older individuals with traumatic injuries may not be treated as aggressively as younger persons. More studies in this area are essential because rural areas of this country contain a disproportionate number of the nation's elderly.

Telemedicine

Some of the legal controversies surrounding telemedicine have already been discussed. These legal issues will continue to be reviewed and refined by state medical licensing boards, the courts, and the United States Congress.

Another important controversy about telemedicine is whether medical information transmitted electronically can be maintained securely and confidentially. Recent rules proposed by the US Department of Health and Human Services would make such information available to a wide array of insurers, government agencies, and other third parties. The desirability and logistics of these issues continue to be discussed.

Other controversies regarding telemedicine include identification of the optimal bandwidth and data-compression modes for transmission of images and how variations in these parameters might influence diagnostic accuracy. Finally, despite its obvious allure and applicability to rural health problems, few good studies have been performed to determine if patients' outcomes are improved by using telemedicine technologies.

References

Baxt WG, Moody P, Cleveland HC, et al: Hospital-based rotorcraft aeromedical emergency care services and trauma mortality: a multicenter study. *Ann Emerg Med* 14:859, 1985.

Berry RF, Barry MH: Evaluation of a personal-computer–based teleradiology system serving an isolated Canadian community. *Can Assoc Radiol J* 49:7, 1998.

Burney RE, Fischer RP: Ground versus air transport of trauma victims: medical and logistical considerations. *Ann Emerg Med* 15:1491, 1986.

Carto TF, Rogers FB, Pilcher DB: Review of care of fatally injured patients in a rural state: 5-year follow-up. *J Trauma* 23:559, 1983.

Deakin C, Davies G: Defining trauma patient subpopulations for field stabilization. *Eur J Emerg Med* 1:31, 1994.

Esposito TJ, Snaddal ND, Hansen JD, et al: Analysis of preventable trauma deaths and inappropriate trauma care in a rural state. *J Trauma* 39:955, 1995.

Falcone RE, Herron H, Werman H, et al: Air medical transport of the injured patients: scene versus referring hospital. *Air Med J* 17:161, 1998.

Furrow BR: An overview and analysis of the impact of the Emergency Medical Treatment and Active Labor Act. *J Leg Med* 16:325, 1995.

Henderson RA, Thomson DP, Bahrs BA: Unnecessary intravenous access in the emergency setting. *Prehosp Emerg Care* 3:312, 1998.

Hotvedt R, Kristiansen IS, Førde OH, et al: Which groups of patients benefit from helicopter evacuation? *Lancet* 347:1362, 1996.

Jacobs LM, Sinclair A, Beiser A: Prehospital advanced life support: benefits in trauma. *J Trauma* 24:8, 1984.

Jones MG: Telemedicine and the National Information Infrastructure: Are the realities of health care being ignored? *J Am Med Inform Assoc* 4:399, 1997.

Leicht MJ, Dula DJ, Brotman S: Rural interhospital helicopter transport of motor vehicle trauma victims: causes for delays and recommendations. *Ann Emerg Med* 15:450, 1986.

Mann NC, Hedges JR, Mullins RJ: Rural hospital transfer patterns before and after implementation of a statewide trauma system. *Acad Emerg Med* 4:764, 1999.

Martin GD, Cogbill TH, Landercasper J, et al: Prospective analysis of rural interhospital transfer of injured patients to a referral trauma center. *J Trauma* 30:1014, 1990.

Morrisey MA, Ohsfeldt RL, Johnson V: Rural emergency medical services: patients, destinations, times, and services. *J Rural Health* 11:286, 1995.

Moyland JA, Fitzpatrick KT, Beyer J, et al: Factors improving survival in multisystem trauma patients. *Ann Surg* 207:679, 1988.

Pendrak RF, Ericson P: Telemedicine and the law. *Healthcare Financial Manage* December:46, 1996.

Rice B: Will telemedicine get you sued? *Med Economics* Nov 24:58, 1997.

Richardson JD, Cross T, Lee D: Impact of level III verification on trauma admission and transfer: comparisons of two rural hospitals. *J Trauma* 42:498, 1997.

Rogers FB, Osler TM, Shackford SR, et al: Study of the outcome of patients transferred to a level I hospital after stabilization at an outlying hospital in a rural setting. *J Trauma* 46:328, 1999.

Rogers FB, Shackford SR, Hoyt DB, et al: Trauma deaths in a mature urban vs rural trauma system. *Arch Surg* 132:376, 1997.

Smith N: The incidence of severe trauma in small rural hospitals. *J Fam Pract* 6:595, 1987.

Studdiford JS, Panitch KN, Snyderman DA, et al: The telephone in primary care. *J Prim Care* 23:83, 1996.

Urdaneta LF, Miller BK, Ringenberg J, et al: Role of emergency helicopter transport service in rural trauma. *Arch Surg* 122:992, 1987.

Part 2

Gastrointestinal Problems

Ravi Moonka

Abdominal Pain

Introduction

In the emergency room evaluation of abdominal pain, the differential diagnosis is infinite, and time for assessment is short. The clinician daunted by these unfriendly circumstances can take solace in two simple observations. First, more than 40% of individuals presenting to an emergency room with acute abdominal pain of less than 1 week's duration will never be assigned a diagnosis. Rather, abdominal pain in these patients will resolve without a diagnosis and without specific therapy. Second, roughly 90% of patients in whom it is possible to make a diagnosis suffer from one of approximately 10 different diseases (Table 5-1).

The challenge, therefore, is not to definitively diagnose each patient, but instead to determine if a patient suffers from one of a well-defined set of disorders with which most clinicians are familiar. Accordingly, this chapter will focus on the common differential diagnosis of acute abdominal pain, emphasizing the diagnostic process rather than surgical procedures.

Key History

Pain Characteristics

LOCATION

Location of pain is the single most important feature of the patient's history. Pain generally localizes to the epigastrium or one of the four quadrants (right upper, left upper, right lower, left lower). While overlap clearly exists between each pain locale, the association of certain diseases with different locations is reliable enough to be the leading principle in diagnosis of abdominal pain. Diffuse pain that cannot be localized is also associated with specific disorders, and these are also discussed in this chapter.

Radiation or migration of pain from one location to another can also have diagnostic value. For example, radiation of abdominal pain into the groin or into the back and shoulder characterizes pain of a ureteral or pancreaticobiliary origin, respectively.

Similarly, migration of pain from the periumbilical area to the right lower quadrant is one of the most discriminating clinical features of appendicitis. This occurs because when the appendix initially becomes inflamed, pain sensation is carried to the central nervous system by sympathetic afferent fibers that refer pain to the midline around the umbilicus. When appendiceal inflammation progresses and makes contact with the parietal peritoneum on the internal surface of the anterior abdominal wall, somatic afferent nerve fibers localize pain to the right lower quadrant, leading to the classic right lower abdominal pain of appendicitis.

ONSET AND DURATION

The timing of the pain can be helpful in arriving at a diagnosis. An abrupt onset, in which the patient can describe the exact time or exact activity associated with the initial pain, is characteristic of pancreatitis, embolic ischemic disease, or rupture of an organ.

The duration of pain is important in that discomfort that has been present for more than a week without change is unlikely to be caused by an intraabdominal emergency. A colicky pain pattern, in which excruciating exacerbations are interspersed with periods of complete or relative relief, is suggestive of a visceral obstruction such as from urolithiasis obstructing a ureter or gallstones in the cystic or common ducts.

GASTROINTESTINAL SYMPTOMS

Vomiting should be characterized by its frequency, the amount and nature of the vomitus, and the association of vomiting with transient relief of pain. These features can be helpful in that vomiting that relieves pain or contains bilious material may indicate bowel obstruction, while

Table 5-1

The Most Common Diagnoses in Emergency Room Patients Evaluated for Abdominal Pain

DIAGNOSIS	DOMBAL[a] PERCENT	BREWER ET AL[b] PERCENT
Nonspecific abdominal pain	43.0	41.3
Acute appendicitis	24.2	2.5
Acute cholecystitis	8.9	3.7
Gastritis or gastroenteritis	—	8.3
Urinary tract infection or pyelonephritis	—	6.9
Small bowel obstruction	4.0	—
Renal colic	3.4	4.3
Peptic ulcer	2.8	2.0
Pancreatitis	2.3	0.9
Constipation	—	2.3
Acute diverticular disease	2.1	—
Other (mostly gynecologic problems)	9.3	12.3

[a]Diagnoses in 6097 patients with acute abdominal pain, from 17 hospitals in 10 countries. (Data used with permission from deDombal FT: Acute abdominal pain—an OMGE survey. *Scan J Gastroenterol* 14:29, 1979.)
[b]Diagnoses in 1000 patients with acute abdominal pain, from a single emergency room in the United States. (Data used with permission from Brewer RJ, Golden GT, Hitch DC, et al: An analysis of 1000 consecutive cases in a university emergency room. *Am J Surg* 131:219, 1976.)

vomitus containing blood suggests peptic ulcer disease, gastritis, or esophagitis.

Changes in bowel habits are usually nonspecific, but can be helpful in diagnosis if there is an absence of bowel movements (suggesting bowel obstruction) or profuse or bloody diarrhea (suggesting diverticular disease or colitis). Alleviating and exacerbating features, especially changes in pain with respect to posture and movement, can point to specific diagnoses, as patients with peritonitis tend to lie still, while those with ureteral colic tend to move about restlessly.

PAST MEDICAL HISTORY

The need to elicit a detailed history about prior abdominal surgery or a history of hepatitis, gallstones, pancreatitis, peptic ulcer disease, and inflammatory bowel disease is self-evident, as symptoms may represent a recurrence of preexisting conditions. For women with lower abdominal pain, a history of delayed menstruation, prior sexually transmitted disease, or use of an intrauterine device (IUD) may indicate ectopic pregnancy. Prior sexually transmitted diseases and/or IUD use also suggest acute pelvic inflammatory disease.

Patients must be asked about their consumption of alcohol, nonsteroidal antiinflammatory drugs, and prednisone, as these substances predispose to gastrointestinal bleeding. A history of cardiac disease is important, since upper abdominal pain or nausea can be a symptom of heart disease (e.g., inferior cardiac ischemia), and patients with dilated cardiomyopathy or arrhythmias are at risk for ischemic bowel disease caused by hypoperfusion or embolic obstruction of the mesenteric circulation.

Key Physical Examination

Initial inspection of the patient can assess the degree of discomfort, the presence of abdominal distention, and the presence or absence of jaundice, all of which are diagnostically useful. As noted, severe discomfort, especially when of sudden onset, suggests obstruction or visceral rupture. Abdominal distention suggests bowel obstruction, and jaundice indicates pancreaticobiliary disease. Pneumonia can occasionally present as upper abdominal pain, mandating auscultation of the lungs. The need to evaluate the patient's heart has been previously stated.

Abdominal Auscultation and Palpation

Auscultation of bowel sounds is generally not helpful, but positioning a stethoscope on the patient's abdomen is a gentle and nonthreatening way to begin the abdominal examination. For patients who can localize their pain, the examination should proceed with gentle palpation in the quadrant opposite the pain. Initiating palpation in the most tender area will alarm the patient, leading to voluntary guarding of the abdominal muscles, which will all but preclude a meaningful examination. This initial palpation will establish the absence of tenderness in the quadrants in which the patient denies pain, so that when tenderness is elicited, it can be clearly said to localize.

GUARDING AND REBOUND TENDERNESS

Supporting the patient's head and bending the knees will promote relaxation of the abdominal wall. A patient who, despite all measures, cannot relax the abdomen is said to have a rigid abdomen, while a patient whose abdomen is initially soft but then tenses to palpation is said to guard. Both are suggestive of intraabdominal pathology that may require surgical intervention.

Because patients can voluntarily tense their abdominal wall, however, guarding can be a deceptive sign. A more reliable indicator of intraabdominal surgical conditions is rebound tenderness, which refers to greater pain with the release of pressure placed on the abdominal wall than with its initiation. It is best elicited by applying gentle but steady pressure to the quadrant for several seconds, followed by sudden release with minimal flourish. This allows the application and release of

pressure to be separated enough in time so that the patient's response can be clearly assigned to one event or the other. It is not necessary to ask if releasing the tension caused pain, as even the most stoic individuals cannot conceal their response to this unexpected discomfort if peritonitis is present.

Simple motion of the body will aggravate severe peritonitis, leading many physicians to assess the patient's reaction to a shake of the bed or tap on the heel. While entertaining, these needlessly indirect and uncontrolled ways of demonstrating peritonitis are positive in only the most obvious cases of intraabdominal inflammation.

Rectal Examination

In most cases, examination of patients with abdominal pain should include a digital rectal examination. The main purposes of the examination are to check the stool for gross blood (suggestive of colitis or severe gastroenteritis), melena or occult blood (indicating upper gastrointestinal bleeding), and to identify areas of tenderness that might help localize and identify the source of pain.

Pelvic Examination

For women with lower abdominal pain, the cervix should be examined for mucopurulent discharge, and cultures for *Chlamydia* and gonorrhea should be obtained. The size of the uterus and adnexa should be assessed, as should the ability of cervical or adnexal manipulation to exacerbate the patient's pain. Because pelvic abscesses do not touch the anterior abdominal wall, disproportionate tenderness on one side of the rectal vault may be the only physical finding to suggest such a diagnosis.

Ancillary Tests

Certain laboratory studies are obtained on nearly all patients presenting to an emergency room with abdominal pain. These include a complete blood count, serum electrolytes, serum amylase, serum creatinine, liver function tests, a urinalysis, and, in appropriate patients, a urine pregnancy test. Imaging tests usually include a chest radiograph and supine and upright plain x-rays of the abdomen.

Patients seen in office practice, especially those for whom there is an obvious explanation for their abdominal pain (e.g., acute urinary tract infection or acute gastroenteritis with diarrhea) do not necessarily require the full laboratory evaluation outlined above. However, it is essential to be alert for the possibility of serious intraabdominal conditions in all patients with abdominal pain and to obtain those tests necessary to confirm or exclude such conditions.

Abdominal Pain Syndromes

Right Upper Quadrant and Epigastric Pain

The most common surgical conditions causing acute right upper quadrant or epigastric abdominal pain are perforated peptic ulcer, biliary colic, cholecystitis, cholangitis, and pancreatitis.

PERFORATED PEPTIC ULCER

Perforation of a peptic ulcer into the duodenum or stomach, while occurring less frequently since the availability of antisecretory therapy (e.g., histamine-2 blockers and proton-pump inhibitors), is still a common cause of the prototypical "acute abdomen."

HISTORY AND PHYSICAL EXAMINATION   Patients may have a history of a previous peptic ulcer, but perforation can be the first sign of ulcer disease. The onset of the pain is severe and abrupt, as the contents of the peritoneal cavity are bathed in gastric acid. Transient improvement may occur as this acid is diluted by peritoneal transudate, but eventually severe diffuse pain returns. Use of alcohol, prednisone, or nonsteroidal antiinflammatory med-

ications is a risk factor for ulcer formation and should alert the clinicians to the possibility of an ulcer.

Examination will generally reveal a patient in extreme discomfort. Because peritonitis is present, the patient has a rigid abdomen and is often reluctant to move.

ANCILLARY TESTS   The diagnosis is most often based on the visualization of free intraperitoneal air on plain abdominal x-rays (Fig. 5-1, A–D). If the presentation is suggestive of a perforated ulcer, but no free air is apparent on plain films, a water-soluble contrast study of the upper gastrointestinal tract will demonstrate extravasation through the perforation into the peritoneal cavity (Fig. 5-2). Barium should not be used as the contrast agent in this setting, as the introduction of barium salts into the peritoneal cavity can lead to an inflammatory reaction that renders subsequent dissection in the area difficult.

TREATMENT   Distal stomach perforations are usually managed by antrectomy, while more proximal ulcers are treated with excision (Fig. 5-3). Because acid overproduction is not thought to play a major role in the etiology of gastric ulcers, a vagotomy is not necessarily performed when gastric ulcers are surgically managed.

Perforated duodenal ulcers can be definitively closed by securing the omentum over the site of perforation (a Graham patch), which is almost always on the anterior aspect of the first portion of the duodenum. Because acid overproduction plays a role in the etiology of duodenal ulcers, some form of vagotomy and an appropriate drainage procedure is often performed concurrently with the Graham patch.

Though the traditional management of perforated ulcers involves surgery, some patients with duodenal ulcer perforations can be managed without an operation when the omentum spontaneously seals off the perforation, thereby achieving the same result as a Graham-patch procedure. In addition, the need for acid-reduction surgery (e.g., vagotomy) has been reduced substantially through the use of medications to reduce acid

Figure 5-1

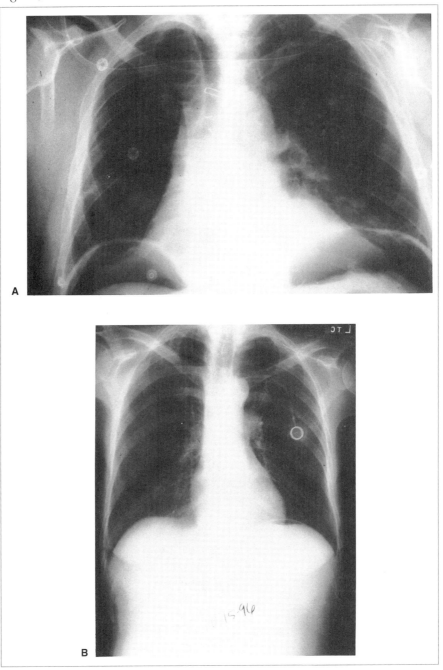

Radiographic appearance of free intraperitoneal air in perforated duodenal ulcer. As shown in **(A)**, free intraperitoneal air is most readily identified beneath the hemidiaphragms, as is seen in this patient with a perforated duodenal ulcer. The x-ray in **(B)** is from a patient with gastric outlet obstruction and a large gastric air bubble that was mistaken for free intraperitoneal air.

Figure 5-1 (continued)

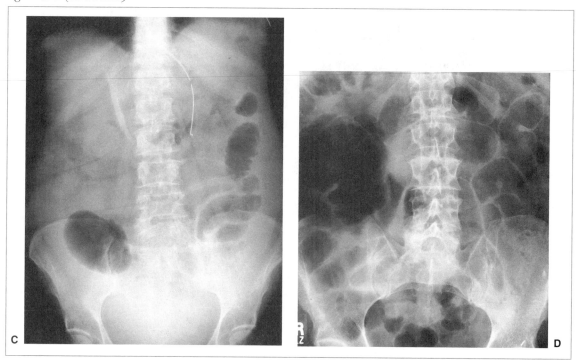

The diagnosis of free air can also be made by a collection of air that outlines the falciform ligament **(C)**, or by visualizing both sides of the wall of the bowel **(D)**.

secretion and antibiotics for treatment of *H. pylori* infection. The safety of this nonoperative strategy can be maximized by limiting it to patients who are not in extremis and in whom a gastrografin upper gastrointestinal contrast study demonstrates a walled-off perforation.

BILIARY COLIC

There are four different ways in which gallstones can cause acute biliary disease, and each is treated differently (Fig. 5-4). The simplest form of calculi-induced disease is biliary colic, in which pain results from contractions of the gallbladder against a gallstone impacted in the cystic duct.

HISTORY AND PHYSICAL EXAMINATION   Patients note the gradual onset of ultimately severe and constant pain in the epigastrium or right upper quadrant that typically occurs soon after a meal, frequently accompanied by nausea and diaphoresis. The pain may also occur only at night, waking the patient from sleep. Discomfort sometimes radiates to the right side of the back, to the midscapular area, or to the right shoulder. These episodes of pain usually last from 1 to 5 hours and then either dissipate on their own or are successfully and definitively treated with injectable narcotics in an acute-care setting. Findings on physical examination are often limited to tenderness in the right upper quadrant or epigastric area.

ANCILLARY TESTS   The diagnosis of biliary colic is confirmed when a right upper quadrant ultrasound reveals gallstones in conjunction with the appropriate history and physical examination.

Figure 5-2

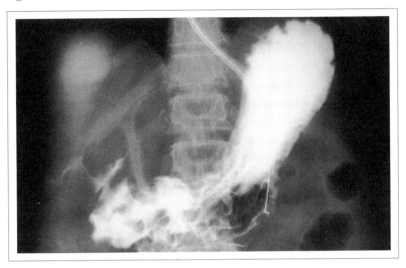

Bowel perforation demonstrated with water-soluble contrast. Although visualizing free intraperitoneal air can usually make the diagnosis of a perforated ulcer, when the diagnosis is unclear, the perforation may be demonstrated using a water-soluble radiographic contrast agent. In this x-ray, contrast can be seen outside the lumen of the duodenum.

TREATMENT   Patients with suspected biliary colic do not require hospital admission in the absence of cholecystitis or other complications. Treatment of the acute pain episode with parenteral narcotics is usually sufficient. Because of the pain involved in biliary colic, most patients will agree, even after a single episode, to a subsequent elective cholecystectomy to diminish the likelihood of recurrent biliary colic.

CHOLECYSTITIS

Cholecystitis represents a more severe form of biliary disease, in which ongoing obstruction of the cystic duct leads to inflammation of the gallbladder.

HISTORY AND PHYSICAL EXAMINATION   The pain pattern of cholecystitis is similar to that of biliary colic, but cholecystitis is usually associated with systemic signs of inflammation such as an elevated temper-

ature and/or an elevated white blood cell count. In addition, cholecystitis does not resolve of its own accord like simple biliary colic, but instead lasts for 24 hours or more.

While rebound tenderness and guarding are rare findings, the patient will often demonstrate a sudden halt to inspiratory effort when the right upper quadrant is forcibly depressed during a deep inspiration (Murphy's sign). In severe cases, one can palpate a tender mass consisting of an omentum-caked gallbladder, which establishes the diagnosis of cholecystitis.

ANCILLARY TESTS   Ultrasound examination (Fig. 5-5) will demonstrate gallstones, plus a thickened gallbladder wall, a localized collection of fluid around the gallbladder, and tenderness directly over the visualized gallbladder (sonographic Murphy's sign). Other imaging modalities such as HIDA scanning or computerized tomography may be needed when the clinical pre-

Figure 5-3

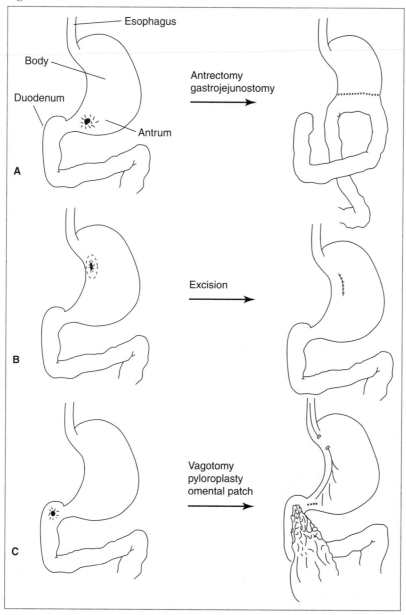

Surgical treatment of perforated gastric or duodenal ulcer. Perforated ulcers of the stomach and duodenum are treated differently depending on their location. Distal (antral) stomach ulcers are treated by antrectomy and gastrojejunostomy, as shown in **(A)**. Proximal stomach ulcers are treated by local excision, as shown in **(B)**. Duodenal ulcers, shown in **(C)**, can be patched with omentum, accompanied by vagotomy, to treat gastric acid hypersecretion, and pyloroplasty.

Figure 5-4

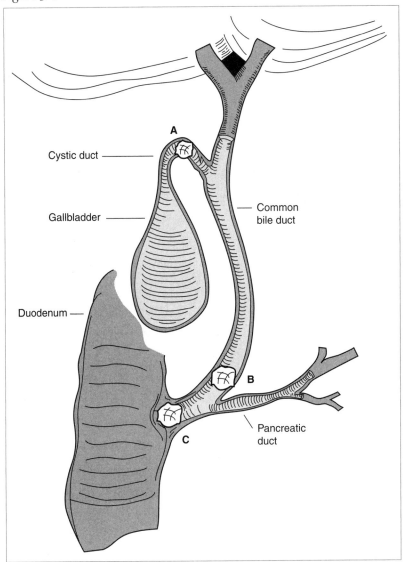

Gallstone disease. Stones in the biliary tree can cause different disease manifestations, depending on the location and irreversibility of the stone's position. Common locations for stones are in the cystic duct **(A)**, common bile duct **(B)**, or at the entry of the pancreatobiliary ducts into the duodenum **(C)**.

sentation suggests cholecystitis but ultrasound is nondiagnostic.

Necrosis of the gallbladder mucosa can cause mild jaundice and hyperbilirubinemia, as conju-gated bilirubin within the gallbladder is able to access the blood system directly. Generally, how-ever, the liver-function tests are normal or only minimally elevated, and substantial derangement of these tests in a patient whose presentation is suggestive of cholecystitis should raise the question of cholangitis or hepatitis.

TREATMENT A patient whose presentation suggests cholecystitis should be admitted to the hospital and treated with a second-generation cephalosporin intravenously. The definitive treatment of cholecystitis is cholecystectomy, which ideally should be performed within 48 hours of admission. On occasion, even more urgent surgery should be considered when a patient has findings suggestive of a gangrenous gallbladder such as air detected in the wall of the gallbladder on ultrasound examination, jaundice or markedly elevated bilirubin, or a markedly elevated temperature or white blood cell count.

In the past, cholecystectomy was often delayed until 6 weeks after the initial episode of cholecystitis. This approach, however, puts the patient at

Figure 5-5

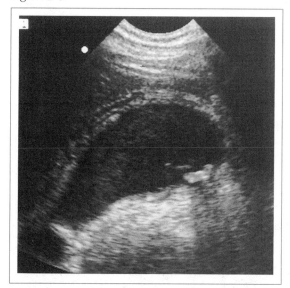

Sonographic appearance of acute cholecystitis. Acute cholecystitis is most often diagnosed by the findings of stones in the gallbladder (note the acoustic shadow), accompanied by thickening of the gallbladder wall and a sonographic Murphy's sign.

risk for another attack during the waiting period and offers no advantage in terms of morbidity and mortality.

CHOLANGITIS

Cholangitis refers to a suppurative infection of the biliary tree. Any obstructive process of the bile ducts can cause cholangitis, but a stone is the most common etiologic agent (Fig. 5-6). The systemic inflammatory response to cholangitis is usually more substantial than that seen in cholecystitis, so the diagnosis is usually more apparent. The mortality of cholangitis and the urgency with which it is treated is correspondingly greater as well.

HISTORY AND PHYSICAL EXAMINATION Cholangitis is classically described by Charcot's triad, which consists of fever, jaundice, and right upper quadrant abdominal pain. Acute hepatitis can present similarly, so laboratory testing is often needed to distinguish the two conditions.

ANCILLARY TESTS Cholangitis can usually be distinguished from hepatitis by the pattern of associated liver-function test abnormalities (Table 5-2). In cholangitis, the alkaline phosphatase, which indicates biliary-tract obstruction, will be elevated disproportionately to the transaminases, while in hepatitis the reverse is true. Cirrhosis can also cause jaundice and liver-function abnormalities, but does not in and of itself cause pain.

Ultrasound is helpful in distinguishing hepatitis from cholangitis. Obstruction of the common bile duct in cholangitis usually occurs at the ampulla, so the resulting dilation of the entire biliary tree is readily discerned sonographically (the normal diameter of the common bile duct is about 1 millimeter for every decade of age). Thus, a dilated biliary tree in the setting of jaundice and abdominal pain confirms the diagnosis of cholangitis. Ultrasound also offers the ability to identify a liver abscess, which is a relatively rare cause of both right upper quadrant pain and an elevated alkaline phosphatase.

Figure 5-6

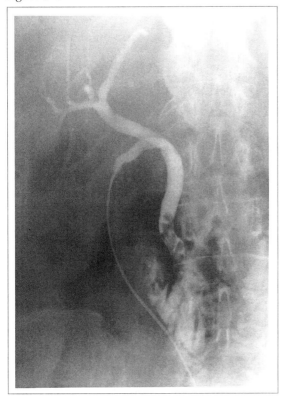

Cholangiogram demonstrating impacted gallstone. Stones impacted in the common bile duct are seen on this intraoperative cholangiogram. Attempts to remove the stones endoscopically failed, necessitating surgery.

TREATMENT Patients with cholangitis should be admitted to the hospital. After a brief period (e.g., overnight for patients admitted in the evening) of hydration and parenteral antibiotics, definitive treatment should be provided.

Definitive treatment of cholangitis requires drainage of the obstructed biliary tree. Drainage can be accomplished surgically or percutaneously under radiologic guidance, but endoscopic sphincterotomy is usually the preferred form of treatment. Gastroenterologists proficient in this technique are able to cut the sphincter of Oddi endoscopically, and then remove common bile duct stones by balloon stripping of the duct. Drainage of the biliary tree subsequently occurs spontaneously through the incompetent sphincter or can be facilitated by a stent placed though the ampulla. Alternatively, a nasobiliary drain can be left in the common bile duct, which allows for intermittent saline flushing.

The gallbladder is removed electively once the patient has recovered fully from the episode of cholangitis. For patients who are poor candidates for surgery, leaving the gallbladder in situ is not usually associated with subsequent biliary complications.

PANCREATITIS

HISTORY AND PHYSICAL EXAMINATION The clinical presentation of pancreatitis is fairly characteristic. Patients complain of the abrupt onset of epigastric pain radiating directly through to the back, associated with nausea and vomiting with minimal production of vomitus. Most cases of pancreatitis in the United States are related either to gallstones or alcohol. Therefore, a history of recent and sub-

Table 5-2

Clues to the Differential Diagnosis of Common Hepatobiliary Problems

PARAMETER	BILIARY COLIC	CHOLECYSTITIS	CHOLANGITIS	ACUTE HEPATITIS
Jaundice	No	Sometimes	Yes	Yes
Fever	No	Yes	Yes	Yes
Transaminase levels	Normal	Normal or ↑	↑	↑↑↑
Alkaline phosphatase level	Normal or ↑	Normal or ↑	↑↑↑	↑
Gallbladder ultrasound	Gallstones	Thickened wall	Biliary tract dilation	Normal

stantial alcohol consumption is important to elicit from patients who have upper abdominal pain.

On physical examination, the patient may prefer sitting up to lying down. Palpation of the abdomen will reveal substantial tenderness in the epigastrium. Ecchymosis of the flank or around the umbilicus is infrequently observed, but is highly suggestive of severe pancreatitis when seen.

ANCILLARY TESTS   In no disease is the association of a single laboratory abnormality with a specific diagnosis as strong as with elevated serum amylase and acute pancreatitis. Serum amylase is an inexpensive and readily available indicator of pancreatitis that has a high positive predictive value in appropriate clinical settings.

Nonetheless, there are circumstances in which the serum amylase is inaccurate. For example, a normal serum amylase level may occur, even in the presence of acute pancreatitis, when patients have a history of alcohol abuse or chronic pancreatitis; this presumably occurs because of loss of pancreatic acini and impaired amylase production. Similarly, the amylase level may be normal when patients present late in the course of pancreatitis, because amylase levels tend to normalize fairly quickly unless there is ongoing pancreatic inflammation.

Serum amylase levels can also be elevated when pancreatitis is not present. Nonpancreatic intraabdominal conditions associated with elevated amylase levels include ischemic bowel, small bowel obstruction, appendicitis, and diverticulitis. Measuring the pancreatic isomer of amylase, apart from its salivary form, can maximize the specificity of amylase levels.

An elevated serum lipase level is more specific than amylase for the diagnosis of pancreatitis and can be helpful when the diagnosis is unclear. However, lipase levels are not widely available on an emergency basis, and they tend to rise later than the amylase level, so they are generally not useful for decision-making at the time of emergency-room evaluation or hospital admission.

Imaging tests, including ultrasound and computerized tomography (CT), can be useful in confirming the diagnosis of pancreatitis and clarifying if gallstones might be the cause. If severe pancreatitis with necrosis is suspected, contrast-enhanced CT is the preferred test.

TREATMENT   Whatever the etiology of an episode of acute pancreatitis, the treatment is initially the same. Ninety percent of all cases of acute pancreatitis will resolve with conservative treatment limited to hydration, pain control, and bowel rest, which should be continued until the patient's pain has resolved and the serum amylase has normalized. Nasogastric suction or drainage, though widely used in treating acute pancreatitis, is not always necessary in mild cases in which patients do not develop gastric distention.

If the patient has gallstones, a cholecystectomy should be performed as soon as the acute pancreatitis has resolved. Patients who have had a single episode of gallstone pancreatitis who are discharged without having had their gallbladder removed are at a 40% risk of having another episode of pancreatitis within the ensuing 6 months.

Severe Pancreatitis   Acute pancreatitis does not always resolve with conservative treatment. Some patients will develop signs of infection, along with pulmonary, circulatory, and/or renal compromise. These patients usually have developed some degree of peripancreatic infection, pancreatic necrosis, or both (Fig. 5-7). In the United States, necrosis occurs in 20% to 30% percent of patients with pancreatitis, and about one-quarter of these patients die. Poor outcomes of patients with pancreatic necrosis are highly correlated with development of infection; in fact, infected, acute, pancreatic necrosis is almost always fatal without treatment. Antibiotic therapy, usually with imipenem-cilastin, can reduce the death rate substantially.

Scoring systems designed to predict prognosis, based on parameters measured on admission to the hospital and characteristics that develop within 48 hours after admission, can help identify patients likely to develop severe disease with necrosis. The Ranson criteria (Table 5-3) are used

Figure 5-7

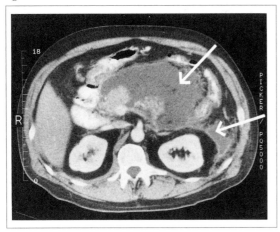

Pancreatic necrosis. A necrotic pancreas with peripancreatic fluid collections (arrows) is seen on CT scan.

most often; the presence of three of more of Ranson's criteria predicts severe disease.

Patients with severe pancreatitis who have gallstones benefit from emergency endoscopic retrograde cholangiopancreatography (ERCP) to ensure adequate biliary drainage. Patients at high risk for severe pancreatitis should undergo early CT imaging to identify necrosis and early transfer to centers with the required surgical expertise to manage such patients. The efficacy of prophylactic or routine antibiotics in improving survival for patients with severe pancreatitis has not been clearly demonstrated, but patients with documented or suspected infections should receive appropriate antibiotic therapy.

Right Lower Quadrant Pain

Appendicitis and appendiceal abscesses are the diagnoses that most readily come to mind when evaluating patients with right lower quadrant abdominal pain. Other diagnoses to consider are those involving the female genital tract, the urinary tract, and gastrointestinal system.

APPENDICITIS

HISTORY AND PHYSICAL EXAMINATION Classically, appendicitis first presents as periumbilical pain, since irritation of the visceral peritoneum of the appendix is referred to this area. Over the ensuing 12 to 24 hours, the pain localizes to the right lower quadrant, as the parietal peritoneum overlying the appendix becomes involved in the inflammatory process.

The patient is usually anorexic and may be nauseous, but repeated emesis is not usually a component of the history. There may be irregularity of bowel movements, but significant diarrhea is more suggestive of gastroenteritis than appendicitis. Since patients with acute appendicitis almost all require care within 48 to 72 hours of the onset of symptoms, pain that has been present for more than a week is unlikely to be caused by simple appendicitis.

On physical examination, the patient may have a low-grade fever or no fever at all. When present, rebound tenderness and rigidity in the right lower quadrant are highly suggestive of appen-

Table 5-3

Ranson's Criteria for Assessing Prognosis of Acute Pancreatitis

Criteria present on admission
Age >55 years
WBC >16,000/cu mm
Serum glucose ≥200 mg %
LDH >700 IU %
AST > 250 Sigma Frankel Units %
Criteria developing within 48 hours
BUN rise >5 mg %
PaO_2 <60
Serum calcium <8.0 mg %
Hct fall >10%
Base deficit >4 mmol
Fluid sequestration >6 liters

SCORING: 0–3 criteria present: 3% mortality rate. 3 or more criteria present: 62% mortality rate.
SOURCE: Data from Ranson JH, Rifkind KM, Turner JW: Prognostic signs and nonoperative peritoneal lavage in acute pancreatitis. *Surg Gynecol Obstet* 143:209–219, 1976.

dicitis. However, these signs may be absent when the appendix lies in the pelvis or posterior to the cecum. As a result, various maneuvers have been designed to elicit appendiceal tenderness in these situations. For example, a retrocecal appendix usually lies in close proximity to the psoas muscle, which runs from the transverse processes of the lumbar spine to the femur and acts as a hip flexor. Therefore, extending the hip tends to stretch the psoas muscle and will cause pain if there is inflammation in proximity to the muscle. To maximize stretching of the psoas muscle, the patient is rolled into the left lateral decubitus position and the hip is extended posterior the plane of the patient's body.

Similarly, a pelvic appendix will tend to lie on the obturator muscle, which acts to externally rotate the hip. Bending the hip and knee at 90 degrees and pushing the thigh medially internally rotates the right hip, this will stretch the obturator and cause an increase in pain if there is nearby inflammation.

In cases of a pelvic appendix, physical signs may be difficult to detect. Tenderness can sometimes be elicited along the right lateral aspect of the rectal vault on digital exam.

A number of European studies have measured the ability of various clinical parameters to predict the presence of appendicitis, providing some insight into the relative significance of various findings (Table 5-4). Unfortunately, no set of signs, symptoms, or diagnostic tests is 100% predictive of the presence or absence of appendicitis.

ANCILLARY TESTS Laboratory evaluation will usually demonstrate either a high-normal or mildly elevated white blood cell count. Plain x-rays of the abdomen will on occasion demonstrate a fecalith, representing a calcified nodule of stool within the lumen of the appendix. Its size, location, and singularity will usually distinguish it from ureteral stones, gallstones, and phleboliths, respectively. In a patient with right lower quadrant pain, the presence of a fecalith generally justifies an operation for appendicitis, so its presence in an ambiguous case can be extremely helpful.

Table 5-4

Scoring System Derived from 830 Patients with Suspected Appendicitis

CLINICAL PARAMETER		SCORE
Gender	Male	8
	Female	−8
White blood cell count	<8.9	−15
($\times 10^9$/L)	9–13.9	2
	>14	10
Duration of pain (hours)	<24	3
	24–48	0
	>48	−12
Progression (worsening) of pain	Yes	3
	No	−4
Migration of pain from umbilicus		
to right lower quadrant	Yes	7
	No	−9
Vomiting	Yes	7
	No	−5
Pain aggravated by coughing	Yes	4
	No	−11
Rebound tenderness	Yes	5
	No	−10
Rigidity	Yes	15
	No	−4
Tenderness outside right		
lower quadrant	Yes	−6
	No	4

SCORING: A total score of −2 or greater correlates with a more than 45% chance of having appendicitis. A score of less than −17 correlates with a less than 16% chance of having appendicitis. Values between −17 and −2 correlate with intermediate probabilities that appendicitis is present.
SOURCE: Reproduced with permission from Fenyo G, Lindberg G, Blind P: Diagnostic decision support in suspected acute appendicitis: Validation of a simplified scoring system. *Eur J Surg* 163:831, 1997.

Other findings on plain x-rays are equally important, but often more subtle. In a normal film, the change in density between the psoas muscle and the fat that abuts its lateral aspect produces bilaterally symmetric diagonal lines, referred to as the psoas shadow. Loss of the psoas shadow on the right implies an increase in the density of the surrounding fat, possibly caused by inflammation from appendicitis.

In toddlers and children with appendicitis, the right lower quadrant pain can produce a temporary scoliosis as the patient attempts to splint the source of the pain. The radiographic finding of scoliosis can, therefore, be useful when evaluating young patients who are unable to either express themselves or to clearly locate the source of their pain.

Great promise surrounds the increasing use of helical CT scanning in the diagnosis of acute appendicitis. This imaging technique has the potential to accurately visualize an inflamed appendix, but its role in general clinical practice requires further investigation.

TREATMENT Since the morbidity of a negative appendectomy is small compared with that of a ruptured appendix, most surgeons err on the side of surgery when dealing with patients who are suspected of having appendicitis. In fact, a "negative" laparotomy rate (i.e., laparotomy performed for appendicitis when appendicitis is not present) of 15% is generally considered acceptable and even desirable in centers that see a reasonable volume of appendicitis. When the diagnosis is less than certain, laparoscopic exploration of the abdomen prior to laparotomy is a reasonable alternative before proceeding with what is expected to be a negative laparotomy.

Appendectomy is performed as soon as possible after diagnosis, to minimize the risk of perforation and the attendant morbidity that accompanies this event. The transverse appendectomy incision is generally centered on McBurney's point, located two-thirds of the way along a line beginning at the umbilicus and terminating at the iliac crest. The appendix is generally removed whether it is normal or diseased. If it is normal, the ovaries, the cecum, and the distal two feet of the ileum are examined to rule out other potential causes of the patient's pain. Obvious abnormalities such as pus or fluid of unclear origin may require a new incision or lengthening of the original incision to investigate and treat the source of the abnormality.

APPENDICEAL ABSCESS

Patients suffering from an appendiceal abscess present and are managed differently than those with simple appendicitis. Patients who have an abscess will generally complain of a longer duration of symptoms than in acute appendicitis, are more likely to have a substantially elevated temperature and white blood cell count, and may on examination demonstrate a mass in the right lower quadrant. Tenderness often precludes vigorous examination of the right lower quadrant, so the absence of a discernible mass by no means rules out an abscess.

If an abscess is suspected, a CT scan of the abdomen is a highly effective diagnostic procedure. CT-guided percutaneous drainage of the abscess can be performed as a therapeutic maneuver (Fig. 5-8).

If there are phlegmonous changes suggestive of an old perforation without discrete abscess formation, the patient's pain and fever will usually respond to parenteral antibiotics. An appendectomy can then be performed under elective conditions 6 to 8 weeks later, once the acute inflammation has subsided. This delayed or "interval" appendectomy is generally considered safer

Figure 5-8

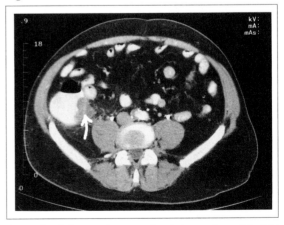

Appendiceal abscess. An appendiceal abscess (arrow) is seen on CT scan. The abscess was drained percutaneously, and an interval appendectomy was performed 6 weeks later.

than one undertaken acutely on tissue obscured by pus and weakened by inflammation.

OTHER CAUSES OF RIGHT LOWER QUADRANT PAIN

Not all right lower quadrant pain represents appendicitis or an appendiceal abscess. In some cases, appendicitis is suspected, but no appendicitis is found at laparotomy. The most frequent diagnostic outcome in such cases is that no specific diagnosis is made (Table 5-5).

In some situations, incorrectly diagnosing another condition as appendicitis is of little consequence, because the alternate condition may also require laparotomy for treatment. Examples of such diagnoses are an acutely inflamed Maeckel's diverticulum or an acutely perforated cecal cancer, both of which can be clinically indistinguishable from appendicitis and both of which require surgery. When performing a laparotomy in such cases, the surgeon may face a more extensive operation than originally planned or may need to extend or change the incision during the course of the operation, but neither of these represents inappropriate outcomes for patients.

Many conditions, however, do require an accurate diagnosis. For example, it is inappropriate to perform a laparotomy on a patient with a readily diagnosed urinary tract infection or a nonsurgical condition of the female reproductive system. In fact, many of the well-defined diseases that lead to unnecessary surgery for an appendectomy involve the ovary (Table 5-5). Conversely, failure to perform surgery can be life threatening in a patient who has a ruptured ectopic pregnancy.

Thus, a variety of other conditions must be considered in patients who have right lower quadrant pain. The most common are ovarian cysts, pelvic inflammatory disease, ovarian torsion, urinary tract disorders, and several gastrointestinal problems other than appendicitis.

CORPUS LUTEUM CYST   The corpus luteum forms from an ovarian follicle following ovulation, and a limited amount of bleeding into the corpus luteum occurs physiologically 3 to 4 days follow-

ing ovulation. Excessive bleeding results in a hemorrhagic corpus luteal cyst, which can lead to the gradual onset of lower abdominal pain. Ultimately, cyst rupture can release blood into the peritoneal cavity and cause the abrupt onset of pain. Cyst rupture is sometimes associated with intercourse or delayed menstruation and can also complicate pregnancy. Because corpus luteum cysts develop following ovulation, they generally do not occur in the first 2 weeks of the menstrual period and should not occur in women using oral contraceptives

Fever and leukocytosis will generally be absent in this disorder, but can be observed in a small percentage of patients. Blood in the peritoneal cavity can result in rebound tenderness, leading to frequent confusion of this disorder with appendicitis. Pelvic examination may reveal an enlarged tender adnexa, especially if the luteal cyst has not ruptured.

Women in whom the diagnosis is suspected can undergo an pelvic ultrasound, which will reveal either an ovarian cyst with complex internal echoes suggestive of blood, or, if the cyst has ruptured, fluid in the cul-de-sac between the uterus and rectum. The presence of blood in the cul-de-sac either on ultrasound or by aspiration (culdocentesis) is also consistent with intraperitoneal bleeding and rules out appendicitis as a cause for the patient's pain.

Life-threatening hemorrhage does occur from corpus luteum cysts and sometimes requires surgery. Usually, however, the bleeding is self-limited, and no treatment is necessary for most patients with a corpus luteum cyst.

PELVIC INFLAMMATORY DISEASE   Pelvic inflammatory disease (PID) is the term used to describe any suppurative inflammation of the ovaries and fallopian tubes. The infection is generally caused by gonorrhea, *Chlamydia*, or gram-negative or anaerobic bacteria and frequently is polymicrobial. Many patients have a history of prior PID, and this can be helpful in making the diagnosis.

Patients with severe disease will describe lower abdominal pain and on examination can demon-

Table 5-5

Diagnoses of Patients Operated for Appendicitis Whose Appendix Was Normal

DIAGNOSIS	THE HONG KONG EXPERIENCE		THE SWEDISH EXPERIENCE	
	NUMBER	(PERCENT)	NUMBER	(PERCENT)
No diagnosis or diagnosis unclear	64	(60)	33	(39.8)
Gastrointestinal disorders				
Small or large bowel				
Colitis, ischemic	2	(0.9)		
Colitis, unspecified			2	(2.4)
Diverticulitis	1	(0.9)	2	(2.4)
Inflammatory bowel disease			3	(1.6)
Meckel's diverticulum	3	(2.8)		
Perforated cecum by foreign body	1	(0.9)		
Periappendicitis			1	(1.2)
Small bowel obstruction			2	(2.4)
Hepatobiliary or pancreatic				
Cholecystitis	1	(0.9)	1	(1.2)
Gallbladder torsion	1	(0.9)		
Gallstones	3	(2.8)		
Pancreatitis	1	(0.9)	2	(2.4)
Other				
Mesenteric lymphadenitis	9	(8.4)	28	(33.7)
Torsion of the omentum	1	(0.9)	1	(1.2)
Gynecologic disorders				
Ectopic pregnancy	1	(0.9)		
Endometriosis	1	(0.9)		
Ovarian cysts	5	(4.7)	6	(7.2)
Ovarian teratoma	1	(0.9)		
Ovarian torsion	2	(1.9)		
Pelvic inflammatory disease	2	(1.9)	2	(2.4)
Infectious disorders				
Infectious mononucleosis	1	(0.9)		
Samonella enteritis	3	(2.8)		
Tuberculous ileitis	1	(0.9)		
Urinary tract infection	1	(0.9)		
Yersinia pseudotuberculosis	1	(0.9)		
Malignant neoplasms				
Appendix, adenocarcinoma	1	(0.9)		
Duodenum, leiomyosarcoma	1	(0.9)		
Liver, metastatic adenocarcinoma			1	(1.2)

SOURCE: Data used with permission from Lau W, Fan S, Yiu, T, et al: Negative findings at appendectomy. *Am J Surg* 148:375, 1984 and Fenyo G, Lindberg G, Blind P: Diagnostic decision support in suspected acute appendicitis: validation of a simplified scoring system. *Eur J Surg* 163:831, 1997.

strate both an elevated temperature and rebound tenderness. Pus in the cervical os and adnexal or cervical motion tenderness can serve to distinguish this disease from appendicitis. Similarly, a wet mount of vaginal secretions that demonstrates a significant number of leukocytes can serve the same function. However, leukocytes are also seen in vaginal secretions of patients who have cervicitis and/or vaginitis, and therefore the presence of leukocytes cannot be relied on as a definitive diagnostic criteria for PID. While positive endocervical cultures for chlamydia or gonorrhea are highly suggestive of a diagnosis of PID and should be obtained in patients suspected of having the condition, culture results are not available during the initial evaluation.

Treatment of PID involves antibiotic therapy, either in or out of the hospital depending on the severity of illness and the patient's reproductive history (more aggressive therapy is often recommended for nulliparous women to diminish the likelihood that PID will lead to scarring of the fallopian tubes with subsequent infertility). Nonetheless, even severe cases of PID associated with adnexal abscess formation can usually be successfully treated with antibiotics alone, obviating the need for surgery.

ECTOPIC PREGNANCY Ectopic pregnancy describes an early embryo that implants not in the uterus, but in the ovary, fallopian tube, or an adjacent intraperitoneal organ or surface. Ectopic pregnancies are prone to rupture, resulting in potentially life-threatening hemorrhage, and are associated with a surgical urgency even greater than that of appendicitis. The patient will describe having missed one or several periods as would occur in a normal pregnancy. A history of tubal ligation, prior episodes of pelvic inflammatory disease, and the use of an intrauterine device are all risk factors for an ectopic pregnancy. Pelvic examination may reveal an enlarged adnexa and an enlarged uterus.

Ectopic pregnancy merits consideration in any women with abdominal pain and a positive urine pregnancy test for the beta subunit of human chorionic gonadotropin (beta-HCG). If the beta-HCG test is positive in a patient with lower abdominal pain, ectopic pregnancy must be ruled out by the visualization of an intrauterine gestational sac by endovaginal ultrasound. Failure to visualize the sac is suggestive either of an ectopic pregnancy or a normal pregnancy that is too early to be seen ultrasonographically. Since an intrauterine sac can be reliably detected when the quantitative beta-HCG level is 1500 mIU/mL, a measurement above this level in a patient with no intrauterine gestational sac is diagnostic of an ectopic pregnancy. The diagnostic evaluation in patients in whom the beta-HCG is less than 1500 requires serial beta-HCG measurements as an outpatient, followed by ultrasonography when the level reaches 1500.

Treatment of ruptured ectopic pregnancy with hemorrhage usually requires an open surgical procedure. If ectopic pregnancy is diagnosed prior to rupture, therapeutic options include medical therapy with methotrexate (which causes death and involution of the developing conceptus), fallopian tube–sparing open or laparoscopic procedures, or laparoscopic or open salpingectomy.

OVARIAN TORSION Ovarian torsion can occur in women of any age and refers to a twisting of the adnexa, resulting in compromise of the blood supply to the ovary. The usual symptoms of torsion are lower abdominal pain, fever, nausea, and vomiting, resulting in frequent confusion with appendicitis. This confusion is especially likely in children, in whom ovarian disorders are not usually considered and in whom appendicitis is common. Torsion is more frequently observed in women with ovarian tumors and in those who have had torsion in the past.

The diagnosis is usually based on pelvic ultrasonography, which demonstrates a complex cystic or solid adnexal mass. Doppler ultrasonography may show an absence or diminution of ovarian blood flow. Confusing ovarian torsion with appendicitis is far from catastrophic, since immediate surgery is needed both for patients with appendicitis and for those with torsion to acheive either detorsion or ovarian resection. A greater concern is that a delay in the diagnosis or the failure to expeditiously operate on a patient misdiagnosed with appendicitis will result in infarction and the loss of a previously viable ovary.

URINARY TRACT DISEASE   The urinary tract is another potential source of confusion in evaluating right lower quadrant pain. In clinical practice, however, urinary tract disease is rarely misdiagnosed as appendicitis. The two most important urinary tract disorders that cause right lower quadrant pain are urinary infection and urolithiasis.

Urinary Tract Infection   A bladder infection will usually cause suprapubic pain, as well as frequent painful micturition of a small volume of often foul-smelling urine. Bladder infections are more common in women than men and are especially frequent in women with diabetes or who are sexually active. The diagnosis is usually made by history or by detecting bacteria and white blood cells in the urine.

Urolithiasis   A kidney stone causing irritation or obstruction of the ureter will on occasion present as right lower quadrant abdominal pain. These patients are usually men, and they may give a history of recent dehydration or prior kidney stones.

Usually the pain, referred to as "renal colic," will arise more in the back than the abdomen and can radiate into the testicle. Unlike a patient with peritonitis who prefers to lie still, a patient with ureteral colic tends to move around, searching in vain for a comfortable position. The pain is excruciating and exceeds even the severe pain associated with appendicitis. Because the history is so distinct, it is unusual for renal colic to be confused with appendicitis

Blood in the urine further increases the likelihood of renal colic, and the culprit stone (usually calcium oxalate) can be seen on the plain abdominal x-rays in the majority of cases. If urolithiasis is suspected, but no stone is seen on plain x-rays,

imaging with ultrasound, or intravenous pyelography, or non-contrast computerized tomography may reveal the diagnosis by demonstrating the stone or by showing dilation or obstruction of the urinary collection system.

GASTROINTESTINAL DISEASE   Several gastrointestinal diseases can be confused with appendicitis. The most common of these are mesenteric lymphadenitis, acute gastroenteritis, and Crohn's disease.

Mesenteric Lymphadenitis   Mesenteric lymphadenitis is the most commonly described diagnosis discovered during the course of a negative appendectomy. While the diagnosis in and of itself is devoid of clinical significance, the presence of enlarged lymph nodes in the ileal mesentery implies the presence of ileal inflammation, which can be difficult to distinguish from appendicitis.

Ileal inflammation (acute ileitis) resulting from bacterial infection is most often associated with either mycobacteria or *Yersinia enterocolitica*. The latter is a common pathogen in Europe, but is limited to localized outbreaks in the United States and is often confused with appendicitis when such an outbreak occurs. Though the diagnosis can be made by serologic studies or by stool culture, the results of these tests are not available during the initial evaluation of patients with abdominal pain. The diagnosis rests, therefore, on epidemiologic recognition of a *Yersinia* outbreak and the liberal use of imaging and endoscopic diagnostic studies to exclude other diagnoses.

Viral Gastroenteritis   In primary-care practice, acute viral gastroenteritis is a more common cause of right lower quadrant discomfort than any of the other diagnoses discussed in this chapter. In most patients who undergo a negative appendectomy, no diagnosis is ever established to explain their pain, and many of these patients probably had viral gastroenteritis. A prominence of vomiting or diarrhea in the patient's history may suggest this diagnosis, as might the presence of other symptoms of viral illness such as rhinorrhea, headaches, myalgias, or arthralgias.

Crohn's Disease Crohn's disease, which causes ileal and segmental colonic inflammation, can be difficult to distinguish from appendicitis. Patients with Crohn's disease may describe a family history of inflammatory bowel disease and, in comparison with patients with acute appendicitis, usually have less severe and more chronic pain, usually accompanied by symptoms of weight loss and diarrhea. The physical examination and laboratory evaluation can be similar to appendicitis, in that any abnormalities in temperature and the white blood cell count are usually not particularly dramatic.

Because medical management of Crohn's disease is often successful, every effort should be made to avoid acute surgical interventions by distinguishing these patients from those with appendicitis—a task that will usually entail some combination of an abdominal CT scan, a small bowel follow-through, or endoscopy. Even in cases in which Crohn's disease has led to local perforation and abscess formation, many surgeons prefer percutaneous drainage followed by elective surgery, so that the extent of small bowel resection can be minimized.

Left Lower Quadrant Pain

DIVERTICULITIS

In many ways, the differential diagnosis of left lower quadrant pain parallels that of the right lower quadrant, with the additional need to consider diverticulitis of the sigmoid colon as a diagnostic possibility. Because it is so common, the diagnosis of diverticulitis is often made on the basis of the history and physical examination alone.

The inflammatory process in diverticulitis can be limited to the sigmoid colon; can rupture through the colonic wall, resulting in an abscess that is contained in a retroperitoneal location; or can rupture through the colonic wall into the abdominal cavity causing diffuse peritonitis.

DIAGNOSIS Patients with diverticulitis are usually (but not always) over 40 years of age. Findings on history and physical examination consist of left lower quadrant pain and tenderness associated with nonspecific gastrointestinal complaints such as constipation, diarrhea, nausea, and vomiting. In some cases, the diagnosis is not clear from the history and physical. Under such circumstances, a CT scan of the abdomen can delineate the presence and severity of diverticulitis.

TREATMENT Both medical and surgical modalities can be used to treat patients who have diverticulitis. Depending on severity, medical treatments can be administered in or out of the hospital.

Medical Treatment Patients with either a fever or an elevated white blood cell count should be admitted to a hospital and treated with intravenous antibiotics, chosen to eradicate both gram-negative rods and anaerobic organisms. Patients without fever and leukocytosis can be managed on an outpatient basis with oral antibiotics that have a similar spectrum of antimicrobial activity.

Patients who do not respond to intravenous antibiotics require a CT scan to determine if they have a diverticular phlegmon, an abscess, or a diagnosis other than diverticulitis. A phlegmon represents a collection of inflammatory tissue that will ultimately respond to antibiotics, though often in a delayed fashion. Abscesses require surgical or interventional radiologic treatments, as described below.

Surgical Treatment Patients who experience recurrent episodes of diverticulitis requiring admission to the hospital generally are treated with elective sigmoid resection. In such cases, objective documentation of diverticular disease is desirable, as the simple presence of diverticuli does not prove that diverticular inflammation (i.e., diverticulitis) is present. CT evidence of diverticulitis that has reasonable sensitivity and specificity include thickening of the wall of the sigmoid colon or stranding of mesenteric and retroperitoneal fat near the sigmoid colon (Fig. 5-9).

Surgical treatments are also appropriate for patients who have a diverticular abscess. The first-choice treatment is percutaneous CT-guided

Figure 5-9

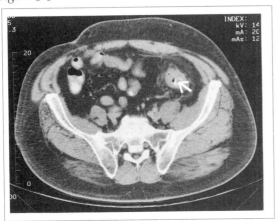

Sigmoid diverticulitis. The CT findings of sigmoid diverticulitis are seen in the thickening of the wall of the bowel (arrow) and in the presence of streaking in the surrounding fat.

drainage. Percutaneous drainage permits delaying sigmoid resection until the surgical field is no longer infected, at which time the affected segment of colon can be removed and primary anastomosis safely performed. If sigmoid colon resection must be performed in the presence of an active abscess, however, most surgeons would resect the abnormal segment of colon and then perform a temporary colostomy. Similarly, if the abscess cannot be drained percutaneously, or if the patient does not respond to antibiotics and percutaneous drainage, then surgery with resection and colostomy is necessary.

On occasion, a perforated diverticula can rupture freely into the peritoneal cavity without abscess formation, resulting in peritonitis. These patients will present with some combination of rigidity, rebound tenderness on examination, or free air visible on plain upright abdominal x-rays, in which case the need to identify and repair the colonic perforation requires emergency surgery.

Diffuse Abdominal Pain

Several surgical conditions result in diffuse, nonlocalized abdominal pain. The most common and

important of these are small bowel obstruction, small bowel ischemia, large bowel obstruction, and colitis.

SMALL BOWEL OBSTRUCTION

Small bowel obstruction is a common cause of abdominal pain that generally can be diagnosed at the time of the patient's initial evaluation. The two leading causes of small bowel obstruction in the United States are adhesions from prior surgery and incarceration of an inguinal or abdominal wall hernia.

HISTORY AND PHYSICAL EXAMINATION   Patients typically report colicky pain, manifest as periods of excruciating cramping pain followed by periods of relative or complete relief. Episodes of vomiting produce a large amount of occasionally foul-smelling vomitus and are often associated with transient relief of pain. In contrast, attempts to eat often lead to an exacerbation of the pain. The patient will usually report an absence of bowel movements, but may also complain of diarrhea in the early stages of obstruction.

On physical examination, the abdomen is generally distended and diffusely tender. Special attention should be paid to surgical scars on the abdomen, as these might indicate the presence of bowel obstruction resulting from adhesions and to sites of potential herniation such as the umbilicus and groin.

ANCILLARY TESTS   Plain abdominal films are usually diagnostic or at least suggestive of obstruction. They show dilated loops of small bowel lying proximal to the obstruction, with an absence or paucity of air and stool in the colon, which by definition lies distal to the obstruction (Fig. 5-10). A distinction is sometimes made between patients with no colon contents (complete obstruction) and those with a small amount of recognizable colon air or stool (incomplete obstruction), though the clinical significance of this distinction is not clear. Air-fluid levels are often present, but are not a specific finding of obstruction. In patients in whom the diagnosis is unclear, either an abdominal CT scan or an upper gastrointestinal contrast study can usually confirm or refute the presence of small bowel obstruction.

TREATMENT   Patients with small bowel obstruction die either from hypovolemia, resulting from extravasation of the intravascular volume into the small bowel, or from perforation, which occurs when distended and twisted loops of small bowel undergo ischemic necrosis.

Hypovolemia is prevented by intravenous rehydration and correction of electrolyte abnormalities. Surgical relief of the obstruction within 12 to 24 hours of admission can prevent necrosis and perforation. An attempt at nonoperative management of small bowel obstruction using naso-

Figure 5-10

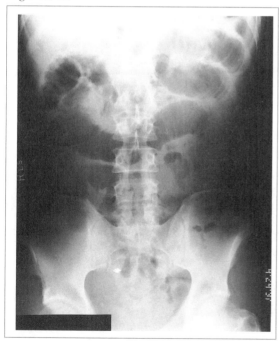

Small bowel obstruction. Plain abdominal x-ray shows the absence of large bowel contents and the presence of dilated loops of small bowel, which together are suggestive of small bowel obstruction.

gastric suction is appropriate in adhesion-related small bowel obstruction in which signs of ischemia, including constant (noncolicky) pain, fever, tachycardia, leukocytosis, and acidosis, are absent. The risk of nonoperative management is failure to diagnose bowel ischemia, and the decision to withhold surgery should always be made in consultation with a surgeon.

ISCHEMIA OF THE SMALL BOWEL

Primary ischemia of the small bowel describes four diseases (Table 5-6). Regardless of the etiology, however, small bowel ischemia is extremely difficult to diagnose because of its nonspecific clinical features.

The pain is usually severe and diffuse and is classically described as being disproportionately great when compared with the findings of physical examination. Abdominal examination reveals diffuse tenderness, but peritoneal signs of rigidity and rebound tenderness are often not present. An important clue to the diagnosis, however, is that, unlike most diseases that cause acute surgical abdominal pain, small bowel ischemia is frequently associated with melena or hematochezia.

Leukocytosis is generally present, but is a nonspecific finding. Acidosis is helpful, but is typically absent early in the course of the disease when it is most treatable.

The test required to make a definitive diagnosis is a visceral angiogram. In addition to diagnosing ischemic bowel disease, angiography is also useful for planning the correct surgical treatment. However, angiography is expensive, not readily available in all hospitals, and not helpful in making any other diagnoses besides that of ischemic bowel. In addition, angiographers are often unwilling to perform angiography in the absence of compelling evidence for ischemic disease, which is difficult to obtain until late in the course of the disease, when outcomes of treatment are poor.

An alternative to angiography is abdominal ultrasonography with Doppler examination of the superior mesenteric artery. This test is especially

Table 5-6

Four Forms of Acute Primary Ischemia of the Small Bowel

| | | FORM OF ISCHEMIA | | |
	ARTERIAL THROMBOSIS	ARTERIAL EMBOLISM	NONOCCLUSIVE MESENTERIC ISCHEMIA	MESENTERIC VEIN THROMBOSIS
Site	Usually SMA, in patient with stenosis or obstruction of celiac artery and IMA	SMA or branch thereof	Spasm of mesenteric arterial circulation, generalized or localized	In situ thrombosis of superior mesenteric vein
Risk factors	Chronic mesenteric ischemia; systemic atherosclerotic disease	Arrhythmias; congestive heart failure; past or concurrent embolism	Critically ill inpatient; norepinephrine; digoxin	Hypercoagulable state; congestive heart failure
Angiographic findings	Occluded SMA, with occlusion or severe stenosis of celiac artery and IMA	Occluded SMA, close to middle colic artery, or occlusion of SMA branch	Abnormal tapering and beading; narrowing of branch origins; slow vessel opacification	Failure to visualize SMV in venous phase of angiogram
Treatment	Resection of bowel; bypass of obstruction	Resection of bowel; operative embolectomy	Bowel resection; intraarterial papaverine	Resection of bowel; anticoagulation; thrombectomy (?)

Abbreviations: SMA, superior mesenteric artery; SMV, superior mesenteric vein; IMA, inferior mesenteric artery.

useful when the indications for angiography are unclear. Unfortunately, Doppler ultrasound is also not available in all hospitals.

If neither angiography nor Doppler ultrasound are readily available, timely exploration by an experienced surgeon is the next best option. The most likely etiology for small bowel ischemia can be determined during surgery based on the distribution of diseased bowel, and appropriate therapeutic interventions can then be undertaken (Table 5-6).

LARGE BOWEL OBSTRUCTION

Patients with large bowel obstruction may complain of diffuse abdominal pain, but they are equally likely to complain of abdominal distention or a failure to move their bowels. Except for massive distention and tympany on percussion, and the possibility of feeling an obstructing tumor on rectal exam, the physical findings of large bowel obstruction are nonspecific.

Plain x-rays of the abdomen, however, are usually extremely helpful. Dilation of the colon proximally to the site of obstruction is usually obvious and can be massive, especially in the cecum. In instances in which sigmoid volvulus is the cause of the obstruction, the plain films can be diagnostic (Fig. 5-11). When the diagnosis of large bowel obstruction is suspected but cannot be confirmed on plain x-rays, an enema with water-soluble contrast media is an easy and safe way to confirm or exclude the diagnosis (Fig 5-12).

Large bowel obstruction almost always requires surgery. The urgency with which surgery must be performed is usually based on the etiology and severity of the obstruction and the association of obstruction with signs of bowel ischemia such as a fever, leukocytosis, and acidosis.

ACUTE COLITIS

A history of bloody or profuse diarrhea and abdominal pain is highly suggestive of some form of acute colitis. The differential diagnosis is fairly

Figure 5-11

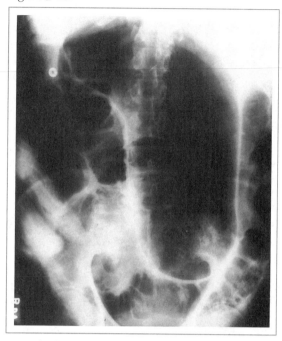

Sigmoid volvulus. The diagnosis of sigmoid volvulus is often apparent from the plain abdominal films in which a large "omega-loop" is present.

limited (infectious colitis, ulcerative colitis, neutropenic colitis), and the history can be extremely helpful.

One of the most common causes of infectious colitis, *Clostridium difficile*, is typically preceded by a course of antibiotics for an unrelated problem. Other infectious causes of colitis may occur in the setting of outbreaks such as shigella, salmonella, and *E. coli*, while others, like amebiasis, occur sporadically. An individual or familial history of inflammatory bowel disease is helpful and suggests ulcerative colitis, while a history of recent immunosuppressive therapy is suggestive of neutropenic colitis.

On physical examination, the patient is usually diffusely tender and distended and may be mildly febrile and have a leukocytosis. Plain x-rays of the abdomen show a distended colon and can also

Figure 5-12

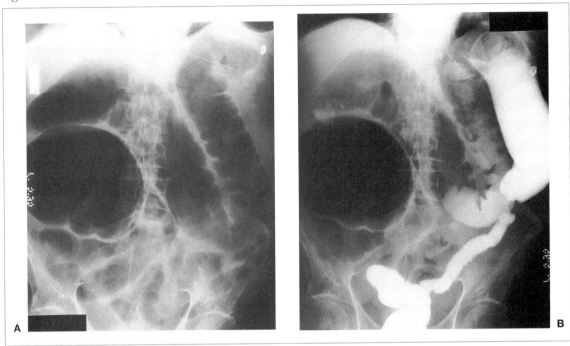

Large bowel obstruction. This patient's plain abdominal films **(A)**, were suggestive of a sigmoid obstruction with dilated colon proximal to the obstruction. The diagnosis was confirmed by a gastrografin (water-soluble contrast) enema **(B)**, which demonstrates an obstructing "apple-core" lesion.

demonstrate mucosal edema, often referred to as "thumbprinting" (Fig. 5-13). Definitive diagnosis usually is made by a combination of history, radiographs, stool cultures, toxin assays, and a gentle flexible sigmoidoscopic examination. Stool cultures can identify infecting microorganisms, and *C. difficile* toxin assay can be used to diagnose antibiotic-associated colitis. Flexible sigmoidoscopy can visually demonstrate findings specific for ulcerative colitis and ischemic colitis and can permit biopsy or culture specimens to be obtained when appropriate.

Management of colitis is usually supportive, involving management of fluid and electrolytes, plus specific pharmacologic therapy for infections or ulcerative colitis. Appropriate medical management will usually resolve the acute problem and obviate the need for surgery. However, failure of severe colitis to respond to medical management is an indication for colectomy.

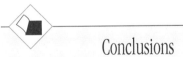

Conclusions

When evaluating patients with acute abdominal pain, clinicians should keep the following principles in mind:

- Almost half of patients with acute abdominal pain will never receive a definitive diagnosis, and in the great majority of these patients, pain

Figure 5-13

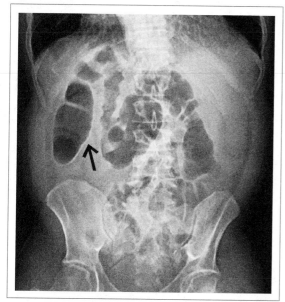

Colitis. "Thumbprinting" (arrow) is a sign of mucosal edema, which can occur in any form of colitis.

ultimately resolves without treatment. For patients in whom a diagnosis is possible, 90% will have pain caused by one of the common conditions discussed in this chapter.

- Perforation of a peptic ulcer can almost always be suspected based on the dramatic nature of the presentation and the visualization of free intraperitoneal air on plain abdominal films.

- Acute biliary disease resulting from gallstones must be categorized as biliary colic, cholecystitis, cholangitis, or pancreatitis if appropriate therapy is to be instituted.

- Diseases that commonly lead to a misdiagnosis of appendicitis are finite and well-defined and should be methodically considered in patients with right lower quadrant pain to avoid preventable diagnostic errors.

- Sigmoid diverticulitis is often diagnosed based on the history and physical examination alone. Failure of diverticulitis to respond to intravenous antibiotics should result in a CT scan

to confirm the presence of diverticulitis and to detect abscesses, perforations, and other complications.

- Generalized abdominal pain is usually caused by diffuse diseases of the large or small bowel. Primary ischemia of the small bowel is especially difficult to diagnose and requires a high index of suspicion if the diagnosis is to be made in time for effective treatment to be administered.

References

Agarwal N, Pitchumoni CS, Sivaprasad AV: Evaluating tests for acute pancreatitis. *Am J Gastroenterol* 85: 356, 1990.

Barnhart K, Mennuti MT, Benjamin I, et al: Prompt diagnosis of ectopic pregnancy in an emergency department setting. *Obstet Gynecol* 84:1010, 1994.

Baron TH, Morgan DE: Acute necrotizing pancreatitis. *N Engl J Med* 340:1412, 1999.

Bohner H, Yang Q, Franke C, et al: Simple data from history and physical examination help to exclude bowel obstruction and to avoid radiographic studies in patients with acute abdominal pain. *Eur J Surg* 164:777, 1998.

Brewer RJ, Golden GT, Hitch DC, et al: An analysis of 1000 consecutive cases in a university hospital emergency room. *Am J Surg* 131:219, 1976.

Chapman AH, McNamara M, Porter G: The acute contrast enema in suspected large bowel obstruction: value and technique. *Clin Radiol* 46:273, 1992.

Crofts TJ, Park KGM, Steele RJC, et al: A randomized trial of nonoperative treatment for perforated peptic ulcer. *N Engl J Med* 320:970, 1989.

Dause EM, Van Beers BE, Goffette P, et al: Acute intestinal ischemia due to occlusion of the superior mesenteric artery detected with Doppler sonography. *J Ultrasound Med* 15:323, 1996.

de Beaux AC, Palmer KR, Carter DC: Factors influencing morbidity and mortality in acute pancreatitis: an analysis of 279 cases. *Gut* 37:121, 1995.

de Dombal FT: Acute abdominal pain—an O.M.G.E. survey. *Scand J Gastroenterol* 14:29, 1979.

Dickson AP, Imrie CW: The incidence and prognosis of body wall ecchymosis in acute pancreatitis. *Surg Gynecol Obstet* 159:343, 1984.

Fenster LF, Lonborg R, Thirlby RC, et al: What symptoms does cholecystectomy cure? Insights from an outcomes measurement project and review of the literature. *Am J Surg* 169:533, 1995.

Fenyo G, Lindberg G, Blind P: Diagnostic decision support in suspected acute appendicitis: validation of a simplified scoring system. *Eur J Surg* 163:831, 1997.

Hallatt JG, Steele CH, Snyder M: Ruptured corpus luteum with hemoperitoneum: a study of 173 surgical cases. *Am J Obstet Gynecol* 149:5, 1984.

Hammarstrom LE, Holmin T, Stridbeck H, et al: Long-term follow-up of a prospective randomized study of endoscopic versus surgical treatment of bile duct calculi in patients with gallbladder in situ. *Br J Surg* 82:1516, 1995.

Hibbard LT: Corpus luteum surgery. *Am J Obstet Gynecol* 135:666, 1979.

Ho HS, Frey CF: The role of antibiotic prophylaxis in severe acute pancreatitis. *Arch Surg* 132:487, 1997.

Jess P, Bjerrgaard B, Brynitz S, et al: Prognosis of acute nonspecific abdominal pain. *Am J Surg* 144:338, 1982.

Lai ECS, Mok FPT, Tan ESY, et al: Endoscopic biliary drainage for severe acute cholangitis. *N Engl J Med* 24:1582, 1992.

Lau W, Fan S, Yiu T, et al: Negative findings at appendectomy. *Am J Surg* 148:375, 1984.

Lo C, Liu C, Fan S, et al: Prospective randomized study of early versus delayed laparoscopic cholecystectomy for acute cholecystitis. *Ann Surg* 227:461, 1997.

Neoptolemos JP, London NJ, James D, et al: Controlled trial of urgent ERCP and endoscopic sphincterotomy versus conservative treatment for acute pancreatitis due to gallstones. *Lancet* 8618:979, 1988.

Nitecki S, Karmeli R, Sarr MG: Appendiceal calculi and fecaliths as indications for appendectomy. *Surg Gynecol Obstet* 171:185, 1990.

Nitecki S, Assalia A, Schein M: Contemporary management of the appendiceal mass. *Br J Surg* 80:18, 1993.

Olinde AJ, Lucas JF, Miller RC: Acute yersiniosis and its surgical significance. *South Med J* 77:1539, 1984.

Pace BW, Bank S, Wise L, et al: Amylase isoenzymes in the acute abdomen: an adjunct in those patients with elevated total amylase. *Am J Gastroenterol* 80:898, 1985.

Paloyan D, Simonowitz D, Skinner DB: The timing of biliary tract operations in patients with pancreatitis associated with gallstones. *Surg Gynecol Obstet* 141:737, 1975.

Phelan MB, Valley VT, Materr JR: Pelvic ultrasonography. *Emerg Med Clin North Am* 15:789, 1997.

Pisarska MD, Carson SA, Buster JE: Ectopic pregnancy. *Lancet* 351:1115, 1998.

Ralls P, Colletti, Lapin SA: Real-time sonography in suspected acute cholecystitis. *Radiology* 155:767, 1985.

Ranson JHC, Rifkind KM, Roses DF, et al: Prognostic signs and the role of operative management in acute pancreatitis. *Surg Gynecol Obstet* 139:69, 1974.

Rao PM, Rhea JT, Novelline RA, et al: Effect of CT of the appendix on treatment of patients and use of hospital resources. *N Engl J Med* 338:141, 1998.

Shust NM, Hendricksen DK: Ovarian torsion: an unusual cause of abdominal pain in a young girl. *Am J Emerg Med* 13:307, 1995.

The Standards Task Force of the American Society of Colon and Rectal Surgeons: Practice parameters for sigmoid diverticulitis—supporting documentation. *Dis Colon Rectum* 38:126, 1995.

Westrom L: Clinical manifestations and diagnosis of pelvic inflammatory disease. *J Reprod Med* 28:703, 1983.

Matthias Stelzner

Chapter 6

Anorectal Problems

This chapter will discuss three of the most common surgical anorectal problems seen in primary-care practice: hemorrhoids, anal fissures, and anal fistulas.

Hemorrhoids

When discussing the pathogenesis of hemorrhoids, one first has to differentiate between "internal hemorrhoids" and "external hemorrhoids," which are fundamentally different in their pathophysiology and treatment.

Pathophysiology

ANATOMY

INTERNAL HEMORRHOIDS "Internal hemorrhoids" are hyperplastic formations of the corpus cavernosum recti (Fig. 6-1). The corpus cavernosum recti, formerly known as the internal hemorrhoidal plexus, is a collection of anal vascular cushions in the upper third of the anorectum. These anal cushions receive their blood supply primarily from terminal branches of the superior hemorrhoidal arteries. Venous drainage from the corpus cavernosum recti occurs through veins that traverse the internal anal sphincter musculature.

The corpus cavernosum recti resembles in its construction other cavernous bodies that are found in the genital organs of males and females. In all of these structures, the primary role of blood is not to provide oxygenation and nutrition. Rather, blood acts as a filling substance to enhance the organ's function, which, in the case of the corpus cavernosum recti, is to swell and thereby contribute to maintaining anal continence.

The finding that internal hemorrhoids are derived from arterially supplied anal cushions explains why hemorrhoidal bleeding is commonly described as "bright-red blood per rectum." This observation was never easy to reconcile with the notion that internal hemorrhoids were varicose anal veins, as was believed in the past.

Internal hemorrhoids are commonly classified by their degree (Table 6-1). In first-degree hemorrhoids, the anal cushions are enlarged and may bleed at the time of defecation. While they project

Figure 6-1

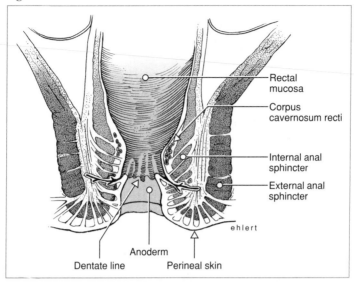

Anorectal anatomy. Note the corpus cavernosum recti, a plexus of vessels that receive blood supply from branches of the superior hemorrhoidal arteries. The vessels in the corpus cavernosum recti form "cushions" that distend with blood and contribute to the anal sphincter mechanism. Internal hemorrhoids occur in these vessels. So-called external hemorrhoids are varicose veins in the anal canal or perianal skin.

into the lumen during anoscopy, they do not prolapse to the outside of the anal canal. Second-degree hemorrhoids prolapse to the outside of the anal canal during defecation, but return spontaneously to within the anal canal after the bowel movement. Third-degree hemorrhoids prolapse with defecation, but can be manually reduced by the patient. Fourth-degree hemorrhoids are continuously prolapsed, remain at the outside of the anal canal, and are irreducible.

EXTERNAL HEMORRHOIDS   "External hemorrhoids" are dilated segments of perianal veins that arise from the inferior hemorrhoidal venous plexus below the dentate line. External hemorrhoids are covered by squamous cell epithelium of the perianal skin or the skin of the anal canal. External hemorrhoids are, therefore, varicose veins similar to those found in the lower extremities in the drainage areas of the saphenous veins. These varicose veins in the perianal area become symptomatic when they are acutely thrombosed.

ETIOLOGY

Many risk factors for the formation of hemorrhoids have been suggested. Clinicians frequently attribute hemorrhoids to constipation, and epi-

Table 6-1

Classification of Internal Hemorrhoids

DEGREE	PROTRUSION OUT OF ANUS	REDUCIBILITY BACK INTO ANUS
First	No	—
Second	During defecation	Reduce spontaneously after defecation
Third	During defecation	Require manual reduction
Fourth	Continuous	Irreducible

demiologic studies link hemorrhoids and constipation. However, the etiology of hemorrhoids is not fully understood, and the reason why hyperplasia of the corpus cavernosum recti occurs with internal hemorrhoids is uncertain.

Several abnormalities of rectal structure and function have been detected in patients with hemorrhoids. For example, it appears that filling and emptying of the corpus cavernosum recti are disturbed in hemorrhoidal disease. In addition, the anal sphincter of many patients with hemorrhoids demonstrates an abnormal and excessive rhythm of contraction. Such an overactive sphincter might contribute to venous congestion and expose the engorged anal cushions to greater sheer forces, leading to inflammation and further enlargement. Furthermore, starting in the third decade of life, the anchoring and supporting tissues holding the hemorrhoidal cushions in place in the anal canal often begin to deteriorate, and disruption of these holding structures is a prerequisite for hemorrhoidal prolapse. Further research is needed to understand the roles and relative importance of these abnormalities in hemorrhoidal disease.

Epidemiology

Symptomatic hemorrhoids are one of the most common afflictions of Western civilization. The problem can occur at any age, but is more common after the third decade of life. It is generally held that at least 50% of persons over the age of 50 years have experienced hemorrhoidal complaints at some time in their life. Johanson and Sonnenberg found in a large epidemiologic study that the point prevalence of symptomatic hemorrhoids in the United States is 4.4%. They found that whites are more commonly affected than blacks, and that a higher socioeconomic status was positively correlated with an increased frequency of hemorrhoids. The reasons for these associations are not understood.

It should be pointed out that, contrary to common opinion among clinicians, there is no evidence for an increased incidence of hemorrhoids among patients with portal hypertension. While patients with liver disease often have bleeding from existing hemorrhoids as a result of their coagulation disorder, several studies have failed to confirm that hyperplastic anal cushions are more common among individuals with portal hypertension and liver disease.

Hemorrhoids are, however, more common in persons who have certain other diseases and conditions. In addition to constipation, as mentioned above, hemorrhoids are also more common in individuals who have diseases associated with diarrhea and in those with spinal cord injuries.

Typical Presentation

The most important symptoms of hemorrhoids are bleeding, itching, rectal pain, and constipation. These symptoms can occur with both internal and external hemorrhoids.

BLEEDING

The classic and most common presenting symptom of patients with hemorrhoids is rectal bleeding. It usually occurs during or immediately following defecation. The extent of blood loss is highly variable. It can range from streaks of blood on the tissue paper to large amounts of blood in the toilet bowl. In rare cases, bleeding can be so severe that it leads to anemia or acute hypovolemia.

ITCHING

Anal itching (pruritis ani) is also frequently associated with hemorrhoids. However, it is unclear if hemorrhoids truly cause pruritus ani. In many cases the itching appears to be a concomitant problem, and, frequently, the pruritus does not resolve following hemorrhoidectomy. Patients for whom hemorrhoidectomy is being considered should be made aware that the procedure may not eliminate anal itching.

PAIN

The rectal mucosa has little innervation, and it is unusual for internal hemorrhoids to cause pain unless the hemorrhoidal plexus is incarcerated, thrombosed, or gangrenous. When present, pain originates from the anal skin, which is very richly innervated. Thus, pain from internal hemorrhoids only occurs in advanced stages of hemorrhoidal disease, when the anal skin is undermined by enlarged anal cushions. Pain occurs from external hemorrhoids when they become acutely thrombosed.

Most commonly, however, pain, particularly severe pain at the beginning of a bowel movement, is not from hemorrhoids. Rather, it should lead the clinician to consider that the patient may have an anal fissure or perirectal abscess.

CONSTIPATION

Hemorrhoids are frequently associated with constipation, and infrequent, hard bowel movements will tend to worsen hemorrhoidal symptoms. Because of these symptoms, patients tend to avoid going to the bathroom, often subconsciously, to avoid exacerbating their hemorrhoidal symptoms, resulting in even harder stools and worsening constipation. This can result in development of painful anal fissures and yet further avoidance of defecation.

Key History

When taking a history from a patient with suspected hemorrhoids, clinicians should focus on the duration of the condition and associated symptoms.

DURATION OF SYMPTOMS

Hemorrhoidal disease is usually a long-standing disorder, and the symptoms tend to come and go over time. There are frequently episodes during which bleeding and/or pain are more severe, followed by a time with fewer or no symptoms. Sudden onset of pain while passing a particularly hard bowel movement is more typically associated with an anal fissure, not with hemorrhoids.

ASSOCIATED SYMPTOMS

In addition to asking about the duration and timing of symptoms, clinicians should ask about the presence of other symptoms that may be associated with hemorrhoids. These include rectal bleeding, symptoms of prolapse, and altered bowel habits.

RECTAL BLEEDING Clinicians should ask questions to assess the extent of bleeding. In making this assessment, one must bear in mind that the amount of blood lost is often overestimated by the patient, because very small amounts of blood in the toilet can turn the toilet water red and make it appear that there has been a substantial amount of bleeding. When the volume of bleeding is in doubt, the patient's hematocrit should be measured to determine how much blood loss has occurred.

SYMPTOMS ASSOCIATED WITH ANAL PROLAPSE In third- and fourth-degree hemorrhoids, the rectal mucosa prolapses out of the anal canal. The anoderm, dislodged from its normal position in the anal canal, can no longer serve its role as a sensing mechanism of the organ of continence, and a variety of associated symptoms occur. For example, patients frequently report incontinence of flatus, liquid stool, or even formed stool. It is important to document even minor signs of incontinence because resolution of incontinence is an important objective of treatment.

Rectal discharge also occurs with third- and fourth-degree hemorrhoids, as mucus is secreted by the prolapsed rectal mucosa. The discharge can result in constant wetness of the perianal skin, which in turn leads to excoriation and itching—a symptom complex sometimes referred to as "wet anus syndrome."

ALTERED BOWEL HABITS All patients with symptoms of hemorrhoids should also be asked about changes in bowel habits. Recent onset of diarrhea or constipation may be a symptom of an early colonic neoplasm. Bowel changes of particular concern include recent onset of frequent, marked diarrhea or subtle changes such as the development of normal, easy bowel movements in a patient who had formerly been constipated. Most patients reporting changes in bowel habits, and those reporting rectal bleeding, will warrant colonoscopy or imaging of the colon to exclude colonic neoplasms.

Key Physical Examination

The diagnosis of hemorrhoids can never be made by history alone. An anorectal examination must be performed in all cases. The key purposes of the examination are to identify that hemorrhoids are present and, if the patient has experienced bleeding, to confirm that hemorrhoids are the cause of the bleeding. A second purpose of the examination is to exclude three conditions that can be confused with hemorrhoids—rectal prolapse, hypertrophied anal papillae, and rectal neoplasms.

When performing the physical examination, clinicians should position the patient in Sims' position (Fig. 6-2), ask the patient if there is any anorectal pain, and assure the patient that the examination will be discontinued if any undue pain should arise. The cause of very painful conditions associated with hemorrhoidal disease is usually apparent on external inspection. The presence of significant pain without any visible perianal abnormalities speaks in favor of an anal fissure and against internal hemorrhoids.

INSPECTION

The examination then begins with inspection of the anorectal area. External hemorrhoids will present as a painful, swollen, dark-colored nodule close to the anal orifice. When patients have hemorrhoidal thrombosis or gangrene, the corpus cavernosum recti is invariably prolapsed into a position below the high-pressure zone of the anal sphincter (Fig. 6-3). The engorged anal cushions are then visible on the outside of the anal canal.

PALPATION

Following the inspection of the anal region, a digital anorectal exam is performed using a water-soluble lubricant applied to the gloved index finger. The patient is informed that the finger will be passed into the rectum, and many patients need to be continually reassured during the examination. As described later in this chapter, in the pres-

Figure 6-2

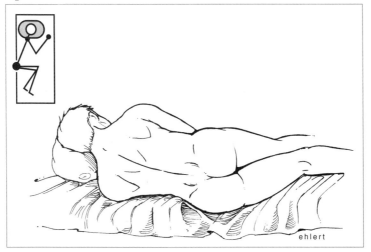

Sims' position. Sims' position is the preferred position for examining the anal canal.

Figure 6-3

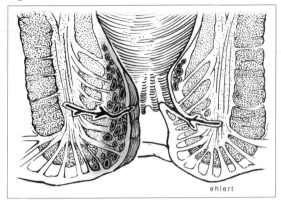

Hemorrhoidal prolapse. The vessels of the corpus cavernosum recti have descended below the high-pressure zone of the anal sphincter muscles and are visible at the anus.

ence of an anal fissure, it is usually not necessary, and often inappropriate because of pain, to perform a rectal examination in the office.

The clinician should examine the rectum and its surrounding structures using an organized approach, sequentially palpating all quadrants of the anorectal canal. There are usually no palpable abnormalities with first- and second-degree hemorrhoids, though on occasion, thickened tissue can be felt in the anal canal. Thickened tissue can often be palpated in third-degree hemorrhoids, and in fourth-degree hemorrhoids the prolapsed rectum will be apparent.

In thrombosed external hemorrhoids (thrombosed perianal veins), palpation reveals a localized pea-sized subcutaneous swelling. It may be hard and tender to palpation, which distinguishes it from internal hemorrhoids.

Perhaps the most important part of the rectal examination is to identify problems other than hemorrhoids that might be causing the patient's symptoms. In particular, the clinician should use palpation to detect rectal masses.

ANOSCOPY

The next step in the physical examination is visual inspection of the anal canal using anoscopy. Many types of anoscopes are available, but a commonly used device is the Hirschmann-style anoscope (Fig. 6-4). Anoscopes with built-in illumination are expensive and unnecessary for most examinations. Instead, a malleable goose-neck lamp or even a simple pocket flashlight can provide sufficient illumination.

When recording pathologic changes in the anal canal, the site should be specified using o'clock descriptions. By convention, the system assumes that the patient is positioned in lithotomy position. This means that a lesion located toward the perineum is in the 12 o'clock position, and lesions located toward the coccyx are in the 6 o'clock position.

During the anoscopic examination, hemorrhoidal nodules will usually protrude into the lumen of the anoscope opening and appear as dark blue cushions. In most cases, evidence of hemorrhoids (hemorrhoidal "nodes") is found at the 3 o'clock, 7 o'clock, and 11 o'clock positions, which correspond to the entry points of the branches of the superior hemorrhoidal arteries supplying the corpus cavernosum recti. However, satellite hemorrhoidal nodes may be also present in other locations. On occasion, such as when

Figure 6-4

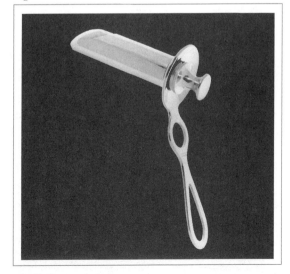

Hirschmann anoscope.

patients have recently experienced hemorrhoidal bleeding, anoscopy may reveal the bleeding site as a small laceration on a hemorrhoidal node.

While the key purpose of the anoscopic examination is to identify the source of bleeding, the examination also serves to differentiate "external hemorrhoids" from "internal hemorrhoids." Since external hemorrhoids are derived from perianal veins, they do not extend above the dentate line.

EXCLUSION OF OTHER CONDITIONS

As noted earlier, an important purpose of the physical examination is to exclude rectal prolapse, hypertrophied anal papillae, and rectal neoplasms. Each of these conditions is commonly confused with hemorrhoidal disease.

RECTAL PROLAPSE   Rectal prolapse is often confused with third- and fourth-degree hemorrhoids, because prolapse of the rectal mucosa (i.e., rectal prolapse) may appear similar to prolapsed hemorrhoids. To make the distinction, the clinician

must recognize that internal hemorrhoids are generally separated from one another by radial sulci that emanate from the center of the anus, permitting individual hemorrhoidal cushions to be identified. Furthermore, third- and fourth-degree hemorrhoids are usually accompanied by some edema and, occasionally, overt inflammatory changes.

In contrast, rectal prolapse has no radial sulci. Instead, the prolapsed rectal mucosa presents as a concentric protrusion of rectal tissue. The three specific characteristics of rectal prolapse that distinguish it from hemorrhoids are characteristic concentric folds, absence of radial sulci between individual hemorrhoids, and the much larger size of the protruding tissue segment. If the rectal prolapse is complete, it can usually be differentiated easily from advanced hemorrhoidal disease (Fig. 6-5).

HYPERTROPHIED ANAL PAPILLAE   Hypertrophied anal papillae (Fig. 6-6) are usually identified by palpation. On a digital rectal exam, they feel like firm nodules arising from the dentate line, and they are smaller in diameter than hemorrhoids.

Figure 6-5

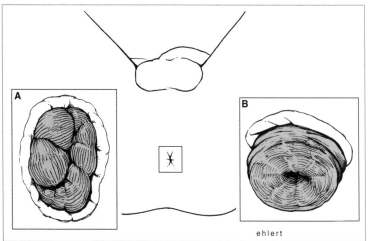

Hemorrhoids versus rectal prolapse. Prolapsed hemorrhoids can be distinguished from prolapsed rectal tissue by the fact that hemorrhoids **(A)** have radial folds between each of the individual hemorrhoidal cushions, creating a stellate appearance, whereas prolapsed rectal tissue **(B)** demonstrates concentric, rather than radial, folds.

Figure 6-6

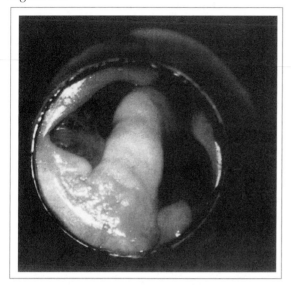

Hypertrophied anal papillae. Hypertrophied anal papillae are smaller than hemorrhoids and are covered by squamous epithelium. They do not connect to the corpus cavernosum recti above the dentate line. (*From Corman ML:* Colon and Rectal Surgery, *3rd ed. Philadelphia, JB Lippincott, 1993, with permission.*)

On anoscopy, hypertrophied anal papillae are covered by squamous cell epithelium, and they do not connect to the corpus cavernosum recti above the dentate line.

RECTAL NEOPLASMS Rectal carcinomas are differentiated from hemorrhoids by their firm texture on palpation. Rectal polyps, however, which are typically less firm than carcinomas, are sometimes mistaken for hemorrhoids when they are palpated in the typical location of hemorrhoids. To avoid misdiagnosing polyps as hemorrhoids, clinicians should keep in mind that as a general rule, any anorectal abnormality that is readily palpable and cannot be attributed to a thrombosed hemorrhoid (which is usually painful) is not likely to be hemorrhoidal tissue.

Furthermore, anoscopy usually provides visual evidence of whether a lesion is hemorrhoidal or neoplastic. Most neoplasms do not have the characteristic dark blue color of hemorrhoids. In addition, the texture of neoplasms is commonly different from that of hemorrhoidal vascular cushions. It may be indurated and/or ulcerated (as with carcinomas) or very soft (as with villous polyps). Nonetheless, in some cases it may be impossible to distinguish hemorrhoids from neoplasms, and biopsy with histologic examination may be necessary to establish the correct diagnosis. When biopsies are necessary, clinicians should keep in mind that the corpus cavernosum recti and hemorrhoids are vascular structures supplied by the arterial circulation. Biopsies of hemorrhoidal tissues can, therefore, be followed by severe arterial bleeding requiring operating room management for placement of a stitch tie to achieve hemostasis.

Ancillary Tests

COLONOSCOPY, SIGMOIDOSCOPY, AND BARIUM ENEMA

In all patients with rectal bleeding who are older than 40 years of age, a complete colon evaluation is imperative to exclude neoplastic disease. This is true even if hemorrhoids appear to be the cause of the bleeding, because hemorrhoids are very common and often exist simultaneously with colorectal neoplasms. In most cases the preferred technique for this evaluation is colonoscopy. If colonoscopy is unavailable, the evaluation can be performed with the combination of sigmoidoscopy and air-contrast barium enema.

If the patient is less than 40 years old, and hemorrhoids are not identified as the certain source of bleeding during anoscopy, the patient should undergo proctosigmoidoscopy. Whether a rigid sigmoidoscope or a flexible sigmoidoscope is used depends on the preference and training of the clinician. Although most recently trained clinicians have more experience with flexible sigmoidoscopy, including retroflexion of the scope to view the rectum, some prefer to use a rigid sigmoidoscope because it is easier to examine the rectum with a rigid sigmoidoscope. When the source of rectal bleeding cannot be identified by anoscopy or proctosigmoidoscopy, colonoscopy or barium enema must be performed.

HEMATOCRIT

Hematocrit should be measured if signs and symptoms of severe rectal bleeding are present. No other blood testing is routinely necessary to diagnose hemorrhoidal disease.

TESTS FOR SEXUALLY TRANSMITTED INFECTIONS

In some patients with hemorrhoids, the hemorrhoids have been caused or aggravated by receptive anal intercourse. When evaluating such patients, who are typically gay males, clinicians should consider performing rectal cultures for *Neiserria gonorrheae* and screening for other sexually transmitted disease such as human immunodeficiency virus (HIV) infection.

Algorithm

As shown in Figure 6-7, evaluation of patients with suspected hemorrhoids includes the examination and ancillary tests described above to confirm the diagnosis and to exclude those conditions that can be confused with hemorrhoids.

Treatment

Treatment of external hemorrhoids depends on the stage of severity (Table 6-2). First-degree hemorrhoids usually require only physical and medical treatments. Second-degree hemorrhoids typically are treated with banding or sclerotherapy. Third- and fourth-degree hemorrhoids most often require surgical hemorrhoidectomy.

External hemorrhoids require treatment when they become thrombosed, a condition that can be extremely painful. Treatment of thrombosed

Figure 6-7

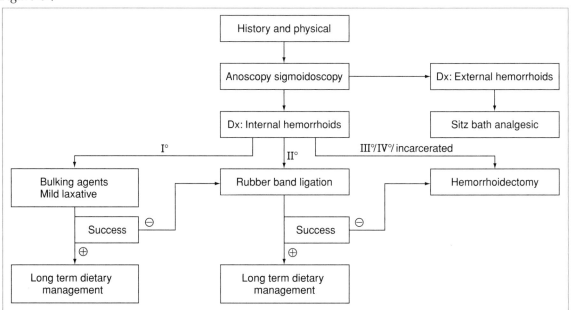

Algorithm for evaluation and treatment of hemorrhoids. Abbreviations: I° = first degree; II° = second degree, etc.

Table 6-2

Treatment of Internal Hemorrhoids

DEGREE	MOST COMMON TREATMENTS
First	Sitz baths
	Stool softeners
	Topical antiinflammatory agents
	Dietary management
Second	Rubber-band ligation
	Sclerotherapy
	Cryosurgery
	Infrared coagulation
	Diathermy
Third	Surgical hemorrhoidectomy
Fourth	Surgical hemorrhoidectomy

external hemorrhoids is a minor surgical procedure performed under local anesthesia.

FIRST-DEGREE HEMORRHOIDS

First-degree hemorrhoids are generally treated with sitz baths, medications, and dietary management.

SITZ BATHS   Sitz baths provide symptomatic relief of first-degree hemorrhoids and also improve anal hygiene. They should be used twice a day and after every bowel movement. While the effect of a sitz bath can be achieved by having patients sit in a bathtub filled with lukewarm water, it is easier for the patient to use a sitz bath device that can be obtained in drugstores or medical supply houses. Such devices are typically plastic bedpans with a mechanism that permits spraying of water onto the perianal area. If the patient can tolerate it, another method that has a similar effect is to have patients use a handheld shower device and spray water onto the perianal area.

Following the sitz bath, the perianal area should be dried by patting it gently with a dry towel. Rubbing with a hand cloth or towel should be strongly discouraged. While patients are often tempted to rub if pruritus is present, the rubbing action will increase irritation.

MEDICATIONS   Medical therapy for first-degree hemorrhoids includes both oral and topical agents. Oral agents are used to soften the stool and decrease constipation. Topical agents are used to decrease anorectal inflammation.

Stool Softeners   Stool softeners such as docusate and bulking agents such as psyllium are used to minimize constipation and straining. To achieve maximal effectiveness, it is important that these stool-softening medications be taken simultaneously with a large glass of water or other liquid. Laxatives, however, because they can be habit-forming, are not appropriate treatments for the often chronic constipation that accompanies hemorrhoids.

Topical Antiinflammatory Agents   Topical hydrocortisone is widely used to treat the inflammation and itching that accompanies hemorrhoids. Hydrocortisone can be administered as a cream (2.5% three times per day) or in suppository form (e.g., Anusol-HC). While generally quite effective, it is important not to use these preparations for prolonged periods (e.g., more than 2 to 3 weeks) to avoid cutaneous steroid side effects.

Another topical preparation often used to treat the inflammation of hemorrhoids is witch hazel extract pads. Witch hazel (*Hamamelis virginiana*) is a shrub native to the United States. The extract from this plant is a nondrying astringent that has been used as a skin toner and hemorrhoidal remedy for centuries. Many patients will experience considerable improvement with this treatment.

DIETARY MANAGEMENT   Standard treatment for hemorrhoids involves dietary modification to decrease the likelihood of constipation by softening and adding bulk to stools. This can be achieved by increasing the fiber content of the diet by consumption of fruits, vegetables, and nonabsorbable fibers such as wheat bran.

There is also evidence that skipping breakfast leads to fewer morning bowel movements and retention of stool leading to constipation. Therefore, a morning routine that includes breakfast and morning stools should be encouraged.

SECOND-DEGREE HEMORRHOIDS

Several treatment options are available for second-degree hemorrhoids, the most common of which are rubber-band ligation and sclerotherapy. Indications for rubber-band ligation and sclerotherapy include bleeding, itching, and other hemorrhoid-related symptoms. Several other forms of nonoperative hemorrhoidal treatment can also be used, including cryotherapy, diathermy, and other modalities briefly discussed later.

RUBBER-BAND LIGATION

Procedure   Prior to performing rubber-band ligation, the patient is prepared with a cleansing enema. An anoscope is then introduced, and a rubber band is placed around the base of the hemorrhoidal cushion, using a special hemorrhoid ligator device (Fig. 6-8). Because of the possibility that a rubber band may break, most clinicians place two rubber bands around the base of each hemorrhoid. In our experience all three hemorrhoids can be banded in one session, except in very sensitive individuals.

If the bands are placed correctly (i.e., above the dentate line), no anesthetic is required and the procedure is painless. Some discomfort may develop, however, in the hours and days following the procedure.

Postoperative Care   Following the procedure, the patient should take bulking agents or stool softeners. Sitz baths may help to relieve the discomfort experienced by some patients.

The banded tissue usually sloughs off about 7 days after the procedure. While a small amount of rectal bleeding is common in the days following the procedure, patients should be aware that more bleeding will occur when the banded tissue sloughs. If bleeding is severe, the patient should seek medical care because operative hemostasis may be required, but this is a rare complication (less than 1% of cases). To decrease the chance of bleeding, many experts recommend that the patient be taken off any anticoagulant medication

and platelet aggregation inhibitors prior to undergoing hemorrhoidal banding.

After the banded tissue has sloughed off, a small ulcer forms at the site. This ulcer heals within 1 or 2 weeks. Patients should return for reevaluation about 3 to 4 weeks after the procedure, at which time anoscopy is repeated.

If additional hemorrhoids remain at follow-up examination, they can be rubber-banded during this same examination, or further banding can be performed at any future date. Patients whose hemorrhoids have completely resolved are informed that they may return for treatment again if symptoms recur, but further follow-up is otherwise unnecessary.

Complications   Moderate discomfort and/or anorectal fullness is commonly experienced after a banding procedure, but severe complications are rare. In addition to pronounced delayed bleeding, as described earlier, serious complications include pain and thrombosis of the ligated hemorrhoidal cushions and sepsis.

Sepsis, including life-threatening infections with clostridia species, has been reported following banding of hemorrhoids. While such incidents are very rare, any postoperative complaints suggesting perianal/perineal infection such as perineal pain, fever, scrotal edema, or difficulties urinating require immediate emergency evaluation.

Outcomes   Results with hemorrhoidal banding are usually very good. A significant improvement of symptoms has been reported by up to 80% of patients in large series. For many patients, even a single treatment session can achieve satisfactory results. If more than three successive treatment sessions are required, however, banding should probably be abandoned, and the patient should be treated with surgical hemorrhoidectomy.

Longer-term outcomes are also good. Studies indicate that when rubber-band ligation is used for treatment of second-degree hemorrhoids, about three-quarters of patients are hemorrhoid-free 5 years after treatment, and more than two-thirds are disease-free after 10 years.

Figure 6-8

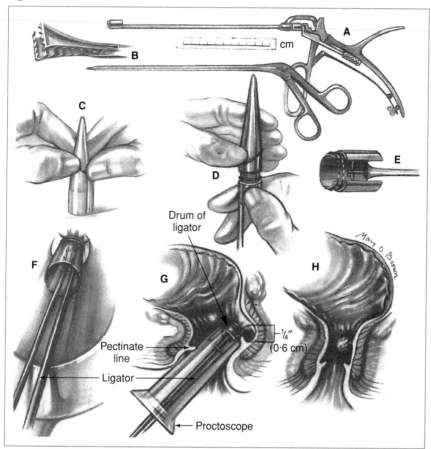

Rubber-band ligation of second-degree hemorrhoids. The ligator device for applying rubber bands to hemorrhoids is shown in **(A)**. Note the drum on the end of the device that will hold the rubber bands and the triggered handle that will release the rubber bands. The forceps device in **(B)** is used to grasp the hemorrhoid to be ligated through the lumen of the drum. To use these devices, rubber bands are first slid onto a cone-shaped applicator **(C)**. The cone-shaped applicator is then attached to the end of the ligator device, as shown in **(D)**, and the rubber bands slid down further onto the drum of the ligator, at which point the cone is removed and the rubber bands are in place on the tip of the ligator **(E)**. In **(F)** and **(G)**, the drum is applied through an anoscope, over and around the hemorrhoid, using the forceps to pull the hemorrhoid through the drum. The trigger is then activated, releasing the rubber band around the hemorrhoid. The devices are removed and the banded hemorrhoids are left to undergo necrosis **(H)**. (*From Goligher JC: Surgery of the Anus and Rectum, 5th ed. London, Bailliere Tindall, 1984. Reproduced with permission of WB Saunders.*)

SCLEROTHERAPY   Sclerotherapy, the injection of hemorrhoids with sclerosing chemicals, can be used to treat both first- and second-degree hemorrhoidal disease, although it is not often used for first-degree hemorrhoids. Original reports of hemorrhoidal sclerotherapy date back to the 1860s, when iron persulfate was injected into prolapsed hemorrhoids. Other agents, including sodium morrhuate and sodium tetradecyl sulfate, had been used for sclerosis of varicose veins and were once used for sclerosis of hemorrhoids based on the erroneous assumption that internal hemorrhoids were varicose veins. These agents are no longer used, however, because they produced large ulcerations and unnecessary bleeding when injected intravascularly.

Procedure   Currently, 5% phenol mixed in almond or vegetable oil is the safest and best sclerosing agent available. Most clinicians inject 3 mL of this solution into each hemorrhoidal site. Injections are performed during anoscopy, using a specialized syringe and needle, by injecting the agent into the submucosa of the lesion. The injected solution produces a mild fibrotic reaction that decreases blood circulation through the lesion, which leads to shrinkage.

Outcomes And Complications   It is generally recommended that patients be treated only once, and that clinicians should proceed to other treatments if the injections are not successful in relieving the patient's symptoms. Overall, approximately 70% of patients with second-degree hemorrhoids will achieve resolution of symptoms after sclerotherapy. Large hemorrhoids with considerable amounts of fibrous tissue are least likely to respond to sclerotherapy. Complications include sloughing of the hemorrhoidal cushion, thrombosis, and injection-site infections.

Meta-analyses comparing different forms of treatment for internal hemorrhoids have shown that rubber banding is preferable to sclerotherapy because of its higher cure and lower complication rates. Others experts, however, have argued that sclerotherapy is still a suitable treatment for first-degree and early second-degree hemorrhoids.

OTHER TREATMENTS   Several other nonoperative techniques have been reported for the treatment of second-degree hemorrhoids. These include cryosurgery, endoscopic elastic-band ligation, infrared coagulation, bipolar diathermy, and Lord's anal dilatation. While these treatment modalities are effective, they are more costly and have no advantages over rubber banding or sclerotherapy for the majority of patients.

THIRD-DEGREE AND FOURTH-DEGREE HEMORRHOIDS

In general, third- and fourth-degree hemorrhoidal disease requires surgical hemorrhoidectomy. On occasion, however, rubber banding can be used to treat early third-degree hemorrhoids when a patient is reluctant or unwilling to undergo surgical hemorrhoidectomy. When taking this approach, patients should be made aware that the success rates with rubber banding of third- and fourth-degree hemorrhoids is not as good as with lower degrees of hemorrhoidal disease. Nonetheless, because rubber banding does not preclude later surgical hemorrhoidectomy, there is no contraindication to attempting rubber banding first, followed by hemorrhoidectomy if banding does not produce satisfactory results.

PROCEDURE   The aim of surgical hemorrhoidectomy is to excise hemorrhoidal tissue. When performing hemorrhoidectomy, the patient is first prepared with a small enema on the morning of the operation, and the anus is infiltrated with a solution of 0.5% bupivacaine with 1:200,000 epinephrine.

The excision is begun at the perianal skin and carried upward in a drop-shaped fashion. The hemorrhoidal plexus is dissected off the external and internal sphincter muscle. Finally, a suture ligature is placed at the stalk of hemorrhoidal pedicle and the hemorrhoid resected.

The hemorrhoidal tissue is removed in the three sectors where the superior hemorrhoidal arteries enter into the corpus cavernosum recti (at 3 o'clock, 7 o'clock, and 11 o'clock positions). Sufficient amounts of anal skin are left between the excision sites to prevent the formation of an anal stricture. Some surgeons will perform a "closed hemorrhoidectomy" and reapproximate the wound edges. Others will leave the wound open to heal by secondary intention.

Compete resection of the corpus cavernosum recti in an attempt to remove all hemorrhoidal tissue ("Whitehead's operation") inevitably leads to incontinence and the "wet anus syndrome." This procedure is no longer used.

POST-OPERATIVE CARE   Follow-up care after hemorrhoidectomy is mainly directed at elimination of postoperative pain and avoidance of constipation. Discharge medications, therefore, include an analgesic for pain, as well as a bulking agent and a stool softener or a stimulant laxative.

The patient is then seen for examination 4 weeks after discharge, at which time rectal examination can usually be accomplished with minimal discomfort. Earlier examinations are unnecessary because they are usually painful and yield little useful information. If an early follow-up examination is performed, it is not uncommon to find an open wound, even after a closed hemorrhoidectomy, because reapproximated wounds may open with the first bowel movement. However, office visits during the first few weeks following the procedure may occasionally be useful to reassure an anxious patient. A specific cause for anxiety is the bleeding that often occurs following the first bowel movement; while this bleeding can be alarming to patients, they should be assured that it is expected and has no harmful consequences.

COMPLICATIONS

Early Complications   Early postoperative complications of surgical hemorrhoidectomy include postoperative hemorrhage and urinary retention and infection.

Early postoperative hemorrhage occurs in about 0.5% of patients. It is almost always the result of inadequate ligation of the hemorrhoid pedicle. Its occurrence requires a return to the operating room for repair and hemostasis.

Postoperative urinary retention requiring catheterization occurs in 4% to 15% of patients who undergo surgical hemorrhoidectomy. Urinary retention is related to perineal edema, infections that may occur following intraoperative catheterization, and possibly excessive intraoperative fluid administration. The occurrence of urinary retention frequently leads to the need for a 24- to 48-hour postoperative hospital stay. If, on the other hand, the patient has minimal pain and no problems with urinary retention, surgical hemorrhoidectomy can be carried out as an outpatient surgical procedure with same-day discharge.

Delayed Complications   Some patients will develop anal skin tags at the sites of the surgical incisions. These skin tags may interfere with proper cleansing of the anus and occasionally are responsible for skin irritation and pruritus. If the patient is symptomatic, these tags can be removed under local anesthesia as an office procedure, simply by excising them with scissors or a scalpel.

Some patients develop anal strictures and/or mucosal ectropions (eversion of the rectal mucosa through the anus). These complications are largely the result of improper surgical technique and, therefore, are potentially avoidable. When they occur, they require extensive plastic surgical repair, which should be performed by surgeons specialized in colorectal surgery.

EXTERNAL HEMORRHOIDS

As with varicose veins in other locations, reassurance of the patient and expectant treatment is usually sufficient for patients with uncomplicated external hemorrhoids. Even when external hemorrhoids are thrombosed and painful, complete resolution of symptoms can be expected over 4 to 7 days. Resolution may be aided by use of a mild laxative; frequent, hot sitz baths; and the administration of a nonconstipating analgesic (i.e., narcotics are constipating and should be avoided).

Many clinicians have been trained to evacuate the underlying clot from within an acutely painful, thrombosed, external hemorrhoid. In most cases, however, such operative treatment is unnecessary and should be discouraged. Nonetheless, many patients "expect" such treatment. It is doubtful that operative treatment hastens the resolution of pain, and the issue has never been rigorously studied.

PROCEDURE   The first step in evacuating the clot from a thrombosed external hemorrhoid is to provide the patient with local anesthesia by injecting the lesion with 1% or 2% lidocaine with epinephrine. Then, a small elliptical incision, oriented radially from the anus, is made through the skin into the thrombosed vein; the ellipse of skin is removed; and the clot is expressed (Fig. 6-9). The wound is left to heal by secondary intention.

POST-OPERATIVE CARE   After evacuating the clot from a thrombosed external hemorrhoid, the patient should receive sitz baths and stool softeners, as described earlier. Pain should diminish rapidly (i.e., within hours), and, with the excep-

tion of some mild bleeding, the patient should be asymptomatic in a matter of days. In the absence of problems, no follow-up examination is required.

Errors

Clinicians make a variety of errors in management of hemorrhoids. These include errors in the diagnostic evaluation and errors in management. Specific technical surgical errors will not be discussed.

DIAGNOSTIC ERRORS

Failure to diagnose cancer is one of the leading causes of malpractice allegations against physicians. Diagnostic failure occurs during the evaluation of hemorrhoids when clinicians inappropriately ascribe rectal bleeding in older patients to hemorrhoids without excluding the possibility that a colorectal neoplasm is the cause

Figure 6-9

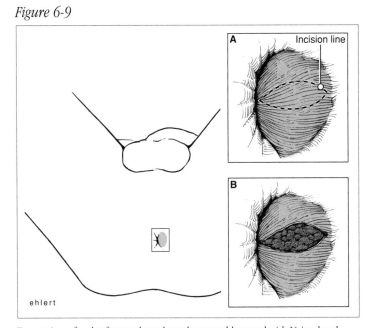

Evacuation of a clot from a thrombosed external hemorrhoid. Using local anesthesia, a small elliptical incision is made **(A)** oriented radially from the anus, and the clot is expressed through the incision **(B)**.

of bleeding. It is important to emphasize that, even if hemorrhoids are visualized on anoscopic examination, and even if these hemorrhoids appear to be the source of bleeding, patients over age 40 should still undergo colonoscopy. Colonoscopy is essential to ensure that the hemorrhoids are not an incidental finding, unrelated to a more proximal neoplastic lesion in the rectum or colon.

TREATMENT ERRORS

As shown in Table 6-2, conservative treatment (i.e., sitz baths, stool softeners, and dietary management) as the sole therapy of hemorrhoids is only appropriate for first-degree hemorrhoids. Nonetheless, many clinicians attempt to manage second-degree hemorrhoids with these conservative measures, but such measures are likely to be unsuccessful. Patients with second-degree hemorrhoids are better treated with rubber-band ligation, and patients with third- and fourth-degree hemorrhoids should be treated with surgical hemorrhoidectomy.

Anal Fissures

Anal fissures are painful tears in the squamous epithelium of the anus (anoderm). In most patients the tear in the anoderm extends to the internal anal-sphincter muscle. Anal fissures can be acute or chronic.

Pathophysiology

The cause of anal fissures is obscure. It is generally held that anal fissures result from constipation and hard bowel movements. This theory assumes that a hard fecal bolus distends and produces a tear in the anal canal. The credibility of this theory is put in question by the fact that anal

fissures can also occur in the presence of frequent defecation and diarrhea, as well as with specific inflammatory conditions affecting the anal rectum such as tuberculosis and syphilis. In addition, anal fissures in atypical locations occur in patients who have inflammatory bowel disease.

About 90% of anal fissures not related to inflammatory bowel disease occur in the posterior midline, and the reason for this is also not certain. There is evidence that the anoderm tears most easily in the posterior midline when overstretched in cadaver experiments, but this does not explain why fissures occur in this location in the presence of diarrhea. It is known that the posterior midline is the least well-perfused segment of the anal canal, and this might also be the reason fissures occur in this location. Beyond this, the reason some fissures in this location resolve well with therapy while others persist and become chronic is unclear. Furthermore, there is no explanation for the fact that fissures occur in other locations in the presence of inflammatory bowel disease. Finally, it is not known why some long-standing anal fissures lead to the development of characteristic skin tags ("sentinel folds"), while others do not.

Studies using sphincter manometry have repeatedly shown that the resting sphincter pressures of patients with anal fissures are significantly elevated compared with pressures in normal controls. However, it is unclear whether this phenomenon is the result of the chronic pain sensations experienced from the fissure, or if the causative factor is in the pathogenesis of fissures. The beneficial effect of muscle-relaxing treatments such as botulinum toxin (see below) suggests that increased sphincter pressure may be causative.

Epidemiology

Anal fissures are fairly common and affect individuals of all ages, including infants and children. They are most frequent between the ages 10 and 40, and the prevalence is roughly equal in men and women.

Key History

While the diagnosis of anal fissures requires physical examination, history can suggest the diagnosis. Questions should be directed at the characteristics of pain, the presence of anal discharge, and the amount of bleeding. The key symptom of anal fissures in adults is anal pain at the onset, during, and/or immediately following defecation. Anal fissures without pain suggest inflammatory bowel disease, most commonly Crohn's disease.

Perianal swelling and, occasionally, mucous discharge can occur. Bleeding can be overt or completely absent. When present, it is often manifest as streaks of blood on the toilet paper.

Key Physical Examination

ACUTE OR PAINFUL FISSURES

Patients who seek care for acute anal fissures have usually had significant pain, and they may be frightened that the examination will cause yet additional discomfort. Thus, reassurance of the patient is essential. The clinician should explain that most likely, the examination will require only inspection of the anus, as the diagnosis of an anal fissure can usually be made by inspection alone. Digital rectal examination or instrumentation of the rectum is not generally needed.

Visual examination is easier if the examiner is committed but gentle. A topical anesthetic jelly (e.g., 4% lidocaine) applied around the anal margin is helpful if the examiner is willing to wait a few minutes for it to take effect. However, if the patient has been adequately reassured, it is often possible to part the buttocks gently without use of anesthetic. Because the patient experiences either pain or fear of pain, the anus is commonly contracted by excessive sphincter activity. Nonetheless, it is usually possible to see a small skin tag at the low portion of the defect in the anal skin.

It is generally unnecessary to perform a rectal examination at this stage of the evaluation. If further workup of an exquisitely painful anorectal problem is necessary and the patient has significant pain, rectal examination and anoscopy can be performed under general anesthesia.

CHRONIC FISSURES

For patients with chronic fissures, pain is commonly not severe, thus permitting digital and anoscopic examinations. Chronic fissures are often accompanied by a sentinel tag on the distal end of the fissure, and hypertrophied anal papillae proximally. Anoscopy will typically reveal a well-circumscribed ulcer or tear of the anoderm, usually in the posterior commissure. An irregularly shaped ulcer or a polypoid lesion usually requires a tissue biopsy to exclude an anorectal neoplasm.

On occasion, patients with an anal fissure will have a narrowing of the anal canal. When this situation is encountered, it may be necessary to use a narrow-caliber anoscope.

EXCLUDING OTHER CONDITIONS

Physical examination also permits diagnosis of other conditions that cause symptoms similar to those of anal fissures. These include thrombosed external hemorrhoids, Crohn's disease, intersphincteric abscesses, rectal tuberculosis, and proctalgia fugax. Thrombosed external hemorrhoids were discussed earlier.

CROHN'S DISEASE   In Crohn's disease, rectal fissures are often located laterally and not in the posterior commissure. The fissures of Crohn's disease are often broader than simple anal fissures, and they may be multiple or associated with fistulas and abscesses. Any fissure with these characteristics, or which does not respond to therapy, should raise the possibility of Crohn's disease.

INTERSPHINCTERIC ABSCESS   Intersphincteric abscesses cause intense anal pain, but neither an anal fissure nor other mucosal or dermal abnormality can be identified, even during an examination under anesthesia. The diagnosis is confirmed by surgical exploration at the site of maximal tenderness.

TUBERCULAR FISSURES   Anal fissures caused by tuberculosis infection are uncommon, but they often appear similar to simple anal fissures and should be considered if a patient has risk factors for tuberculosis, especially if an otherwise uncomplicated–appearing anal fissure fails to resolve with standard therapy. Occasionally, tubercular fissures will have a unique appearance, with ulcerations in the anal canal that have livid, undermined edges. The diagnosis of tubercular fissures requires demonstration of acid-fast bacilli in cultures or biopsy specimen.

PROCTALGIA FUGAX   Proctalgia fugax is an ill-defined functional pain syndrome of unknown cause in which patients experience anorectal pain for no identifiable reason. If the patient has no hemorrhoids, an intersphincteric abscess has been excluded, sigmoidoscopy is normal, and there are no fissures, then proctalgia fugax is often the presumed diagnosis. However, clinicians should bear in mind that, given the current state of knowledge, proctalgia fugax is a diagnosis of exclusion. A computerized tomographic scan of the pelvis and neurologic workup should be considered to exclude pelvic masses or neuropathic causes of the pain, and interval reevaluation may be necessary to avoid overlooking such conditions.

Ancillary Tests

Except in children, it is desirable to perform a proctosigmoidoscopic examination of patients who have anal fissures. In surgical practices, 5% to 10% of patients will have additional abnormalities found on proctosigmoidoscopy such as distal proctitis, adenoma, condyloma, melanosis coli, metaplastic polyps, Crohn's disease, or tuberculosis. The prevalence of such conditions in primary-care practice is undoubtedly much lower, though no data exist to support this contention. A complete colon examination with barium enema or colonoscopy is not indicated for patients with visible anal fissures unless there is strong evidence for inflammatory bowel disease or a colorectal neoplasm.

Algorithm

The algorithm in Figure 6-10 shows the basic approach to diagnosis and treatment of anal fissures. When a fissure is clearly identified on examination, treatment with analgesics, bulking agents, and laxatives may be all that is needed. If treatment is unsatisfactory, or if the diagnosis is unclear, the patient should be examined under anesthesia; if a fissure is found, lateral internal sphincterotomy is usually the preferred treatment.

Treatment

NONSURGICAL TREATMENT

CONSERVATIVE THERAPY   Up to 40% of anal fissures will heal with conservative therapy alone. Because most patients with anal fissures are constipated, conservative therapy is mainly directed at the normalization of bowel habits. A bulk laxative such as methylcellulose or psyllium should be prescribed. It is important to stress, especially in older patients, the necessity of ingesting enough water (usually 8 oz or more) with the bulk laxative to make the laxative function properly.

Application of local anesthetic agents (e.g., 2% lidocaine jelly) to the anus may be effective in relieving pain, particularly for patients who have acute fissures. Sitz baths are advantageous in some patients.

MUSCLE-RELAXING THERAPY   The realization that hypertension of the anal sphincter is present in patients with chronic anal fissures has led to the use of two medical treatments aimed at decreasing sphincter tone—nitroglycerine ointment and injections of botulinum toxin.

Nitroglycerin Ointment   Nitric oxide is an inhibitory neurotransmitter in the internal anal sphincter. It is also a by-product of the degradation of nitroglycerin. Thus, when nitroglycerin ointment is applied topically to the anus and anal canal, the resulting production of nitric oxide results in re-

Figure 6-10

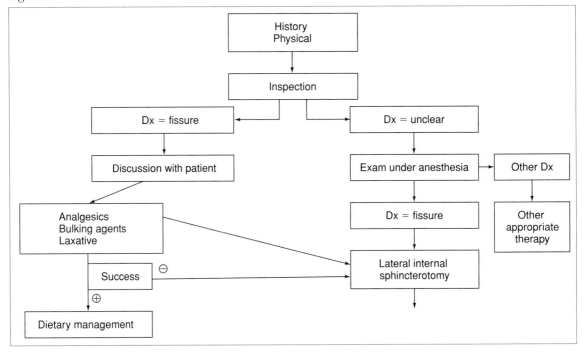

Algorithm for diagnosis and treatment of anal fissures.

laxation of the anal sphincter. The result is healing of anal fissures in about 60% of patients treated with nitroglycerin ointment. Relapses are infrequent, even when patients are followed for more than 1 year.

The treatment regimen that has been found successful in published studies is the application of 0.2% nitroglycerin ointment by fingertip to the anus and anal canal, twice daily for 6 weeks. About 1.2 g of ointment is needed for each application, or about 100 g for a 6-week course of treatment. About 20% of patients will experience moderate-to-severe headaches after application of the ointment; headaches last about half an hour and can be relieved with oral analgesics.

Botulinum Toxin Botulinum toxin, produced by the bacterium *Clostridium botulinum*, acts on neuromuscular junctions to block release of acetylcholine. When injected into the internal anal sphincter,

botulinum toxin produces long-lasting (3 months) but reversible paralysis of some muscle fibers of the sphincter, reducing sphincter pressure and permitting chronic anal fissures to heal.

Botulinum toxin A is diluted in saline to a concentration of 50 U/ml, and injections are performed through a 27-gauge needle without sedation or local anesthesia. The internal anal sphincter is palpated, and 0.2 mL of the solution is injected into each side of the anterior midline of the internal anal sphincter. This treatment results in healing of chronic anal fissures in more than 95% of patients, with a relapse rate of close to zero at 1 year.

SURGICAL TREATMENT

If symptoms recur or persist despite nonsurgical therapy, definitive surgical treatment should be offered. The options include anal sphincter dilation and internal sphincterotomy.

ANAL SPHINCTER DILATION   Anal sphincter dilation has been used for over a century and is a successful treatment for anal fissures, achieving healing of fissures in 90% to 95% of patients. After induction of deep intravenous anesthesia, the anal sphincter is dilated manually or with an anal speculum to about 5 cm in diameter. The dilation can be performed as an outpatient procedure, and the patient can return home a few hours after the procedure, with a prescription for acetaminophen to use as an analgesic.

Sphincter dilation has fallen into disfavor in the United States in recent decades, because anal incontinence may result in the small percentage of patients in whom dilation is performed too forcefully.

LATERAL INTERNAL SPHINCTEROTOMY   Lateral internal sphincterotomy is currently the procedure of choice for the operative treatment of anal fissures. The procedure involves division of a portion of the internal anal sphincter in the 3 o'clock or the 9 o'clock position. The success rate for healing of fissures is 92% to 98%.

Lateral internal sphincterotomy requires no preoperative bowel preparation and can be performed under local or regional anesthesia. The patient is positioned in prone jack-knife position, and a 3-cm lateral circumferential incision is made to approach the internal sphincter. The intersphincteric plane is identified by palpating the depression between the internal and external sphincters, and this plane is opened by dissection with scissors. The internal sphincter is then divided up to the dentate line, and the skin wound is left open.

Patients who undergo lateral internal sphincterotomy can be discharged on the day of the operation. They should receive a prescription for bulk laxatives and nonconstipating analgesics. Further follow-up is unnecessary unless symptoms recur.

While some impairment of anal continence for flatus and liquids may occur after the procedure, this problem is nearly always temporary. Other potential complications include hematoma for-

mation and low anal fistulas, but both are exceedingly rare.

Errors

Probably the most common errors in the management of anal fissures are failure to examine for anal fissures, inappropriate performance of rectal examinations, and failure to consider the diagnosis of Crohn's disease.

FAILURE TO EXAMINE FOR ANAL FISSURES

Some clinicians assume that hemorrhoids are the cause of a patient's rectal pain or bleeding and overlook or even fail to examine a patient for the possibility that bleeding is caused by an anal fissure. This error leads to unnecessary treatments of hemorrhoids and delay in relieving a patient's pain.

INAPPROPRIATE RECTAL EXAMINATIONS

As noted earlier, digital rectal and anoscopic examinations are generally not appropriate for patients with acute, painful anal fissures. In addition to exacerbating pain, such examinations cause anal distention and may worsen the anodermal defect of the fissure. If these patients require examinations such as anoscopy or colonoscopy, sedation or examination under anesthesia should be considered.

FAILURE TO CONSIDER CROHN'S DISEASE

Some clinicians assume that all anal fissures are caused by constipation and fail to consider the possibility that they may be caused by Crohn's disease, thereby delaying the diagnosis of inflammatory bowel disease. As discussed, clinicians should always consider the possibility of Crohn's disease when patients have fissures in atypical locations, fissures that are painless or have an atypical appearance, or fissures that do not respond to usual therapy.

Anal Fistulas

An anal fistula is a granulating sinus tract that connects the anal mucosa to the perineum. Most are caused by infection, but the presence of an anal fistula may also indicate the presence of Crohn's disease.

Pathophysiology

There is overwhelming evidence that common anal fistulas are the result of pyogenic infections in the anal glands and the lymphatic system draining those glands. Once an anal gland has become infected, a small abscess is formed in the intersphincteric plane. This abscess leads to swelling and fibrosis, occluding the exit site of the anal gland at the crypt line. Unable to exit through the gland orifice, the purulent process then expands through

tissue spaces down toward the perineum, or less commonly, upward or laterally, leading to formation of perianal abscesses or fistulas. However, while most fistulas occur as a result of an abscess, not all abscesses are complicated by a fistula.

Anorectal abscesses occur in different spaces with different frequency (Fig. 6-11). Because of this, fistulas can take a myriad of courses and have unpredictable exit sites on the perianal skin.

Epidemiology

While most primary-care clinicians will encounter only a few anorectal fistulas over the course of their career, they are commonly seen in general surgical practice. There is a male dominance of about 5 to 1 in most reported series. Affected patients are usually between 30 and 60 years of age. Recent studies indicate that anal fistulas and abscesses are more frequent in persons infected with the human immunodeficiency virus.

Figure 6-11

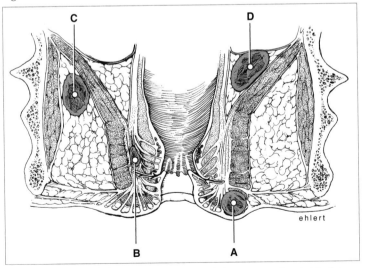

Locations of anorectal abscesses. Most anorectal abscesses are located in the perianal area or intersphincteric areas, shown in this figure as **(A)** and **(B)**, respectively. Anorectal abscesses may be associated with anal fistulas. Other locations for perirectal abscesses include the ischiorectal **(C)** and supralevator **(D)** areas.

Typical Presentation

Patients with anal fistulas commonly have a history of anorectal abscesses or repeated episodes of perirectal sepsis requiring surgical drainage, and the development of a fistula is often preceded by episodes of pain and perianal swelling from an abscess. However, not all patients with anorectal abscesses and fistulas are aware that they have an infection, and the most frequent presenting complaint of patient with an anal fistula is anal discharge of fecal or mucous material.

Anal fistulas and abscesses may be confused with perianal hidradenitis or pilonidal sinus infections. Hidradenitis can be diagnosed by culturing gram-positive organisms from the fistula/abscess drainage. Pilonidal sinuses can be distinguished from an anal fistula by the fact that pilonidal sinuses characteristically drain into the posterior midline, whereas fistulous openings may occur anywhere around the anus.

Key History

Patients with known or suspected anal fistulas should be asked about recent episodes of perianal discharge and whether there have been previous fistula operations or drainage procedures for abscesses.

Patients with a history of anal fistulas, especially those with multiple fistulas caused by Crohn's disease, have often suffered considerable damage to their anal sphincter apparatus if multiple fistulotomies were performed in the past. Therefore, the history should include an assessment of the patient's anal continence.

Key Physical Examination

Inspection of the perianal region will usually demonstrate an external opening and occasionally some perianal excoriation. During inspection, the clinician may notice the presence of scarring from previous surgical drainage operations. Absence of

an external opening, however, does exclude the presence of an anal fistula because in about 20% of fistulas, an external opening cannot be identified on clinical examination.

When fistulas are chronic, the fistulous tract may become fibrotic, in which case it is easily detected by palpation. Subsequent anoscopy provides an opportunity to inspect the anal crypts, in which a bead of pus can characteristically be seen emerging from the internal opening of a fistula.

Attention should be paid to identifying additional external openings of fistulas that may be located at a distance from the anus. In rare cases, they have been located as far away as the iliac crest. Examination for distant fistulous openings is important because if they are not identified during the office evaluation, they may also be overlooked during subsequent examinations under anesthesia, when only the perianal area may remain undraped.

Attempts at passing probes during the examination in the office are strongly discouraged. Not only is probing exquisitely unpleasant for the patient, there is also a risk that the probe might create additional fistulas.

Ancillary Tests

For most common anal fistulas, additional tests are unnecessary, and the diagnosis can be made based on history, physical examination, and, sometimes, examination under anesthesia. However, when patients have complex and recurrent fistulas, particularly those that have undergone previous operative treatment, imaging techniques may be needed to identify the number and course of fistulas. Imaging tests are also needed when Crohn's disease is suspected.

Appropriate imaging techniques include contrast fistulography and intraanal and perianal ultrasound. Because the accuracy of these tests depends very much on the examining radiologist, results need to be discussed in detail between the surgeon and radiologist, and radiologic findings should be correlated with findings on physical examination. Contrast imaging or ultrasound examinations are not appropriate as routine diagnostic procedures before referring the patient to a surgeon.

Treatment

Treatment, as outlined in Fig. 6-12, should be performed only by a surgeon experienced in management of anal fistulas. Fistulotomy (i.e., the surgical opening of the fistulous tract) can be performed as a primary procedure or a delayed procedure. If the anal fistula was preceded by formation of an anal abscess, fistulotomy should not be performed during the drainage procedure for the abscess, because such "primary fistulotomy" may lead to inferior functional results (i.e., impaired continence). Such patients should be advised at the time of abscess drainage that they will require a second-stage fistulotomy procedure

several weeks after the incision and drainage of the abscess.

PROCEDURE

When fistulotomy is performed, preoperative preparation for the fistulotomy involves administration of an enema. The fistulotomy is then performed under general anesthesia. Fistulous tracts that run below the anorectal ring are treated simply by identifying the fistulous tract using probes and laying the tract open. Fistulous tracts that run outside the external anal sphincter or near the anorectal ring require external drainage and fistulectomy with closure of the defect in the gut.

Sometimes during surgery, complex fistulous tracts cannot be identified by probing alone. In this situation, it is useful to use methylene blue–stained milk as a contrast agent to identify the course of the fistula. Surgically created external

Figure 6-12

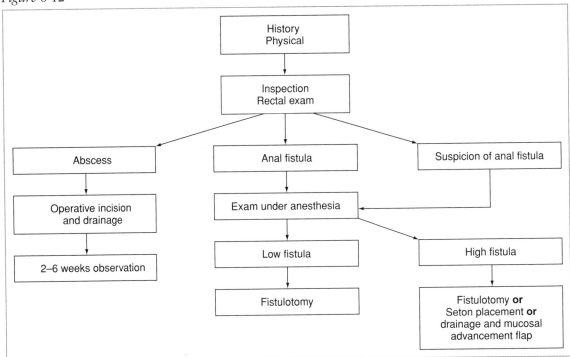

Algorithm for diagnosis and treatment of anal fistulas.

drainage wounds are deliberately conical to facilitate healing from within outward, thereby preventing the pocketing of pus. The wound cavities are initially gently packed with gauze.

POSTOPERATIVE CARE

External drainage wounds are allowed to heal by secondary intention. The packing is removed after 48 hours, and patients instructed to use the head of a shower hose to cleanse the granulating area twice daily and after every bowel movement. It is essential that the surgeon inspect the wound regularly. The wounds should remain clean, and the pocketing of pus or the bridging of skin must be prevented.

Gross incontinence following a correctly performed fistulotomy is exceedingly rare. A temporary, minor decrease in continence function, on the other hand, is relatively common. Reassurance of the patient and follow-up visits with the treating surgeon are important during the postoperative period. The patient needs to be aware of the fact that healing of the perianal wounds can take several weeks and sometimes a few months.

Errors

It is essential that clinicians avoid the error of inserting probes into anal fistulas during an office examination because, as noted earlier, probing may result in creating additional fistulous tracts. It may also be painful. A second potential error is the failure to consider Crohn's disease as the cause of an anal fistula.

References

Brisinda G, Maria G, Bentivoglio R, et al: A comparison of injections of botulinum toxin and topical nitroglycerin ointment for the treatment of chronic anal fissure. *N Engl J Med* 341:65, 1999.

Delco F, Sonnenberg A: Associations between hemorrhoids and other diagnoses. *Dis Colon Rectum* 41:1534, 1998.

Ho YH, Lee J, Salleh I, et al: Randomized controlled trial comparing same-day discharge with hospital stay following haemorrhoidectomy. *Aust N Z J Surg* 68:443, 1998.

Ho YH, Seow-Choen F, Tan M, Leong AF: Randomized controlled trial of open and closed haemorrhoidectomy. *Br J Surg* 84:1729, 1997.

Ibrahim S, Tsang C, Lee YL, et al: Prospective, randomized trial comparing pain and complications between diathermy and scissors for closed hemorrhoidectomy. *Dis Colon Rectum* 41:1418, 1998.

Johanson JF, Sonnenberg A: The prevalence of hemorrhoids and chronic constipation. An epidemiologic study. *Gastroenterology* 98:380, 1990.

Keighley MRB, Williams NS: *Surgery of the Anus, Rectum and Colon*, 1st ed. London, WB Saunders, 1993.

Klosterhalfen B: Anatomic nature and surgical significance of anal sinus and anal intramuscular glands. *Dis Colon Rectum* 34:156, 1991.

Kunimoto M, Nishi M, Sasaki K: The relation between irregular bowel movement and the lifestyle of working women. *Hepatogastroenterology* 45:956, 1998.

Lacerda-Filho A, Cunha-Melo JR: Outpatient haemorrhoidectomy under local anaesthesia. *Eur J Surg* 163:935, 1997.

MacRae HM, McLeod RS: Comparison of hemorrhoidal treatment modalities. A meta-analysis. *Dis Colon Rectum* 38:687, 1995.

Sadahiro S, Mukai M, Tokunaga N, et al: *Gastrointest Endosc* 48:272, 1998

Savioz D, Roche B, Glauser T, et al: Rubber-band ligation of hemorrhoids: relapse as a function of time. *Int J Colorectal Dis* 13:154, 1998.

Stelzner F: Hemorrhoidectomy—a simple operation? Incontinence, stenosis, fistula, infection and fatalities. *Chirurg* 63:316, 1992.

Trowers EA, Ganga U, Rizk R, et al: Endoscopic hemorrhoidal ligation: preliminary clinical experience. *Gastrointest Endosc* 48:49, 1998.

Wesselmann U, Burnett AL, Heinberg LJ: The urogenital and rectal pain syndromes. *Pain* 73:269, 1997.

Whitehead WE: Functional anorectal disorders. *Semin Gastrointest Dis* 7:230, 1996.

Wrobleski DE: Long-term evaluation of rubber-ring ligation in hemorrhoidal disease. *Dis Colon Rectum* 23:478, 1980.

Yuhan R, Orsay C, DelPino, et al: Anorectal disease in HIV-infected patients. *Dis Colon Rectum* 41:1367, 1998.

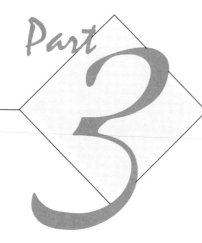

Part 3

Oral and Nasal Problems

Todd G. Dray

Chapter 7

Peritonsillar Abscess

Introduction

Peritonsillar abscess, also referred to as "quinsy," is an abscess that involves the deep fascial space in the neck adjacent to the tonsils. Peritonsillar abscesses are encountered more frequently than other head-and-neck abscesses, and, in fact, they have an incidence rate similar to that of dental abscesses. Peritonsillar abscesses are seen predominantly in adolescents and young adults, although they sometimes occur in children and geriatric-aged individuals.

Pathophysiology

Anatomy

The peritonsillar space is actually a potential space between the capsule of the tonsil and the

Table 7-1

Bacteria Commonly Involved in Peritonsillar Abscess

MICROORGANISM	APPROXIMATE FREQUENCY (%)
Aerobes (25%–50%)	
Group A beta-hemolytic streptococci	29–53
Streptococcus milleri	25–30
Streptococcus viridans	10–15
Haemophilus influenzae	5–11
Staphylococcus aureus	2–5
Anaerobes (48%–75%)	
Prevotella species	32–38
Peptostreptococcus species	15–27
Fusobacterium species	10–30
Bacteroides species	0–25
Actinomyces species	0–25
Arcanobacterium species	Rare

Note: Reported prevalence of various microorganisms in peritonsillar abscess varies widely in the literature. Figures reported in this table are approximations based on published reports.

superior constrictor muscle of the pharynx. The peritonsillar space communicates with the parapharyngeal space, which is itself a potential space located lateral to the superior constrictor muscle (Fig. 7-1). Peritonsillar abscesses develop when a bacterial infection in the parenchyma of the tonsil extends through the tonsillar capsule into the potential peritonsillar space, filling it with purulent exudate.

As with all deep neck–space abscesses, untreated peritonsillar abscesses may spread to other fascial spaces. While spread of peritonsillar abscess is rare in immunocompetent individuals who receive adequate treatment, when it occurs, it may result in serious complications. These complications include involvement of major vascular structures such as the carotid artery and jugular vein and, in rare cases, mediastinitis and necrotizing fasciitis.

Microbiology

Most peritonsillar abscesses are polymicrobial—generally, a mixture of anaerobic and aerobic organisms, with anaerobes predominating. Species of *Prevotella* and *Peptostreptococcus* are the most common anaerobes, while group A beta-hemolytic streptococcus and *Streptococcus milleri* are the most common aerobes (Table 7-1). Patients with peritonsillar abscesses frequently report recent oropharyngeal infections, with the incidence of such antecedent infections ranging from 11% to 56%. The microbiology of these antecedent infections is generally not determined, however, and it may be similar or dissimilar to the microbiology of the peritonsillar abscess.

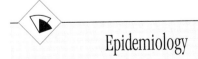

Epidemiology

The overall incidence rate for peritonsillar abscess is approximately 30 per 100,000 persons per year for individuals between 5 and 59 years of age, with a total of about 45,000 cases annually

Figure 7-1

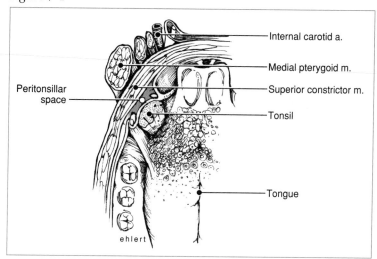

Internal carotid a.

Medial pterygoid m.

Superior constrictor m.

Peritonsillar space

Tonsil

Tongue

ehlert

Anatomy of peritonsillar abscess. The peritonsillar space is actually a "potential" space in which purulent material collects in peritonsillar abscess. Note the peritonsillar space is adjacent to other structures, including the parapharyngeal space, the medial pterygoid muscle, and the superior constrictor muscle. Inadequately treated peritonsillar abscesses can spread to these other structures.

in the United States. The typical primary-care physician seeing about 6000 patient-visits per year will therefore encounter the condition infrequently. However, the incidence of peritonsillar abscess may be rising, related to the recent decrease in the rate of tonsillectomies, but no good data are available to support this possibility. Death from peritonsillar abscess is rare in immunocompetent individuals, with mortality rates well below 1%.

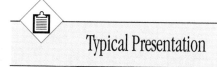

Typical Presentation

Patients with peritonsillar abscess typically present to clinicians with complaints of fever, sore throat, and trismus (painful opening of the mouth). Fever can be low grade, but the temperature is more typically elevated to 102° to 104°F. Sore throat is often severe and accompanied by extreme difficulty swallowing and, sometimes, drooling because of the difficulty swallowing oral secretions. Most patients also describe ipsilateral ear pain.

Patients diagnosed with peritonsillar abscess typically report having developed a sore throat 3 to 7 days prior to seeking medical care for the abscess. It is unusual for a peritonsillar abscess to exist when sore throat has been present for a shorter period, as several days are needed for loculation of pus to develop in the peritonsillar space. Over the 3 to 7 days, patients often report progressively worsening pain, even if antibiotics were prescribed when the sore throat began. Because of the painful swallowing, patients' food and fluid intake has often been decreased in the days prior to seeking medical care.

In very young children such as those under 5 years, the symptoms may be less clear-cut. The most common presentation in this age group is high fever, poor oral intake, drooling, and, if the child is able to describe it, trismus.

Key History

When taking a history from patients with suspected peritonsillar abscess, questions can be grouped into three categories. The first category contains questions suggesting the diagnosis—that is, whether the patient has a peritonsillar abscess. The second contains questions regarding the degree of toxicity of the patient. The third category contains questions regarding whether airway compromise might be present.

Questions Suggesting the Diagnosis of Peritonsillar Abscess

Clinicians should first ask questions to determine if patients have symptoms suggestive of peritonsillar abscess. These questions are shown in Table 7-2. While throat pain and difficulty swallowing are almost always present, the key to the diagnosis is the presence of trismus, as peritonsillar abscesses rarely exist in the absence of trismus.

Questions Indicating the Degree of Toxicity

Questions about the degree of toxicity are important because toxicity is common in peritonsillar abscess and, if present, it corroborates the diagnosis. Furthermore, the degree of toxicity provides an indication of the severity of systemic illness and concomitant dehydration. Thus, clinicians should ask about the presence of fever or chills, the amount of oral fluid intake over the preceding 24 hours, and the presence of light-headedness or orthostatic dizziness.

Questions Regarding Airway Compromise

Although life-threatening airway symptoms are unusual in straightforward peritonsillar abscess,

Table 7-2

Useful Questions for Patients with Suspected Peritonsillar Abscess

QUESTION	USUAL RESPONSE/FREQUENCY WITH PERITONSILLAR ABSCESS
How long has the throat pain been present and has it progressively worsened?	Progressive worsening over 3–7 days is the norm. Peritonsillar abscess is unlikely with shorter duration of throat pain.
Is the throat pain diffuse or is it localized to one side?	Throat pain is typically diffuse, though may be worse on one side. Isolated unilateral pharyngeal findings suggest peritonsillar cellulitis.
Is it painful to swallow (odynophagia)?	Very common in peritonsillar abscess, but also occurs with severe pharyngotonsillitis in the absence of abscess.
Is it painful to open and close the mouth?	Painful opening of the mouth (trismus) is almost always present in peritonsillar abscess.
Has the voice changed to a "hot potato voice?"	Typically occurs in peritonsillar abscess, but may also occurs with severe pharyngotonsillitis in the absence of abscess.
Is ear pain (otalgia) present?	Common.
Have there been any previous peritonsillar abscess or recurrent tonsillitis episodes?	Suggests increased risk of peritonsillar abscess.

clinicians should always ask about them. A few simple questions concerning difficulty breathing or shortness of breath are usually sufficient. If the patient reports difficulty breathing, it is useful to know if the difficulty occurs in the upright or supine position, as patients with peritonsillar abscess have more difficulty breathing when supine. Such individuals can be positioned upright to lessen symptoms.

Key Physical Examination

As with the history, physical examination is directed at diagnosing peritonsillar abscess, estimating the degree of toxicity and dehydration, and assessing adequacy of the airway.

Physical Findings Indicative of Peritonsillar Abscess

Peritonsillar abscess is diagnosed with an examination of the throat. There is typically a triad of findings, which are as follows: (1) unilateral enlargement of the tonsil toward the midline, referred to as "medialization" of the tonsil; (2) unilateral, soft-palate fullness or fluctuance; and (3) deviation of the uvula away from the side of the abscess. These findings are emphasized in Table 7-3 and illustrated in Figure 7-2. In rare instances, bilateral peritonsillar abscesses may be present, and they represent a threat to the airway.

Table 7-3

Diagnostic Triad of Physical Findings in Peritonsillar Abscess

Unilateral, medialized tonsil
Soft-palate fullness
Deviated uvula

Figure 7-2

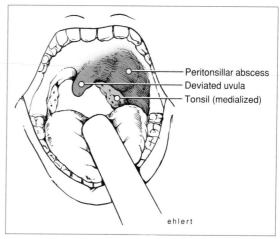

Clinical appearance of peritonsillar abscess. The patient's left tonsil is enlarged and "medialized," the adjacent soft palate is inflamed and full, and the uvula is deviated away from the abscess.

Tonsillar exudate and inflammation associated with soft-palate erythema (unilateral or bilateral), but without unilateral medialization of the tonsil and deviation of the uvula, indicate peritonsillar cellulitis rather than abscess. This is especially true if trismus is absent.

In addition to examining the throat, clinicians should also examine the ears and neck of patients with suspected peritonsillar abscess. The ears are examined to diagnose or exclude a coexisting otitis media. The neck is examined to detect the unilaterally enlarged and tender jugulodigastric (anterior cervical) lymph nodes that are usually present on the same side as the abscess.

Physical Findings Indicating Toxicity or Airway Compromise

Objective measurement of toxicity relies on the vital signs. Tachycardia correlates well with degree of toxicity. Significant tachycardia (heart rate >120 beats per minute) or orthostatic hypotension suggests more marked toxicity and dehydration and generally indicate the need for hospital admission, intravenous hydration, and parenteral antibiotics.

Findings suggestive of airway compromise include stridor, wheezing, tachypnea, and an anxious appearance because of dyspnea. The voice may be changed, with either a "hot potato" voice or muffling of the voice, but these changes do not specifically indicate airway compromise. Rather, such voice changes are common in peritonsillar abscess and are simply caused by the increased bulk of the tonsils and soft palate.

Ancillary Tests

The diagnosis of peritonsillar abscess relies on history and physical examination. In most cases, laboratory tests add little to the diagnosis or evaluation of patients.

Throat Culture

When evaluating a patient with a peritonsillar abscess, many physicians obtain a throat culture to exclude group A beta-hemolytic streptococcal pharyngitis. Such cultures add little to diagnosis and management, however, because the microbiology of peritonsillar abscess dictates that all patients are treated with antibiotics, and the recommended antibiotics all have antistreptococcal activity.

Culture and Sensitivity of Abscess Fluid

Culture and sensitivity of purulent fluid aspirated or drained from a peritonsillar abscess are not necessary unless the patient is immunocompromised, because in immunocompetent individuals the infection is almost always polymicrobial, and

the causative organisms can be reliably predicted (Table 7-1). Furthermore, clinical series have demonstrated that obtaining a culture of peritonsillar abscess fluid does not influence the outcome for patients.

Blood Tests

Complete blood counts are often obtained, but they usually do not aid in diagnosis, although the leukocyte count is sometimes useful as an indicator of severity of infection in hospitalized patients. Blood cultures should be obtained if there is suspicion of bacteremia or sepsis. In some cases testing for infectious mononucleosis (acute Epstein-Barr virus infection) is in order, as this infection may precede development of the abscess and may explain a longer-than-usual persistence of malaise and fatigue following treatment of the abscess.

Other Tests

Other testing is appropriate if the diagnosis is in question, if other head and neck abscesses are suspected, or if there is concern that pharyngotonsillar enlargement is caused by a malignancy. Recent reports suggest that intraoral ultrasound can detect abscesses in the peritonsillar space if the volume of pus exceeds 10% of the inflamed and indurated area. Computerized tomography (CT) is useful for identifying a peritonsillar abscess in very young children (under 5 years of age).

Peritonsillar abscess is unusual in older patients, and malignancy should be suspected in older patients with a history of tobacco use whose pharyngotonsillar enlargement is not accompanied by symptoms or signs of toxicity. The malignancies can be primary head-and-neck cancers or metastatic cancers from other organs (e.g., renal cell carcinoma). The most useful test for excluding malignancy is flexible fiberoptic nasopharyngoscopy with biopsy, and the best test for excluding sites of abscess is CT scanning.

Algorithm

The algorithm in Figure 7-3 shows that the diagnosis of peritonsillar abscess depends on the history and physical examination and especially on the triad of physical findings described earlier (Table 7-3). If peritonsillar abscess is present, antibiotics should be prescribed, and the abscess should be drained, usually with needle aspiration. Details of management, as outlined in the algorithm, depend on whether the patient is toxic or dehydrated and on whether the patient is immunocompromised.

Figure 7-3

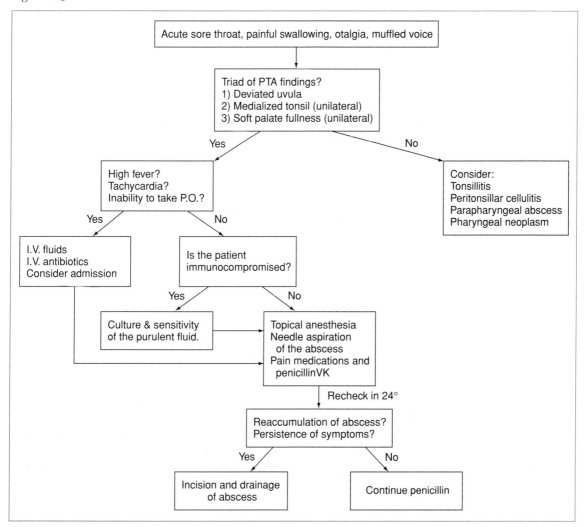

Algorithm for diagnosis and management of peritonsillar abscess (PTA).

Treatment

Standard treatment for peritonsillar abscesses involves antibiotic therapy *and* drainage of the purulent abscess fluid. Because of the possibility that the infection may spread through fascial planes to adjacent structures in the neck, relying solely on antibiotic therapy is not appropriate.

Antibiotics

Most authorities indicate that the antibiotic of choice is penicillin. Penicillin provides effective coverage for both group A beta-hemolytic streptococcus and the anaerobes commonly involved in peritonsillar abscesses. Broad-spectrum antibiotics such as sulbactam-ampicillin and others have not been shown to offer any advantage over penicillin.

Penicillin can be administered orally as penicillin V; the dose for adolescents and young adults is 500 mg four times per day. For patients who are toxic, unable to tolerate oral medications, and/or require hospitalization, intravenous penicillin G is the appropriate antibiotic. Clindamycin is a suitable alternative for patients who are allergic to penicillin. Some experts recommend that metronidazole be administered along with penicillin, especially if the clinical response to penicillin is not satisfactory.

Drainage of the Abscess

In the early 1900s, abscess tonsillectomy (i.e., removal of the tonsil during the acute phase of the abscess) was advocated as the preferred treatment for peritonsillar abscess. However, relying on abscess tonsillectomy resulted in delay of effective treatment. The procedure also carried risk and, in today's medical economic climate, is expensive. Consequently, other forms of drainage were popularized.

Two methods are currently used to drain peritonsillar abscesses: the first is needle aspiration; the second is surgical incision and drainage. While incision and drainage has been the most common technique of abscess drainage used in the United States, there has been controversy about whether this technique is superior to simple needle aspiration of the abscess. A recent comprehensive study of peritonsillar abscesses reported that abscesses resolve in 94% to 96% of patients who undergo needle aspiration as the initial and only method of abscess drainage (though occasional reports describe lower success rates). In addition to being effective, needle aspiration is relatively simple, does not require special equipment, and is inexpensive compared with surgical incision and drainage. For these reasons, needle aspiration is now the preferred technique for draining a peritonsillar abscess.

TECHNIQUE OF NEEDLE ASPIRATION

Needle aspiration is straightforward and can be performed after minimal training. Topical anesthesia is required and can be administered by spraying 2% lidocaine into the oropharynx or by having the patient gargle a 4% lidocaine solution. Clinicians should inform patients that despite the use of anesthesia, a sharp pain may be noted in the throat on insertion of the needle, and that they must remain absolutely still during the procedure even if pain occurs. The area of soft-palate fullness is then aspirated with an 18-gauge needle attached to a small (5 to 10 cc) syringe (Fig. 7-4).

Other than the possibility that aspiration may not fully drain the abscess, the only important complication of needle aspiration is injury to the carotid artery—obviously a serious complication. This complication can be avoided if one keeps in mind that the carotid artery is located 2 cm laterally from the tonsil. Thus, when needle aspiration is performed correctly, the needle should be positioned in the anterior-posterior plane, and lateral progression of the needle should be avoided.

Figure 7-4

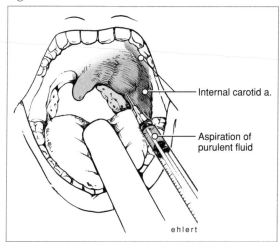

Needle aspiration of peritonsillar abscess. The needle should be of sufficient caliber (18 gauge) to permit flow of purulent material. It is inserted into the area of palatal fullness adjacent to the tonsil. The carotid artery is located 2 cm lateral to the peritonsillar space; therefore it is important to avoid lateral insertion or direction of the needle

Follow-Up Evaluation

Following needle aspiration and 24 hours of antibiotic therapy, reevaluation is mandatory. All patients whose abscesses have been adequately drained should be much improved on their 24-hour follow-up visit. Resolution of both trismus and the unilateral oropharyngeal findings indicates that abscess drainage has been successful. In these cases antibiotics should be continued for 10 days, and a follow-up evaluation at 10 to 14 days after treatment should be scheduled to confirm resolution of the infection.

If the trismus and the unilateral, soft-palate fullness are still present at the 24-hour visit, referral for incision and drainage is necessary. Incision and drainage, usually performed by an otolaryngologist, should bring dramatic improvement in symptoms. Following drainage of a large abscess (10 to 20 cc of purulent material), relief of pain is often immediate.

Long-Term Monitoring, Treatment, and Prognosis

For the majority of patients, there are no long-term problems following treatment for peritonsillar abscess. However, approximately 15% to 20% will experience a subsequent peritonsillar abscess at some point in their life. If recurrent peritonsillar abscess or recurrent tonsillitis occurs, tonsillectomy is usually recommended.

Education

Information About Cause

Patients who develop peritonsillar abscesses are usually concerned that an otherwise "normal" sore throat has turned into a severe infection, often requiring hospitalization, and that this may represent an immune-system defect. Thus, clinicians should reassure patients about the cause of peritonsillar abscess, typically by telling them that they have a bacterial infection that spread out of the tonsil and developed into a pocket of infection. It is important to emphasize that in otherwise healthy patients, peritonsillar abscess does not represent a problem with the immune system and that, with proper treatment, resolution of the infection without future recurrence is the expected outcome for the majority of patients.

Information About Needle Aspiration

Patients should understand that drainage of the abscess is important to prevent the abscess from spreading further into other areas of the head or neck and causing serious complications. They should also understand that needle aspiration is usually followed by slight oral bleeding and pain, but that serious complications (i.e., carotid artery injury) are extraordinarily rare.

Information About Self-Treatment

Patients should be aware that when being treated for peritonsillar abscess, it is important to ensure good fluid intake to maintain hydration. Depending on the degree of throat pain, a soft, solid diet or a liquid diet may be needed. Fevers can be controlled with acetaminophen.

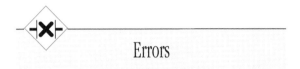

Errors

Physicians make two common errors in diagnosis and treatment of peritonsillar abscess. One involves inaccurate diagnosis, and the other involves inappropriate treatment.

Inaccurate Diagnosis

Otolaryngologists report that many patients referred to them by other physicians for treatment of a peritonsillar abscess do not, in fact, have a peritonsillar abscess—that is, there has been a false-positive diagnosis. This error can be avoided by focusing the diagnosis on the timing of symptoms, the presence of trismus, and the triad of oropharyngeal findings (Table 7-3). Occasionally, the diagnosis may be in doubt despite attention to these key diagnostic features. When this occurs, the clinician can perform a diagnostic needle aspiration to confirm or exclude the presence of abscess.

Inappropriate Treatment

Some clinicians opt for a "trial of antibiotics" to see if patients with suspected peritonsillar abscess

will improve without the need for abscess drainage. This approach to treatment is inappropriate, as it increases the risk that infection will spread to adjacent structures and spaces. Treatment of peritonsillar abscess always requires drainage of the abscess either by needle aspiration or by incision and drainage.

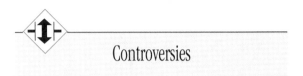

Controversies

The principal controversies in the management of patients with peritonsillar abscess are whether and when a tonsillectomy should be performed. Most otolaryngologists agree that tonsillectomy is necessary in children not able to undergo a local drainage procedure (i.e., needle aspiration or incision and drainage) and in patients for whom these procedures fail to resolve the abscess. Tonsillectomy is also widely recommended for patients who develop recurrent peritonsillar abscesses, although the procedure is typically performed after the (acute) recurrent infection has resolved. Interestingly, there are reports of peritonsillar abscess following tonsillectomy.

There is more controversy about performing a tonsillectomy as treatment for acute peritonsillar abscesses. A substantial minority of otolaryngologists recommend tonsillectomy during the acute phase of peritonsillar abscess, but this approach is more expensive than local drainage techniques, and it probably delays adequate drainage of the abscess. Others recommend routine tonsillectomy following an acute peritonsillar abscess, but only after the acute abscess has subsided. This approach may lack rationale, particularly in children, for whom the recurrence of peritonsillar abscess without tonsillectomy may be as low as 15% over many years. The majority of otolaryngologists do not perform tonsillectomy either during or after an acute peritonsillar abscess, unless the patient has experienced a recurrent abscess.

Emerging Concepts

Although incision and drainage is currently the most common initial procedure performed for drainage of peritonsillar abscess, the evidence cited earlier indicates that needle aspiration yields comparable satisfactory results. Thus, the major emerging concept in managing peritonsillar abscess is that the abscess can be adequately treated by needle aspiration, with incision and drainage reserved only for the small percentage of patients for whom needle aspiration does not result in adequate abscess drainage.

References

Apostolopoulos NJ, Nikolopoulos TP, Bairamis TN: Peritonsillar abscess in children. Is incision and drainage an effective management? *Int J Pediatr Otorhinolaryngol* 31:129, 1995.

Bonding P: Tonsillectomy a chaud. *J Laryngol Otol* 87:1171, 1970.

Brook I, Frazier EH, Thompson DH: Aerobic and anaerobic microbiology of peritonsillar abscess. *Laryngoscope* 101:289, 1991.

Cannon CR, Lampton LM: Peritonsillar abscess following tonsillectomy. *J Miss State Med Assoc* 37:577, 1996.

Friedman NR, Mitchell RB, Periera KD, et al: Peritonsillar abscess in early childhood. Presentation and management. *Arch Otolaryngol Head Neck Surg* 123:630, 1997.

Green KM, Pantelides E, de Carpentier JP: Tonsillar metastasis from a renal cell carcinoma presenting as a quinsy. *J Laryngol Otol* 111:379, 1997.

Greinwald JH Jr, Wilson JF, Haggerty PG: Peritonsillar abscess: an unlikely cause of necrotizing fasciitis. *Ann Otol Rhinol Laryngol* 104:133, 1995.

Herzon FS: Peritonsillar abscess: incidence, current management practices, and a proposal for treatment guidelines. *Laryngoscope* 105:1, 1995.

Herzon FS: Permucosal needle drainage of peritonsillar abscesses — a five year experience. *Arch Otolaryngol Head Neck Surg* 110:104, 1984.

Jousimies-Somer H, Savolainen S, Makitie A, Ylikoski J: Bacteriologic findings in peritonsillar abscesses in young adults. *Clin Infect Dis* 16 (suppl 4):S292, 1993.

Kerzon FS: Harris P Mosher Award thesis. Peritonsillar abscess: incidence, current management practices, and a proposal for treatment guidelines. *Laryngoscope* 105(suppl 74):1, 1995.

Kew J, Ahuja A, Loftus WK, et al: Peritonsillar abscess appearance on intra-oral ultrasonography. *Clin Radiol* 53:143, 1998.

Kieff DA, Bhattacharyya N, Siegel NS, Salman SD: Selection of antibiotics after incision and drainage of peritonsillar abscesses. *Otolaryngol Head Neck Surg* 120:57, 1999.

Lilja M, Raianen S, Jokinen K, Stenfors LE: Direct microscopy of effusions obtained from peritonsillar abscesses as a complement to bacterial culturing. *J Laryngol Otol* 111:392, 1997.

Mitchelmore IJ, Prior AJ, Montgomery PQ, Tabaqchali S: Microbiological features and pathogenesis of peritonsillar abscesses. *Eur J Cin Microbiol Infect Dis* 14:870, 1995.

Nielsen TR, Clement F, Andreassen UK: Mediastinitis—a rare complication of a peritonsillar abscess. *J Laryngol Otol* 110:175, 1996.

Ophir D, Bawnik J, Poria Y, et al: Peritonsillar abscess — a prospective evaluation of outpatient management by needle aspiration. *Arch Otolaryngol Head Neck Surg* 114:661, 1988.

Prior A, Montgomery P, Mitchelmore I, Tabaqchali S: The microbiology and antibiotic treatment of peritonsillar abscesses. *Clin Otolaryngol* 20:219, 1995.

Szuhay G, Tewfik TL: Peritonsillar abscess or cellulitis? A clinical comparative paediatric study. *J Otolaryngol* 27:206, 1998.

Wolf M, Even-Chen I, Kronenberg J: Peritonsillar abscess: repeated needle aspiration versus incision and drainage. *Ann Otol Rhinol Laryngol* 103:554, 1994.

Yilmaz T, Unal OF, Figen G, et al: A comparison of procaine penicillin with sulbactam-ampicillin in the treatment of peritonsillar abscess. *Eur Arch Otorhinolaryngol* 255:163, 1998.

Todd G. Dray

Nasal Bleeding and Fractures

This chapter will review two common conditions involving the nose. Both of these conditions, epistaxis and nasal fractures, are common. They are generally seen as acute problems in emergency rooms, urgent-care centers, primary-care clinicians' offices, and in the offices of otolaryngologists.

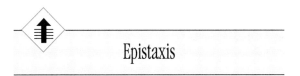

Epistaxis

Introduction

Epistaxis is bleeding that originates from the nasal mucous membranes or paranasal sinuses and is identified clinically as blood in the oropharynx and/or coming from the nares. Epistaxis is often differentiated into anterior and posterior epistaxis, based on the anatomic location or vascular system from which the bleeding originates. From a functional standpoint, however, anterior and posterior epistaxis are best differentiated by the treatment required to control bleeding. Cauterization and anterior nasal packing generally control bleeding from anterior epistaxis, while posterior nasal packing, internal maxillary artery ligation, embolization, or other measures are used to stop posterior epistaxis.

Pathophysiology

About 90% of epistaxis originates from Kiesselbach's plexus, a rich network of anastamotic blood vessels located on the anterior nasal septum. Vessels in Kiesselbach's plexus link the anterior ethmoidal, superior labial, sphenopalatine, and greater palatine arteries (Fig. 8-1). The remaining 10% of epistaxis originates from vessels, vascular abnormalities, or neoplasms in other portions of the nasal mucous membrane or the paranasal sinuses.

Any condition causing turbulent nasal airflow, which dries and traumatizes the nasal mucosa, or

which causes elevated vascular pressures, predisposes to epistaxis. The major etiologies of epistaxis may be categorized as local, systemic, hematologic, or genetic.

Local factors include mechanical trauma; neoplasms; or inflammation caused by upper respiratory infections, allergic rhinitis, chemical irritants (e.g., cocaine), or intranasal foreign bodies. Systemic disorders include coagulopathy related to renal or liver disease, atherosclerotic disease (which causes fragile blood vessels), and hypertension. Epistaxis caused by hematologic disorders occurs in conditions causing thrombocytopenia or platelet dysfunction such as idiopathic thrombocytopenic purpura. Platelet dysfunction also may be caused by medications such as aspirin, which more than doubles the relative risk of hospitalization for epistaxis. The most common genetic disorder responsible for epistaxis is Osler-Rendu-Weber disease, also known as hereditary hemorrhagic telangiectasia, in which patients have numerous telangiectasias of the nasal and oral mucous membranes. These telangiectasias are fragile and susceptible to rupture, and when nasal mucous membranes are involved, epistaxis occurs.

Epidemiology

Approximately 10% of the population of the United States will have at least one episode of epistaxis in their lifetime. While epistaxis can occur in children and adults of any age, men in the fifth decade of life are the group most commonly affected. Children with perennial allergic rhinitis are another frequently affected group. Epistaxis occurs more commonly during the winter, when the temperature and humidity fall, leading to dryness and inflammation of the nasal mucous membranes.

Typical Presentation

Patients who present with epistaxis have often experienced recurrent or minor episodes of nasal

Figure 8-1

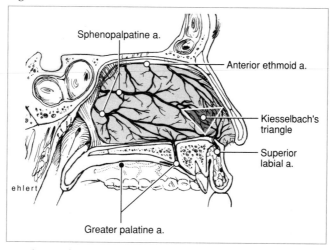

Sagital view of the nasal septal blood supply. The anterior ethmoidal, superior labial, sphenopalatine, and greater palatine arteries converge in an anastamotic network in an area of the anterior septum known as Kiesselbach's triangle.

bleeding in the past. Nonetheless, patients seeking medical care for epistaxis are often anxious, even if the bleeding is of low volume. In fact, anxiety is of such a degree that many patients, even those who do not have chronic hypertension, are hypertensive at the time of presentation for epistaxis.

As noted earlier, the site of bleeding in 90% of patients is Kiesselbach's plexus in the anterior nasal septum. In the vast majority of cases, bleeding is unilateral, and patients usually report that bleeding began with drainage of blood from one nostril. Even with a unilateral bleeding site, however, it will often become bilateral if the bleeding persists. This is because the nostril on the affected side becomes occluded with coagulated blood, and blood then enters the opposite nasal cavity through the nasopharynx.

Rarely, patients will present with profuse bleeding and demonstrate signs and symptoms of hypovolemia such as pallor, diaphoresis, lightheadedness, tachycardia, and hypotension. These patients may be critically ill, requiring fluid resuscitation and management in an intensive-care unit. Patients with severe epistaxis and hemodynamic instability may have bleeding from a site other than the anterior nasal septum—typically from the posterior part of the nasal chamber.

Key History

When taking a history from patients with epistaxis, clinicians should ask questions to determine if the patient is hemodynamically stable, if there are underlying conditions contributing to epistaxis, and to identify the site of bleeding.

QUESTIONS TO ASSESS HEMODYNAMIC STABILITY

If patients have profuse epistaxis, initial history should be directed at detecting hemodynamic instability. Specifically, clinicians should ask about the duration and amount of bleeding and about symptoms of lightheadedness, shortness of breath, or angina pectoris. Obviously, if the patient is overtly unstable, resuscitation and efforts to control the bleeding should take precedence over history taking. If necessary, history may be obtained from members of the patient's family.

QUESTIONS TO DETECT UNDERLYING MEDICAL CONDITIONS

The next line of questioning should be directed at detecting underlying conditions that might be causing or aggravating epistaxis. These include hypertension, renal or liver disease, and the other conditions noted above. In addition, clinicians should ask about use of medications that may predispose to bleeding such as coumadin, aspirin, or nonsteroidal antiinflammatory drugs. However, the occurrence of epistaxis does not necessarily contraindicate continued use of such drugs, including coumadin, as small case series have demonstrated that with appropriate indication for and monitoring of coumadin therapy, the drug can be safely continued in patients who have had episodes of epistaxis.

It is also important to ask about symptoms suggesting the possibility of a neoplasm or intranasal infection. Such symptoms include unilateral nasal pain, chronic nasal obstruction or drainage, and diplopia.

QUESTIONS TO IDENTIFY THE SITE OF BLEEDING

Two items in the history are particularly useful for identifying the site of bleeding. The first is to ascertain the side on which the bleeding started, as this is usually the side of the bleeding site. The second is to determine if the patient was upright (i.e., sitting or standing) when the bleeding began and, if so, whether blood first flowed through the nose or into the throat. If the first sensation of bleeding was into the throat, the possibility of a posterior bleeding site is increased.

It is also helpful to ask patients about any history of previous epistaxis or nasal surgery. Because epistaxis is often recurrent, this information may provide clues about the site of the present episode of bleeding.

Key Physical Examination

Physical examination of patients with epistaxis has the same objectives as the history—assessment of hemodynamic stability, detection of underlying conditions that predispose to epistaxis, and identification of the site of nasal bleeding.

ASSESSING HEMODYNAMIC STATUS

Measurement of vital signs is usually sufficient to assess hemodynamic status, although in some cases it is useful to check for orthostatic hypotension by measuring blood pressure and pulse in the supine and upright positions. As noted earlier, many patients with acute nasal bleeding will be hypertensive when they present for care.

DETECTING UNDERLYING MEDICAL CONDITIONS

Assuming the patient is hemodynamically stable, the clinician should perform a brief examination of the skin to detect petechiae, purpura, or telangiectasias. In particular, when patients have unexplained recurrent nosebleeds, they should be carefully examined for evidence of hereditary hemorrhagic telangiectasia, as the lesions in this condition can be treated with a variety of modalities, including lasers, embolization, and surgical procedures.

The eyes should also be examined to detect proptosis, which would indicate the possibility of orbital invasion from a sinonasal neoplasm.

IDENTIFYING THE SITE OF BLEEDING

The patient should be in a comfortable sitting position, and the clinician should use a light source adequate to visualize the entire nasal cavity. Either a headlamp or a reflecting head mirror will provide sufficient lighting; an otoscope fitted with a plastic nasal speculum is not an appropriate light source. It is essential for the examiner to observe body-fluid precautions, which includes wearing gloves, protective eyewear, and a waterproof gown.

The first step in the examination is to remove clots from the nasal cavity using a Frazer suction device and bayonet forceps. The clinician should then attempt to visualize the site of bleeding by direct examination of the nasal cavity; this should occur prior to instituting measures to stop the bleeding. Visualization is facilitated by the use of a bivalve nasal speculum and a good light source, and by applying vasoconstrictive agents (phenylephrine 0.25% or cocaine 4%) to slow the bleeding. Finally, the oropharynx should be examined (with the patient upright) to assess the degree of posterior flow; in the absence of a clearly identified anterior bleeding site, significant posterior flow indicates the possibility of a posterior source of bleeding.

Ancillary Tests

Regardless of age and medical condition, hemoglobin and hematocrit levels should be performed for any patient who has severe epistaxis, defined as epistaxis requiring an emergency room visit or nasal packing. Such patients should also undergo coagulation studies, including a prothrombin time (PT), partial thromboplastin time (PTT), bleeding time and a platelet count. If the patient has an identifiable source or cause of bleeding, and if control of epistaxis is readily obtained, no further testing is necessary.

When patients have unexplained, recurrent epistaxis, additional studies should be performed to exclude nasopharyngeal or sinus neoplasms as the source of bleeding. In general, sinus x-rays and/or nasal endoscopy are the preferred tests. Computerized tomography or magnetic resonance imaging of the skull base should be performed in teenage males with severe epistaxis to exclude a juvenile nasopharyngeal angiofibroma.

Algorithm

The algorithm in Figure 8-2 outlines the approach to patients with epistaxis. For patients with active bleeding and an identifiable bleeding site, an attempt should be made to stop the bleeding with cauterization. Nasal packing is used if bleeding cannot be controlled with cauterization, or if the bleeding site cannot be identified. For patients who are not actively bleeding, an attempt should still be made to identify and treat the site of bleeding.

Treatment

MILD EPISTAXIS

For patients with mild epistaxis, the appropriate intervention is to advise patients to squeeze their nostrils together, holding firm pressure at the junction of the bony nasal dorsum and the soft, cartilaginous nasal tip for 10 to 15 minutes. In most cases, this will control the bleeding. After the bleeding has stopped, examination is performed to identify and treat the site of bleeding, as described below.

PERSISTENT OR SEVERE EPISTAXIS

If the bleeding persists following pressure, or if the bleeding is sufficiently rapid that simple nasal pressure is not appropriate, the nasal cavities should be examined as described above. Once the clots have been suctioned, any visible bleeding site on the septum or turbinate can be treated with cauterization, as described below. If the site of bleeding cannot be identified, or if the bleeding is not controlled with cauterization, nasal packing is required. Patients with severe epistaxis, or those with cardiovascular conditions in whom epistaxis causes hemodynamic instability, should be transferred to an emergency room or intensive-care unit for management.

CAUTERIZATION   Silver nitrate ($AgNO_3$) cauterization is the most common method used for controlling anterior epistaxis. Electrical cauterization can also be used to control both anterior and posterior epistaxis, but cauterization for posterior epistaxis requires endoscopic visualization.

Prior to applying $AgNO_3$, topical anesthesia (2% lidocaine) is administered. $AgNO_3$ is typically supplied on the tip of a wooden applicator. Con-

Figure 8-2

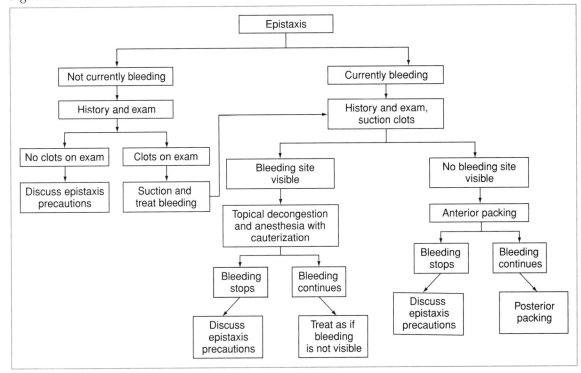

Algorithm for evaluation and treatment of epistaxis.

tact of the applicator tip with the moist nasal membranes causes dissolution of $AgNO_3$ from the applicator onto the nasal membranes. The $AgNO_3$ applicator tip is firmly applied to the bleeding site for 20 to 30 seconds. After bleeding stops, bacitracin or other antibiotic ointment should be used to cover the cauterization site for at least 5 days.

It is essential to emphasize that cauterization should not be performed on both sides of the same region of the nasal septum. Such bilateral cauterization carries a risk of causing tissue necrosis and septal perforation.

ANTERIOR NASAL PACKING   If the site of persistent epistaxis cannot be identified, or if cauterization does not control the hemorrhage, then anterior nasal packing should be performed. Adequate anesthesia of the nasal mucosa is essential before

anterior packing, and this is accomplished by inserting cotton pledglets soaked in a 4% cocaine solution or 2% lidocaine.

Vaseline gauze (¼ inch) coated with antibiotic ointment is the usual packing material. While holding the nares open with a bivalve nasal speculum, the gauze strips are packed tightly in a layered fashion from the posterior choana to the anterior nare (Fig. 8-3). A bayonet forceps is typically used for insertion of the gauze.

If anterior nasal packing cannot be accomplished with Vaseline gauze, pre-fashioned Merocel nasal packs may be used, although they are less reliable in controlling hemorrhage.

Inflatable balloon packs can also be used to control hemorrhage. They are inserted into the nasal cavity and then inflated with saline. These devices can be useful in the short term such as while preparing materials for gauze packing of the nose. Inflatable devices are a second choice to packing for definitive control of hemorrhage, because they cause internal and external nasal injury more frequently than other methods.

Regardless of the material used, packing material should be removed in 3 to 5 days, depending on the severity of the bleeding. Antibiotics (first-generation cephalosporins for antistaphylococcal coverage) are administered to lessen the risk of toxic shock syndrome from an intranasal foreign body and sinus infection from occlusion of sinus ostia by the nasal pack.

Complications of anterior packing include pain, persistent bleeding, sinusitis, displacement of the pack anteriorly or posteriorly, and toxic shock syndrome. By coating the packing material with antibiotic ointment and administering appropriate antibiotics, the risk of infection is minimized, although several cases of toxic shock syndrome have occurred despite these precautions.

POSTERIOR NASAL PACKING If epistaxis does not stop with anterior nasal packing, if anterior packing cannot be performed for anatomic (nasoseptal deviation) or technical reasons, or if the epistaxis is profusely draining into the oropharynx and is obviously posterior in origin, then a posterior nasal pack should be inserted.

Many different posterior packing techniques are available, but perhaps the most simple and effective relies on a Foley catheter to apply pressure to the sphenopalatine area. Alternative packing materials include gauze, which is technically difficult to insert, and commercially produced pneumatic (balloon) nasal catheters.

To install a Foley catheter for posterior packing, a 14-Fr Foley catheter is coated with antibiotic ointment, inserted with the balloon deflated through the nostril that is the source of bleeding, and passed into the nasopharynx. The balloon is then inflated incrementally with small volumes of saline, up to a maximum of 15 cc or until the bleeding stops, as gentle traction is placed on the catheter (Fig. 8-4A). Next, standard anterior packing is performed, maintaining the traction on the Foley catheter (Fig. 8-4B). The catheter is then secured in place with a clamp at the nasal orifice.

Patients should receive an antistaphylococcal antibiotic (e.g., first-generation cephalosporin) while the packing is in place. The nasal packing is left in place for 3 to 5 days, at which time the

Figure 8-3

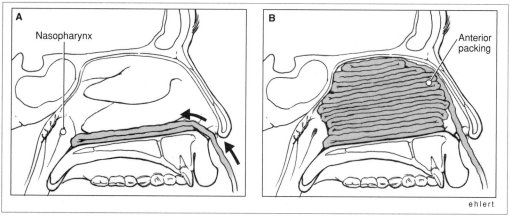

Anterial nasal packing. Approximately 72 inches of one-quarter inch Vaseline gauze is layered into the anterior nasal cavity **(A).** The initial entry and placement of the first few layers of gauze into the nasal cavity is illustrated **(B).** The anterior nasal cavity fully packed with gauze is shown.

Figure 8-4

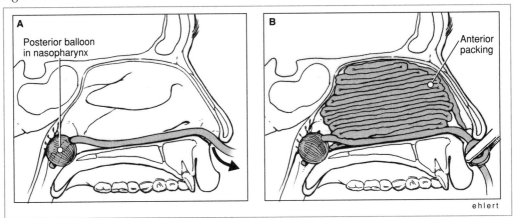

Insertion of foley catheter nasal pack **(A).** A foley catheter is inserted through nostril on the side of the bleeding. The balloon is passed into the nasopharynx and inflated **(B).** The anterior nasal packing is shown in place after installing the Foley catheter posterior pack.

posterior packing is removed first. If no bleeding occurs after removing the posterior pack, then the anterior packing may be removed.

Complications of posterior packing include those seen with anterior packing plus eustachian-tube dysfunction and difficulty swallowing. In addition, because the posterior location of the pack has the potential to interfere with airway function, some patients will experience aspiration, hypoventilation, hypoxia, and hypercapnia. Therefore, hospitalization, often with cardiac and oxygenation monitoring, is required for patients with posterior nasal packing. Patients with posterior nasal packs should also receive humidified oxygenation and medications for pain, as needed.

SPECIAL CONSIDERATIONS When epistaxis occurs in patients who have platelet deficiencies or other disorders of coagulation, nasal packing should be performed with a material that does not require removal. Use of such packing materials avoids disruption of clots at the bleeding site that might occur when standard packs are removed. These special packing materials include Gelfoam sponges, surgical Oxycel, and Avitene (microfibrillar collagen). Standard packing materials (Vaseline gauze, bal-loons) should only be used if these materials fail to control bleeding.

OTHER TREATMENTS

A variety of other procedures are available for treating patients with refractory posterior epistaxis. The long-standing standard treatment has been ligation of the internal maxillary artery, which has a success rate in the range of 90%. As described later under "Emerging Concepts," however, several newer and less-invasive procedures have become available that have success rates similar to those of internal maxillary artery ligation, but with similar or lower morbidity and cost.

Long-Term Monitoring, Treatment, and Prognosis

Patients should receive instructions about "epistaxis precautions" that should be taken in the week immediately following cauterization or unpacking. These precautions include avoidance of activities or medications that might cause recurrence of bleeding (Table 8-1), plus routine use of ointments and saline to provide moisture for the nasal mucosa.

Patients who have had posterior nasal packing should have an endoscopic nasal evaluation approximately 1 week following removal of packing. The purpose of the examination is to exclude iatrogenic complications such as synechiae, ulceration, or infection.

No long-term monitoring is required for patients who have undergone cauterization or anterior packing. The general prognosis is good, assuming risk factors such as aspirin use, hypertension, mucosal drying or trauma, foreign bodies, and coagulopathies have been eliminated or controlled.

Education

In addition to discussing the epistaxis precautions outlined in Table 8-1, patients should understand that, while a single cause of the bleeding often cannot be identified, there are many factors that contribute to the risk of nosebleeds. If these factors can be avoided or minimized, the chance of recurrent nosebleeds can be reduced.

First, patients should understand that smoking, drinking alcohol, and using platelet-inhibiting medications such as aspirin and nonsteroidal anti-

Table 8-1

Epistaxis Precautions: Instructions for Patients After Treatment of Nosebleed

Activities to do
Moisturize nasal mucous membranes by   applying ointment or saline
Activities to avoid
Straining and heavy lifting
Blowing the nose
Substances to avoid
Smoking
Alcohol
Aspirin
Nonsteroidal antiinflammatory drugs

inflammatory drugs increase the risk of nosebleeds; these substances should be avoided, if possible. Second, they should know that nasal trauma (including nose picking) causes nosebleed and should also be avoided. Third, dry-air home heating during the winter dries the nasal mucous membranes and increases the risk of epistaxis; use of humidifiers may reduce the degree of nasal drying. Finally, uncontrolled hypertension increases the likelihood of epistaxis, and one recent study suggests that there is an association between epistaxis and the *severity* of hypertension in hypertensive patients. Thus, patients with hypertension should comply with their treatment regimens to ensure maximal likelihood of control.

Patients should be instructed that if nosebleeds recur, 10 to 15 minutes of continuous nasal pressure, as described earlier, should be applied. If bleeding is not controlled with nasal pressure, patients should seek medical attention.

Errors

Clinicians make several errors in diagnosis and management of epistaxis. Some have already been discussed such as cauterizing both sides of the nasal septum or using an otoscope when attempting to visualize the site of bleeding. Other errors include inattention to hemodynamic status, failure to achieve adequate visualization of the nasal cavity, inadequate packing, and incorrectly diagnosing bilateral epistaxis.

INATTENTION TO HEMODYNAMIC STATUS

Faced with patients who have active, high-volume, nasal bleeding, most clinicians will appropriately assess vital signs, secure intravenous access, and initiate fluid replacement or resuscitation. In some instances, however, high-volume bleeding may have occurred prior to presentation, with relatively less bleeding when the patient is being examined. In such patients, clinicians may fail to recognize the degree of bleeding that may have taken place and that the patient may be hypovolemic or even hypotensive. This is of particular concern for older patients who have posterior epistaxis as a result of hypertension and atherosclerosis, as such patients are at risk for developing cardiopulmonary symptoms when faced with epistaxis-induced circulatory insufficiency.

FAILURE TO ACHIEVE ADEQUATE VISUALIZATION

Visualizing the site of bleeding in a patient with active epistaxis can sometimes be difficult and can be impossible if appropriate examination techniques and equipment are not used. Adequate lighting and suction are essential, and examination is facilitated by the aid of an assistant. Attempting an examination without proper equipment increases the likelihood that the bleeding site will not be identified and, therefore, that the patient will require nasal packing rather than cauterization of a specific bleeding site.

INADEQUATE PACKING

Clinicians who have limited experience inserting anterior nasal packs often fail to insert a sufficient quantity of Vaseline gauze to achieve tamponade of bleeding. In general about 72 inches of Vaseline gauze should be inserted during anterior packing.

INCORRECTLY DIAGNOSING BILATERAL EPISTAXIS

Most cases of epistaxis are unilateral. After an anterior pack is inserted to control unilateral bleeding, however, residual blood in the posterior nasal cavity is unable to drain through the packed nares. This residual blood may flow through the nasopharynx into and out of the contralateral nostril, and the clinician may incorrectly assume that there is a bleeding site in that contralateral nasal cavity. This assumption may lead to unnecessary insertion of a second nasal pack. To avoid this error, clinicians should be aware that unilateral epistaxis can mimic bilateral epistaxis and that they should not treat bleeding in the contralateral side unless bleeding is profuse or unless a specific bleeding site can be identified or significant bleeding persists.

Emerging Concepts

Several new treatment options have become available for treatment of epistaxis, and each is beginning to see increased use. These procedures are particularly useful for patients with heavy bleeding that cannot be controlled with standard cauterization or packing techniques. Each offers an alternative to open, transantral ligation of the internal maxillary artery, which is the traditional surgical treatment for refractory epistaxis. These new treatments include endoscopic ligation of the internal maxillary artery, endoscopic cauterization of posterior epistaxis, and selective embolization.

ENDOSCOPIC LIGATION OF THE INTERNAL MAXILLARY ARTERY

The sphenopalatine and nasopalatine branches of the internal maxillary artery terminate in the posterolateral nasal wall behind the middle meatus. There they are accessible to ligation with endoscopic equipment. Endoscopic ligation of these branches of the internal maxillary artery has been carried out with success rates (control of epistaxis) of approximately 90%.

ENDOSCOPIC CAUTERIZATION OF POSTERIOR EPISTAXIS

Recent reports indicate that posterior epistaxis can be controlled in 82% to 92% of individuals using monopolar cauterization through an endoscopic nasopharyngoscope. This approach has been used with success as a first-line treatment for epistaxis and may obviate the need for hospitalization and nasal packing.

SELECTIVE EMBOLIZATION

Selective embolization is a major advance in controlling bleeding from a posterior site. Embolization, usually with substances such as Gelfoam, is carried out during catheterization and angiographic evaluation of the nasal circulation. It has low morbidity and mortality rates, and it provides definitive treatment for posterior epistaxis in more than 90% of patients. In comparison with ligation of the internal maxillary artery, which is the "standard" surgical procedure for uncontrollable epistaxis, embolization is equally effective and can reduce the length and cost of hospitalization. Although embolization has been in use since the early 1990s, it is still less widely available than internal maxillary artery ligation.

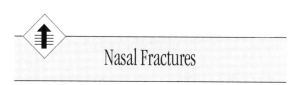

Nasal Fractures

Introduction

Because the nose has a prominent position and protrudes from the face, it is predisposed to blunt trauma, including fractures. Fractures can be nasal fractures (i.e., fractures of the bony framework of the nose) or septal fractures (disruptions of the bony-cartilaginous nasal septum), or both. Nasal

Figure 8-5

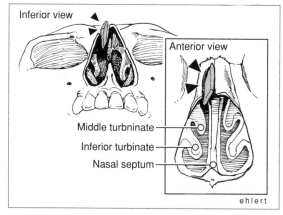

Unilateral nasal fracture. The figure shows anterior and inferior views of a nasal fracture, with the fragment of bone displaced medially.

Figure 8-6

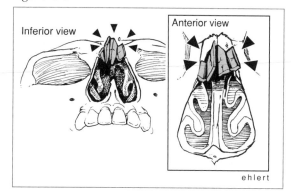

Bilateral nasal fractures. Anterior and inferior view of a bilateral nasal fracture, with bony fragments displaced inferiorly and medially.

fractures may be open or closed and unilateral or bilateral (Figs. 8-5 and 8-6). Open nasal fractures are those that communicate with an open wound.

Most nasal fractures can be restored to proper alignment with appropriate assessment and treatment at the time of injury. However, many nasal and septal fractures are unrecognized at the time of injury, or their severity is underestimated. The result is that a high percentage of septorhinoplasty procedures are performed to correct nasal obstruction and septal deviation from previously unrecognized fractures.

Pathophysiology and Epidemiology

Nasal fractures are the third most common type of fracture, with an incidence exceeded only by fractures of the clavicle and wrist. The most common causes of nasal fractures in urban areas are interpersonal violence, motor vehicle accidents, or sports. In rural areas, the common causes are work accidents, sports, and other leisure activities.

Typical Presentation

Patients with acute nasal fractures typically present following trauma to the face with epistaxis, nasal and facial pain, swelling, and deformity. If significant swelling is present, however, any deformity caused by the fracture may be camouflaged by the swelling.

Patients who present after the acute fracture (delayed presentation) typically demonstrate ecchymosis and may have a nasal deformity. Their epistaxis, swelling, and pain have usually resolved.

Key History

The most important concern in questioning a patient who has an obvious or suspected nasal fracture is to identify the mechanism of trauma and the presence of any associated injuries. If the injury resulted from major trauma such as a motor vehicle crash, the history should be part of a multisystem survey directed at detecting life-threatening injuries that require immediate attention.

When injuries appear limited to the nose, history should be focused on detecting symptoms that might indicate trauma to structures adjacent to nose. Symptoms that suggest such injuries include double vision (which indicates a possible orbital fracture), change in occlusion of the teeth (indicating maxillary or mandibular fractures), or clear nasal drainage (suggesting the possibility of a fractured cribriform plate with leakage of cerebrospinal fluid through the nares). Abscess of the nasal septum should be suspected, especially in children, when patients report an acute onset of nasal obstruction with a recent (but not acute) history of trauma to the nose.

In addition to asking about symptoms of associated injuries, it is important to ask if there has been a change in the appearance of the nose and if there is a history of previous nasal trauma or surgery. The responses to these questions will help determine if an apparent nasal deformity is new or preexisting.

Key Physical Examination

After excluding life-threatening injuries with a systematic trauma survey, the purposes of the physical examination are to detect injuries in structures adjacent to the nose and to define the nature and extent of the nasal trauma. Signs of injury to structures adjacent to the nose are shown in Table 8-2.

EXTERNAL NASAL EXAMINATION

Evaluation of the nose should include an external and internal examination. External examination involves a visual assessment of whether there is an identifiable nasal deformity. Ideally, the

Table 8-2
Physical Examination Signs of Injuries Associated with Nasal Fractures

SIGN	POSSIBLE SIGNIFICANCE
Drainage of clear fluid from nose	L:eakage of cerebrospinal fluid through cribriform plate fracture
Drainage of clear fluid from ear	Leakage of cerebrospinal fluid through basilar skull fracture
Raccoon eyes (ecchymosis around orbits)	Basilar skull fracture
Battle's sign (ecchymosis behind ear)	Basilar skull fracture
Hearing loss	Temporal bone fracture
Trismus	Zygomatic fracture
Dental or jaw tenderness	Dental injury or fractures of the maxilla or mandible
Neck tenderness	Cervical spine injury

appearance of the nose should be compared with its appearance in preinjury photographs of the patient.

It is sometimes difficult to identify a nasal deformity in the presence of significant edema, especially when bilateral edema is symmetric. In such cases it is often useful to reexamine the nose 3 to 5 days after the acute injury, when edema has subsided, to see if a deformity can be identified.

INTERNAL NASAL EXAMINATION

Internal examination should proceed in a fashion similar to that described for patients with epistaxis. In fact, many patients with nasal fractures have active epistaxis or coagulated blood in the nostrils. Thus, the examination should be conducted following the application of a topical decongestant (4% cocaine or 0.25% phenylephrine), with adequate lighting, availability of suction, and a bivalve nasal speculum. If epistaxis is present, the site of bleeding should be identified and treated.

The examiner should seek lacerations, ecchymosis, or hematomas, all of which point toward a nasal fracture. A septal hematoma appears as a soft fluctuant swelling on one or both sides of the septum. It is essential to identify septal hematomas because if they are not treated, they may become infected, resulting in septal abscess, and pressure exerted by the hematoma may cause ischemia and necrosis of the adjacent nasal septum.

Ancillary Tests

Nasal x-rays are not particularly useful in diagnosing or excluding nasal fractures. Approximately half of patients with nasal fractures have x-rays that are read as normal (i.e., falsely negative). X-rays may also be falsely positive, when abnormalities from earlier nasal fractures or natural suture lines in the nasal bones are misinterpreted as acute fractures.

Photographs of the nose, on the other hand, are useful both clinically and medicolegally. Photographs of the patient's nose, when compared with preinjury photographs, can be used to diagnose the deformity of a nasal fractures. Prereduction photographs of the nose can be useful for documenting the extent of the original injury in the event that a patient is not happy with the postreduction appearance of the nose.

If associated injuries are suspected, because of factors such as leakage of cerebrospinal fluid or the others findings noted above, imaging with computerized tomography or magnetic resonance is recommended to identify the nature and severity of the injury.

Algorithm

The algorithm in Figure 8-7 outlines the clinical approach to nasal fractures. Fractures are identified clinically based on the presence of deformity and/or comparison with preinjury photographs. Fractures are treated by closed reduction unless they are severe or complicated, in which case open reduction is performed. Septal hematomas must be detected and treated if present.

Treatment

Management of nasal fractures involves treatment of epistaxis and septal hematoma if present, repair of lacerations, and reduction of fractured bone to restore the normal appearance of the nose. Treatment of epistaxis is described earlier in this chapter, and lacerations are repaired in standard fashion.

The discussion that follows applies to treatment of nasal fractures in adults and adolescents. Nasal fractures in children require special consideration because facial growth centers can be disrupted by nasal fractures, and bone fragments in children become immobile within a matter of days. Thus, most experts recommend that nasal fractures in children be managed by a maxillofacial surgeon who specializes in the care of such injuries and that reductions be accomplished within 4 to 5 days of injury.

Figure 8-7

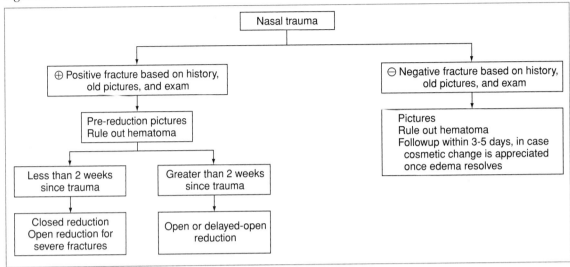

Algorithm for evaluation and management of nasal fractures.

DRAINAGE OF SEPTAL HEMATOMA

When a septal hematoma is identified, incision of the septal mucosa and drainage of the hematoma is indicated. Incision requires topical anesthesia, which is administered by the same technique describe earlier for epistaxis control. The incision should be about 5 to 10 mm long and is accomplished with a number 15 scalpel blade. Content of the hematoma can be expressed manually or removed with suction or a cotton-tipped applicator.

To prevent reaccumulation of the hematoma, it is necessary to insert an anterior nasal pack. Anterior packing is accomplished by the methods described earlier in this chapter. Antistaphylococcal antibiotics should be prescribed to patients who are treated with nasal packs.

If the hematoma is abscessed, cultures should be obtained and antibiotics prescribed. The most common infecting organisms are *Staphylococcus aureus, Streptococcus pneumoniae,* and group A beta-hemolytic streptococcus, but anaerobes may also be identified. Many experts recommend clin-

damycin therapy until results of cultures are available, at which time the antibiotic regimen can be modified based on the culture results.

CLOSED REDUCTION OF NASAL FRACTURES

Nasal fractures can be treated with closed or open reduction. Closed reduction is appropriate for minor fractures of the nasal bones or nasoseptal framework, but only if nasal deviation is less than half of the width of the nasal bridge. Closed reduction should be carried out within 2 weeks of injury. More severe fractures, or those that come to attention long after injury, require open reduction (maxillofacial surgery). Indications for open and closed reductions are shown in Table 8-3.

ANESTHESIA

Assuming the patient is an adult or a cooperative teenager and that the injury is less than 2 weeks old, closed reduction of nasal fractures can be performed under local anesthesia in an office setting. Many techniques and injections are available to anesthetize the nasal framework and mucosa. One common and easily used method is applying 5 to 6 cc of 4% cocaine solution on cotton or surgical pledglets to the nasal mucosa for 10 to 15 minutes. The pledglets should be applied bilaterally to both the anterior and posterior portions of the nasal cavity. This method of anesthesia avoids injections, and it does not distort the appearance of the nose, which often occurs with skin injections and complicates the evaluation of postreduction results.

Some authorities combine local anesthesia with intravenous sedation using medications such as midazolam. With the combined use of local anesthesia and intravenous sedation, patients report reduction of nasal fractures to be less painful than repair of dental caries.

MANIPULATION OF THE FRACTURE

A Boies elevator is used for closed reduction. From the outside of the patient's nose, the distance from the nostril rim to the site of deviation of the nasal bridge is measured with the elevator.

Table 8-3

Indications for Open and Closed Reduction of Nasal Fractures

Indications for closed reduction

Unilateral or bilateral fracture of the nasal bones and fracture of the nasoseptal frame work, if nasal deviation is less than half of the width of the nasal bridge

Absence of indications for open reduction

Indications for open reduction

Fractures with nasal deviation greater than half of the width of the nasal bridge

Extensive fracture-dislocations of the nasoseptal bones

Open septal fractures

Persistent cosmetic change of the nose after closed reduction

The elevator is then inserted into the nasal cavity on the depressed side of the nose, up to the measured distance, and the depressed fragment(s) is elevated by exerting upward pressure (Fig. 8-8). If the opposite nasal bone is also displaced outwardly, it is simultaneously moved into its normal position by blunt medial pressure as the contralateral depressed fragment is elevated. If deformity cannot be corrected with closed reduction, the patient should be referred to a maxillofacial specialist for open reduction.

POSTREDUCTION CARE

The patient should apply ice to the fracture for 24 hours after the injury. Many clinicians recommend using an external nasal splint (i.e., a plaster of Paris splint) for 1 week for fixation and stabilization after closed reduction of nasal fractures, or longer if the patient will be participating in athletic activities that might result in nasal injury. A recent randomized controlled trial, however, showed no benefit from plaster of Paris splinting.

Adults and teenagers should be evaluated 5 to 7 days after the injury, so that the nature of any remaining cosmetic deformity can be appreciated after the swelling has receded. If possible, patients should bring preinjury photos to their follow-up appointment. If deformity is present, and the injury occurred less than 2 weeks previously, re-reduction can be carried out.

Common minor complications of nasal fractures include pain, which is usually minimal, and a limited amount of bleeding. The most important complication, however, is persistent nasal deformity, which emphasizes the need for a postreduction evaluation.

Long-Term Monitoring, Treatment, and Prognosis

The usual outcome is correction of the nasal deformity by closed reduction, but a small percentage of patients will require open reduction to

Figure 8-8

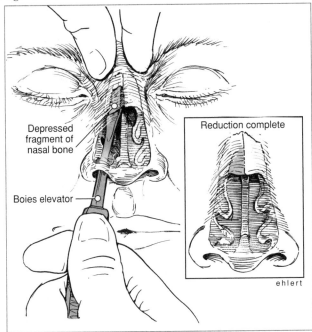

Reduction of a nasal fracture. The clinician has inserted a Boies elevator into the nostril on the side of the fracture and is using the elevator to manipulate the displaced bone fragment into proper position.

correct the deformity. Once the deformity is corrected and the fracture healed, no special long-term monitoring is needed.

Education

When evaluating individuals who have an acute nasal fracture, clinicians should counsel them about options for treatment. Three treatment options are available. The first option is to do nothing and accept whatever cosmetic deformity may be present. The second is a closed reduction, which can be performed acutely or within 2 weeks of the injury. The third is to perform an open reduction (a maxillofacial surgical procedure). Closed reduction is usually the recommended approach, assuming

indications for closed reduction are present (Table 8-3), because of the high success and low complication rates of closed reduction.

Subsequent to closed reduction of nasal fractures, patients should be told that after resolution of swelling, some persistent cosmetic deformity may be noticed. If this occurs, a repeat reduction may be performed if the patient seeks care within 2 weeks of the initial injury.

Errors

Most nasal fractures are obvious, and, with three exceptions, clinicians make few errors in diagnosis and treatment. One error is inappropriately relying on x-rays to determine if a fracture is present. As discussed earlier, x-rays have significant false-positive and false-negative rates for diagnosing nasal fractures. Therefore, diagnosis of a nasal fracture is a clinical diagnosis, not a radiographic diagnosis.

A second error is not reviewing preinjury photographs of the patient's nose, which is especially important for patients who have had prior nasal trauma or surgery. Failure to consider the preinjury appearance of the nose can result in inappropriately attributing nasal deformity to an acute injury when, in fact, the injury might have been preexisting.

The third error is failure to diagnose septal hematomas, which sometimes occurs because of difficulty conducting a thorough nasal examination in an uncooperative patient, or because of difficulty visualizing the nasal cavity. Because an untreated septal hematoma can result in abscess or ischemic necrosis of the septum, it is essential to visualize the septum in all patients with suspected nasal fractures.

References

Bailey BJ: Nasal fractures, in Bailey BJ (ed): *Head and Neck Surgery—Otolaryngology*. Philadelphia, JB Lippincott, 1993, pp. 991–1007.

Canty PA, Berkowitz RG: Hematoma and abscess of the nasal septum in children. *Arch Otolaryngol Head Neck Surg* 122:1373, 1996.

Cullen MM, Tami TA: Comparison of internal maxillary artery ligation versus embolization for refractory posterior epistaxis. *Otolaryngol Head Neck Surg* 118:636, 1998.

Frikart L, Agrifoglio A: Endoscopic treatment of posterior epistaxis. *Rhinology* 36:59, 1998.

Galletta A, Amato G: Hereditary hemorrhagic telangiectasia (Osler-Rendu-Weber disease). Management of epistaxis and oral hemorrhage by Nd-Yag laser. *Minerva Stomatol* 47:283, 1998.

Ginsburg CM, Leach JL: Infected nasal septal hematoma. *Pediatr Infect Dis J* 14:1012, 1995.

Ginsburg CM: Nasal septal hematoma. *Pediatr Rev* 19:142, 1998.

Houghton DJ, Hanafi Z, Papakostas K, et al: Efficacy of external fixation following nasal manipulation under local anaesthesia. *Clin Otolaryngol* 23:169, 1998.

Josephson GD, Godley FA, Stierna P: Practical management of epistaxis. *Med Clin North Am* 75:1311, 1991.

Lepore ML: Epistaxis, in Bailey BJ (ed): *Head and Neck Surgery—Otolaryngology*. Philadelphia, JB Lippincott, 1993, pp. 428–446.

Lubianca-Neto JF, Bredemeier M, Carvalhal EF: A study of the association between epistaxis and the severity of hypertension. *Am J Rhinol* 12:269, 1998.

Newton CR, White PS: Nasal manipulation with intravenous sedation. Is it an acceptable and effective treatment? *Rhinology* 36:114, 1998.

Pritikin JB, Calarelli DD, Panje WR: Endoscopic ligation of the internal maxillary artery for treatment of intractable posterior epistaxis. *Ann Otol Rhinol Laryngol* 107:85, 1998.

Srinivasan V, Patel H, John DG, Worsley A: Warfarin and epistaxis: should warfarin always be discontinued? *Clin Otolaryngol* 22:542, 1997.

Tay HL, Evans JM, McMahon AD, MacDonald TM: Aspirin, nonsteroidal anti-inflammatory drugs, and epistaxis. A regional record linkage case control study. *Ann Otol Rhinol Laryngol* 107:671, 1998.

Tseng EY, Narducci CA, Willing SJ, Sillers MJ: Angiographic embolization for epistaxis: a review of 114 cases. *Laryngoscope* 108:615, 1998.

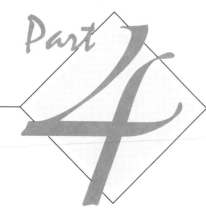

Part

4

Traumatic Injuries

Sarvesh Logsetty and
David M. Heimbach

Burns

Introduction

Of all the ailments for which patients seek medical care, few are as shrouded in folklore and misconception as are burns. From toothpaste to pepper to mayonnaise, there is a myriad of home remedies for burns, and understanding of the mechanisms of burn injury by clinicians and the public is often poor.

In reality, burn care is a simple matter much of the time, requiring the specialized care of a burn center only rarely. For most burns, patients do not seek medical care, and when they do, the vast majority of burn injuries can be treated in an outpatient setting. Primary care clinicians can and should provide care for most burns.

To adequately manage burns, clinicians must be able to determine the nature of the injury, the extent of the injury (both in area and depth), and the presence of confounding factors that might affect outcome unfavorably. After recognizing these factors, decisions can be made about the need for dressings, analgesics, fluids, transfer to a burn center, and potential surgical interventions.

Epidemiology

Although it is estimated that approximately 2 million people are burned each year, only about 70,000 are admitted to a hospital. Most individuals with burns are treated as outpatients, heal without any need for surgical intervention, and have no complications or sequelae. The majority of admitted patients are first seen and assessed by emergency physicians, whose early interventions can decrease the deleterious effects of the injury. Nearly nine of every ten burns originate from unintentional trauma, with only about 10% related to assault or suicide.

Pathophysiology

Skin plays an important role as the main barrier protecting the body from entry of noxious microorganisms and chemicals. Beyond being merely a physical barrier, skin also functions to prevent uncontrolled water and electrolyte loss and is an essential component of temperature regulation. When large areas of skin are lost or damaged, patients become dehydrated and hypothermic and are susceptible to rapid and fulminant infections.

Skin is also a prime organ of sensation. This must be taken into consideration when determining the need for analgesia during burn treatment.

Epidermis

The epidermis is the outermost layer of the skin. It consists of rapidly reproducing epithelial cells that create a permanent outer cover for normal skin, as well as for healing wounds. The most superficial layer of the epidermis consists of dead horny cells (*stratum corneum*). The middle layer contains live epidermal cells (*stratum lucidum*), and in the bottom layer are basal cells (*stratum germinativum* or basal-cell layer). The basal layer is the layer of proliferation, where all the reproductive activity of the epidermis takes place.

The epidermis turns over approximately every 28 days—basal cells drift upward and then slough from the *stratum corneum* in about a month. If cells do not slough, they heap up and become calluses, especially on the soles and palms. The pigment cells (melanocytes) reside in the basal layer.

The epidermis varies in thickness from 0.05 mm on the eyelid to several millimeters in calluses of the hand or foot. Protrusions of the epidermis extend into the dermis by way of the skin appendages—hair follicles, sebaceous glands, and apocrine and eccrine sweat glands. Some of the apocrine sweat glands in the axilla and groin actually extend all the way into the subcutaneous fat. When the sheetlike cover of the epidermis is burned away, if some of these dermal skin appendages remain alive, the resultant wound eventually heals as these cells of these dermal appendages grow superficially and laterally to cover the remaining viable dermis.

Dermis

The dermis is the stromal tissue that supports the epidermis and the skin appendages. Contrary to common perception, there are no native "dermal cells." Rather, normal dermis is composed of highly structured and organized collagen; wandering cells (leukocytes, macrophages, fibroblasts, endothelial cells); blood vessels; elastic fibers; and a gluelike substance, glycoseaminoglycan (GAG), which is also known as "ground substance." When the structured collagen and GAG of the dermis are removed by injury, the framework onto which new collagen is laid down is lost. The result is that new collagen is laid down haphazardly, resulting in scar, not new dermis—that is, the dermis heals by scar formation, not by creation of new dermal cells.

Healing Buds

Epithelial overgrowth cannot commence until all the dead dermis (eschar) is gone because epithelial cells require a live base on which to sit and migrate. Removal of eschar is accomplished by daily cleansing (debridement) and/or by bacterial collagenases that dissolve the denatured collagen holding the dead dermis in place. Then, the epidermal cells from skin appendages grow out of those appendages and spread along the raw dermal surface to meet the cells coming out of neighboring appendages.

When they are migrating, the spreading epidermal cells produce a characteristic appearance of epidermal "buds" (also referred to as "pearls;"). Epidermal buds appear as white dots in a red background of granulating dermis. Since the bottoms of appendages are at varying levels in the dermis, the deeper the burn, the fewer the remaining skin appendages and the farther apart they are. Thus, the deeper the burn, the farther the epithelial cells must migrate upward and laterally to join with others, and the longer it will take the surface to reepithelialize. Furthermore, the deeper the burn, the more of the dead dermis that must come off before epithelial migration can even begin.

Epidermal Healing of Deep Versus Superficial Burns

Deep burns seem to heal from hair follicles instead of from sweat glands. This occurs despite there being many more sweat glands than hair follicles, and despite sweat glands extending deeper into the dermis. The reason is that cells at the base of sweat glands are a type of epidermal cell that cannot de-differentiate into keratinized squamous cells. Thus, when only deep fragments of sweat glands remain after a deep burn, they are unable to generate the cells needed to begin the healing process; new epithelial cells must originate from the less numerous hair follicles instead.

On the other hand, the cells lining the superficial channel of the sweat glands do grow out as an epithelial cover, so more shallow burns can heal from epidermal cells generated by these more numerous sweat glands. This explains why very shallow burns seem raw one day and suddenly healed the next, while deep burns develop scattered hair islands that heal slowly; with shallow burns there is a massive growth of epidermis from millions of sweat gland ducts.

Epidermal Cell Migration—Implications for Healing

Epithelial cells migrate under a variety of stimuli, but regardless of the stimulus, the total distance they can migrate laterally is about 1 cm, growing at a rate of about 1 mm a day. Thus, a round wound 2 cm in diameter will heal from the epithelial edges in 10 days or so.

Because of the limit on lateral epidermal-cell migration, wounds larger than 2 cm must heal by contraction of the edges pulling together to make the wound smaller. If the edges of such a burn cannot pull themselves together (as would take place over an immobile object such as the tibia, heel, or skull), the wound becomes a chronic ulcer and never closes. Epidermal cells continue to duplicate, but, rather than spreading laterally, they begin to heap up vertically. Thus, one can recognize a healing wound that is unable to close by its heaped-up epidermal edges. If the edges do eventually approximate themselves (as over a joint), the wound will close by contraction, but will invariably limit full joint motion, leaving the patient with a limitation of motion (a contracture). Wounds larger than 2 cm therefore heal at least in part by contraction, which sometimes leads to a contracture across a joint.

Typical Presentation

In office-based settings, burn patients either present immediately after the injury or, if the burn is small, after treatment failure at home. Patients will report using a wide variety of home remedies to treat burns before presenting to a clinician. These home remedies range from toothpaste to butter to naturopathic salves.

One effective treatment that patients often do not use is the application of cold water to stop the burning process. Application of cold water probably works by temporarily inhibiting thromboxane release in the burned tissues. Cold water is effective, however, only if it is applied within the first minutes after injury. By the time the patient presents to a clinician, it is too late for cold water to be effective.

Neither patients nor clinicians should apply ice to burned skin, as the resultant vasoconstriction can decrease perfusion and transform a partial-thickness burn into a full-thickness burn. In addition, large burns should not be immersed in cold water for fear of inducing heat loss from the burned skin, resulting in systemic hypothermia.

Key History

While physical examination of burned patients yields more information than history in terms of guiding management decisions, several aspects of the history are nonetheless useful. Specifically, its is important to know the mechanism of the burn (e.g., chemical, electrical, etc.) because, as described later, different mechanisms of injury have different diagnostic and therapeutic implications. It is also useful to collect information about a patient's medical history, medication regimen, and drug allergies, as such information may influence treatment considerations. Finally, tetanus immunization status should be determined because burns, other than superficial (first-degree) burns, are tetanus-prone injuries.

Key Physical Examination

The principal purpose of examining burned skin is to determine the severity of the burn. The severity of a burn is measured by two parameters: size and depth. Knowledge of these characteristics helps communicate the nature of the burn to others and permits the institution of rational therapy.

Burn Size

Burn size is measured by the total body surface area (TBSA) involved in the burn, and it is estimated by the "rule of nines." According to the rule of nines, upper extremities correspond to 9% of TBSA each, lower limbs 18% each, the chest and abdomen together are 18%, the back 18%, the head and neck 9%, and the perineal region 1%. Areas that are noncontiguous may be measured by assuming that the patient's palm (not the examiner's palm) is equal to 1% of the TBSA.

The measurements for estimating TBSA must be modified when describing burns in children younger than 4 years of age, because young children's heads are proportionately larger than those of adults. A newborn's head accounts for 18% of the TBSA and the lower limbs 14% each. For each year of age, subtract 1% from the surface area of the head and add 0.5% to each lower limb. This continues until the child is nine years of age, at which time the rule of nines can be used.

Burn Depth

Burn depth is also an indicator of the severity of the injury. It should be noted, however, that the appearance of a burn changes as skin cells either repair themselves or die, and hence decisions about the correct depth, and the treatment decisions it implies (i.e., surgery versus no surgery), may need to wait for a few days after the injury.

The traditional classification of burn depth has been to describe first-, second-, and third-degree burns. While this system is commonly used, it is also commonly misunderstood by clinicians. Therefore, the current recommendation is to describe burns as superficial, superficial partial-thickness, deep partial-thickness, or full-thickness. This classification conveys more information than simply labeling burns as first-, second-, or third-degree and can be more precise in guiding treatment.

SUPERFICIAL BURNS

Superficial burns (traditionally known as first-degree burns) involve only the superficial epidermis. Because the dermis is unscathed and the epidermis is structurally intact, there is no blis-

tering, no need for dressings, and no need for surgery. On examination, these burns look like sunburns and, like sunburns, will peel in 2 to 3 days as the dry, top layer of the epidermis sloughs. Superficial burns heal without scarring.

FULL-THICKNESS BURNS

At the other end of the spectrum from superficial burns are full-thickness burns. On physical examination, full-thickness burns are insensate, white or smoke-stained, and dry (Fig. 9-1). They look and feel like leather.

Because all the skin appendages are burned away, such burns can only heal by epithelial migration from the periphery and by wound contraction. Except for very small burns, full-thickness burns will not heal without surgical intervention (i.e., skin grafting) (Fig. 9-2). Therefore, most patients with a full-thickness burn should be referred to a burn center or an appropriately trained surgeon.

A variation of a full-thickness burn is the so-called "fourth-degree burn," which extends through skin into the fat and sometimes into the deep structures under the investing fascia. These burns can result from electrical burns, molten metal burns, contact burns from mufflers, flame burns of victims who are trapped or unconscious, and some immersion scalds. Deep decubitus ulcers that extend into deep tissues are effectively

Figure 9-1

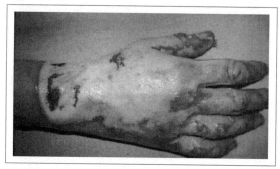

Full-thickness burn. Typical full-thickness burn with a white, dry appearance. (See also color plate.)

Figure 9-2

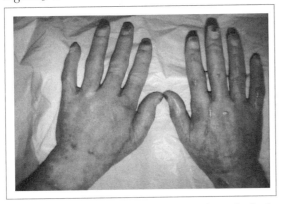

Skin graft on full-thickness burn. This figure shows the final outcome of a full-thickness burn treated with a skin graft. Both the cosmetic and functional results are good. (See also color plate.)

fourth-degree burns, even though they are not caused by thermal injury. The severity of fourth-degree burns is greater than the surface TBSA would indicate, and specialized management is almost always required.

PARTIAL-THICKNESS BURNS

Partial-thickness burns are often confusing to identify. They can be classified as superficial or deep, but are better thought of as representing a continuum from mild injuries that may heal with

Figure 9-3

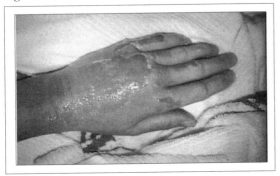

Superficial partial-thickness burn. The burned skin is moist and homogeneously pink and will blanch on application of pressure. (See also color plate.)

Figure 9-4

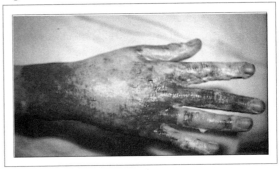

Deep partial-thickness burn. The burned area is a mixture of pale skin and a bright-red reticular pattern that does not blanch on pressure. (See also color plate.)

optimal care to deep burns that are the equivalent of full-thickness injuries.

A superficial partial-thickness burn (Fig. 9-3) is moist, homogeneously pink, and sensitive to touch and blanches on application of pressure. In contrast, a deep partial-thickness burn (Fig. 9-4) is dry and less sensitive to touch and pain and may be either pale or have a bright-red reticular pattern that does not blanch. If a large area of deep partial-thickness burn is identified, or if a burn initially thought to be superficial partial-thickness does not heal within 3 weeks, referral to a burn surgeon is in order. While such burns may heal spontaneously in longer than 3 weeks, they are likely to do so with severe scarring, uncontrollable itching, and contracture formation.

Treatment

Wound Management

SUPERFICIAL BURNS

Patients with superficial burns will benefit from the use of a moisturizing lotion. Superficial burns will heal without scarring, but the burned areas will be more sensitive to subsequent sunburn, so patients should be advised to use sunblock.

PARTIAL-THICKNESS AND FULL-THICKNESS BURNS

Partial-thickness and full-thickness burns need to be covered with antimicrobial dressings. The simplest antimicrobial dressing is silver sulfadiazine cream covered by dry gauze. For individuals allergic to sulfonamides, small burns can be dressed with a single layer of petroleum-impregnated gauze. Dressings need be changed once daily, and in most cases patients can perform their own dressing changes (or have dressings changed by a family member).

Almost invariably, either from fear, pain, or because of advice from family and friends, patients do not wash their burn. Therefore, perhaps the most important advice for patients is to wash burns daily with soap and water. It must be remembered, however, that for deep burns, dressings are only a temporizing measure until a burn surgeon can see the patient and assess the need for surgery.

Finally, tetanus immunization and tetanus immune globulin should be administered to those patients for whom it is indicated. Standard recommendations such as those from the Advisory Committee on Immunization Practices that are outlined in Chapter 10 (Table 10-1) can be used to direct tetanus prophylaxis.

Antibiotic Therapy

All burns are associated with a region of erythema around the burn. This area is called the "zone of hyperemia," and it is a normal consequence of the inflammatory process that follows a burn—it does not signify the presence of an infection.

On the other hand, if the erythema is distant from the burn region, extends in a lymphangitic fashion up a limb, or is visibly progressing beyond marked lines, then cellulitis is likely and antibiotics should be used. The most common organisms in burn-associated infection in outpatient settings are the gram-positive aerobes, *Streptococcus pneumoniae* and *Staphylococcus aureus*. Antibiotics such as a first-generation cephalosporin or dicloxacillin are therefore the usual antibiotics of choice.

In the absence of infection, antibiotics should not be prescribed because they provide no benefit to the patient and place the patient at risk of developing an antibiotic-resistant infection. Sometimes, however, there is confusion about whether a patient has "normal" burn erythema or cellulitis. This confusion is further compounded by the frequent presence of fever and leukocytosis in burn patients as a response to circulating inflammatory mediators. If there is doubt about the presence of infection, perhaps the most useful measure is to mark out the area of redness on the patient's skin and then reassess at 12- to 24-hour intervals to see if the area of redness is expanding. Cultures of the blood and skin may be appropriate in some cases, but are not often useful with small burns in outpatient settings. The routine prophylactic use of antibiotics in burn patients is not recommended, regardless of the burn size.

Pain Management

Burns hurt, and burn treatments hurt. Thus, most burned patients will require measures for treatment of pain. In addition, the pain experienced by many burned patients results in anxiety, which, in turn, may further aggravate the perceived severity of pain.

There are two types of burn pain. The first is background pain—that which is present throughout the acute and healing phases of the burn. The second is the pain that occurs during procedures, as described below.

Both types of pain require analgesic treatment, and it is important to ensure that the patient is receiving adequate pain relief—using nonnarcotic and narcotic analgesics, as needed. Analgesic use should be reassessed at each visit to ensure that doses are sufficient. Once the wound is healed, however, and the dressing changes are reduced in frequency and less painful, analgesic therapy can be weaned and ultimately eliminated. In general, a reduction of 10% every other day will be suitable for most patients. Once the burn is healed, there should be no need for further analgesics.

BACKGROUND PAIN

Background pain is always present in burned patients, and its range of fluctuation is relatively small. Although patients may acclimate to its presence and report its severity as somewhere in the middle of a 10-point scale, it is not always tolerable for them. As time passes, tolerance to any given level of pain may vary, and analgesia may be required.

The constant nature of background pain calls for a constant level of analgesia. This can be accomplished by regularly dosed medications or by the use of long-acting, slow-release medication. While nonnarcotic analgesics such as nonsteroidal antiinflammatory drugs may provide sufficient control of background pain for some patients, narcotics are a reasonable alternative and should not be avoided because of fears of abuse or addiction. If started at a dose sufficient to relieve pain and tapered and discontinued once the wound is healed, there is no realistic addiction potential. Unless patients were opioid-dependent before being burned, they will not become so by the liberal, appropriate use of narcotics during the acute phase of burn management.

PROCEDURAL PAIN

Procedural pain is the pain that occurs when something is done to the patient—wound cleansing, dressing changes, occupational and physical therapy, etcetera. Procedural pain is often the worst pain the patient has ever encountered, and a variety of adjectives have been used to describe it: excruciating, horrible, intolerable, ghastly, horrendous, gruesome, sickening, detestable, monstrous, and loathsome.

Dressing changes can be very painful, as burns are extremely sensitive to exposure to air, and a wound that is comfortable while covered can become very painful when the dressing is removed. At these times a short-acting, potent, narcotic analgesic is in order, with instructions for the patient to take the medication 30 to 60 minutes before commencing dressing changes or other painful activity.

ANXIETY

For many patients, the direct pain of the burn is made worse by high levels of anxiety. Anxiety reflects fear of pain, fear of painful dressing changes, and/or fear of having to face the change in body image that may have occurred as a result of the burn.

It is important to recognize this anxiety and treat it as required. Anxiolytics may be needed in exceptional cases, but, more often, all that is needed is reassurance and an explanation of the process of the evolution of the burn. Rarely does the average patient require anxiolytic medications to treat pain, *per se*. Similarly, patients should not receive excessive amounts of analgesics simply because they are anxious.

Management of Large Burns

Patients with large burns should be assessed and treated as victims of major trauma. The ABCs (airway, breathing, and circulation) must be followed to ensure that the patient is stable. Once the patient has been stabilized, burns may be examined in detail and specific therapy instituted.

AIRWAY

Airway protection and maintenance are of paramount importance in burn victims. Endotracheal intubation is often needed; indications for intubation fall into two main categories: emergent and prophylactic.

EMERGENT   As with any trauma patient, immediate endotracheal intubation is required when patients cannot protect their airway because of impaired consciousness, if there is direct trauma to the airway, or when hoarseness or stridor are present.

PROPHYLACTIC   There are specific considerations for burn patients that make intubation appropriate even in the absence of acute airway compromise. This is because smoke inhalation injury is more a chemical injury than a thermal injury, and evidence of thermal burn may not be evident—even in an injured airway. Specifically, the airway in burned patients may be initially patent and the patient in no respiratory distress; however, the airway may actually be injured and may ultimately become compromised by edema as fluid resuscitation takes place and the airway tissue responds to the burn injury. Once airway edema develops, endotracheal intubation can be extraordinarily difficult. Each year many patients die because an endotracheal tube was not already in place when airway edema developed.

Thus, it is important not only to recognize the signs of acute airway compromise but also the signs suggesting that airway injury has occurred and that prophylactic intubation is needed. The most important signs of airway injury are (1) burn injuries or edema across the neck and/or (2) evidence of intraoral burns. Signs of intraoral burns can be detected by examining the burn victim's mouth. If the mucosa looks dry and red or has blisters, the patient is at risk for respiratory compromise and should be intubated as quickly as possible.

Other patients may also need prophylactic endotracheal intubation, although there may be time for a brief general assessment of the patient before intubation is performed. Such patients are those with a history of inhaling smoke or toxic gases and those with very large burns, especially involving the head and neck. With this group, intubation should be considered as a necessary prophylactic measure, but time is less critical, and it is often appropriate to perform a controlled intubation with sedation. Such individuals must be monitored closely while not intubated, however, and intubation should not be delayed for an inordinate period while pursing laboratory investigations and other examinations.

Finally, prophylactic intubation is often indicated for patients being transferred to a burn center. Transport time, the mode and nature of injuries, and the comfort of the transport personnel with the care of the patient are important considerations when deciding about intubation prior to transport. It is often useful to make this decision in conjunction with the transport team and the accepting physician at the burn center. When in doubt, however, the patient should be intubated; it is far easier to remove an endotracheal tube than to insert one during the transportation process.

BREATHING

Once the airway is secured, the next step is to assess the patient's oxygenation. All intubated patients with burns should receive 100% oxygen until examination and laboratory data support a change in the level of oxygen administration. If there is any suspicion of carbon monoxide (CO) inhalation, the patient should continue to receive 100% oxygen until carboxyhemoglobin levels are known to be normal. Often, metabolic acidosis noted on measurement of arterial blood-gas assay is the first indication of carbon monoxide poisoning.

CARBON MONOXIDE   Patients in closed-space fires are at risk for carbon monoxide poisoning, and their carboxyhemoglobin level should be measured early in the assessment process. CO has an affinity for hemoglobin 200 times that of O_2, resulting in failure of hemoglobin's oxygen-carrying capacity and central nervous system hypoxia. Levels of carboxyhemoglobin of 30% or more (in the fire) portend a significant risk of permanent central nervous system injury. It is possible to generate a CO level of more than 30% after about 3 minutes in a moderately smoky fire.

One can estimate the level of CO in the fire from a knowledge of the half-life of CO in the blood—about 1 hour when patients are receiving 100% O_2. Thus, if a patient is intubated at the scene of a fire and has a carboxyhemoglobin of 15% in the emergency room an hour after rescue and intubation, the patient probably had a CO level of about 30% in the fire.

Many clinicians recommend use of hyperbaric oxygen therapy for patients with CO inhalation, but use of this therapy for CO inhalation is controversial. There are no controlled data to prove that hyperbaric oxygen therapy has a beneficial long-term effect on outcome for patients with CO inhalation. Furthermore, it often takes 2 to 4 hours to get the patient into a hyperbaric oxygen chamber, by which time the CO levels will have gone through two to four half-lives on 100% O_2 and, therefore, will have fallen to nontoxic levels. Finally, there are potential risks to using hyperbaric oxygen, because burn care, resuscitation needs, and critical monitoring are compromised while the patient is in the hyperbaric chamber. In fact, there are reports of patients experiencing cardiac arrest and other medical catastrophes while in a hyperbaric chamber, and treatment in such a situation is extraordinarily difficult.

SMOKE INHALATION Without associated cutaneous burns, smoke inhalation has a low morbidity and mortality. With associated cutaneous burns, however, the mortality rate for any given burn is about doubled when smoke inhalation has also occurred. Even among those who survive, such individuals have a substantial risk of needing artificial ventilation. In fact, the combination of (1) exposure to a closed-space fire, (2) carboxyhemoglobin levels >10% (back-calculated to time of rescue), and (3) carbonaceous sputum (not saliva) in association with burns of ≥10% TBSA indicate more than a 90% chance of needing ventilator support.

Contrary to common opinion, facial burns or singed nasal hairs are only risk factors for, but not evidence of, smoke inhalation. As noted, this is because smoke inhalation is basically a chemical, not a thermal, injury. Thus, it is important to monitor respiratory function for evidence of airway injury. Respiratory function can be followed by serial analyses of arterial blood gases and by using the P/F ratio. The P/F; ratio is calculated by dividing the arterial PaO_2 by the FiO_2 (e.g., a PaO_2 of 80 torr on room air and an FiO_2 of 0.20 creates a P/F ratio of 400). If the P/F ratio is less than 300, the patient has smoke injury that will require ventilator support.

In addition to ventilator support, patients with smoke inhalation require more fluids than patients with the same-sized burns but no smoke inhalation. Occasionally, the total fluid requirements can double those predicted by the Parkland formula (described below). Finally, steroids should not be used, as the rate of death and infectious complications are increased when steroids are used. In fact, one double-blinded study showed twice the mortality and three times the rate of infectious complications among burn patients who received steroids.

CIRCULATION

The goal of fluid resuscitation is to maintain circulating volume in the simplest, safest, and cheapest manner. Ideally, 48 hours after the burn the patient should be alert and in neither cardiac, pulmonary, nor renal failure.

This goal can be difficult to achieve, because capillary permeability, caused by a number of acute inflammatory mediators released during cellular destruction, is increased in burned patients—a process that does not begin to abate until 12 or more hours after the burn event. Systemic effects of capillary permeability are limited to the area of the burn itself when the burn is less than about 20% of TBSA. With larger burns, however, capillary permeability is increased on a bodywide basis. The deeper the burn, the worse the capillary leak. Smoke inhalation aggravates the capillary leak in the lungs, which will significantly increase the fluid requirements during resuscitation.

FLUID RESUSCITATION

Small Burns Because small burns are not associated with systemic increases in capillary permeability, most patients, including children, with small burns (generally less than 15% TBSA) can be resuscitated with oral fluids. If emergency personnel have already inserted an intravenous infusion, however, it should remain in place until it is certain that the patient will tolerate oral fluids.

Large Burns For larger burns (>15% TBSA), intravenous fluids should be administered using the Baxter (or Parkland) formula. This is achieved by administering lactated Ringer's solution started at a dose of 4 mL/kg per percent TBSA burned, at a rate such that the first half of the calculated 24-hour fluid total is given in the first 8 hours and the remainder over the subsequent 16 hours.

Because children have a high volume-to-surface-area ratio, the volume of resuscitation fluid calculated by the burn formula is often similar to their normal, daily, maintenance-fluid requirement. For children, therefore, it is necessary to administer their maintenance fluids *in addition to* the resuscitation fluids calculated by the Baxter formula. For children up to about the age of 3, the usual calculated daily maintenance fluids should be administered (as 5% dextrose in ¼ normal saline) over 24 hours at a constant rate by way of a "piggyback" infusion into a lactated Ringer's intravenous line, and the lactated Ringers solution should be administered according to the Baxter formula described above. This intravenous setup permits bolus administration of lactated Ringer's solution if signs of hypotension or oliguria develop, without altering the maintenance-fluid administration rate.

MONITORING FLUID STATUS Adequacy of fluid administration is assessed by monitoring urine output through an indwelling urethral catheter. Urine output of 30 mL/hour is acceptable for adults; for children 1 to 1.5 mL/kg per hour is sufficient. It is important to average the urine output over 2- to 3-hour periods, instead of increasing and decreasing fluids in response to hourly urine output.

One of the major causes for giving fluids in excess of volumes calculated with the Baxter formula is the mistaken belief that a urine output of >50mL/hour is required. This misconception leads to fluid overload with associated pulmonary edema and other complications. In the absence of myoglobinuria, the rate of fluid administration should be decreased if hourly urine output exceeds 50 mL.

INTRAVENOUS ACCESS Standard peripheral-vein intravenous catheters are generally the preferred route for fluid administration, even if they are inserted through the burn. Saphenous vein and other cutdowns are not recommended because the incidence of phlebitis and subsequent suppurative infection is very high.

For burns of less than 40% of TBSA, and in the absence of smoke inhalation, central venous lines are not usually necessary. Central lines may be needed, however, with burns greater than 40% of TBSA, for patients with severe smoke inhalation, or for elderly patients with preexisting cardiopulmonary problems. Swan-Ganz catheters may be appropriate for patients with cardiopulmonary disease, but they should only be used if the patient is not responding normally to the fluid resuscitation plan.

REFERRAL TO A BURN CENTER

In general, patients with deep burns, large burns, circumferential burns of the extremities or chest, or burns in specialized areas (e.g., face, hands, feet, genitalia, perineum, or major joints) should be referred to a burn center. The American Burn Association's guidelines for referral are shown in Table 9-1.

Table 9-1

Indications for Referral to a Burn Center

Burns larger than 10% TBSA in patients less than 10 years of age
Burns larger than 10% TBSA in patients older than 50 years of age
Burns greater than 20% TBSA in all other age groups
Burns involving the face, hands, feet, genitalia, perineum, or major joints
Full-thickness burns larger than 5% TBSA in patients of any age
Chemical burns
Electrical burns
Inhalation injury

Abbreviations: TBSA, total body surface area.

Special Considerations

Chemical Burns

The depth of a chemical burn is determined by the type and strength of the chemical and by the length of time the tissue is exposed to the chemical. Therefore, the sooner the affected area is washed to remove the chemical, the better. Ideally, irrigation with large quantities of water or saline should begin immediately after the injury.

As a general rule, the use of neutralizing agents is not recommended. The chemical neutralization process can liberate a significant amount of heat and can therefore exacerbate the injury.

The one situation in which neutralizing agents *should* be used, however, is for hydrofluoric (HF) acid burns. HF acid is found in industrial solvents and is used by auto detailers. HF acid burns are of serious concern because the fluoride ions in HF acid have a high affinity for calcium. HF acid penetrates deep into tissues and can bind a large amount of calcium in a short amount of time, resulting in acute hypocalcemia. Patients with HF acid burns often require care in an intensive-care unit, ideally in a burn center, with frequent monitoring of serum calcium levels and calcium replacement as needed. Topical application of calcium gel as soon as irrigation is finished may slow progression of the disease and provide relief from the severe pain by binding HF acid in the tissues. If the pain persists, intraarterial calcium infusion should be considered.

Asphalt Burns

Asphalt burns (Fig. 9-5, *A-C*) are relatively common among roofers and road workers. Asphalt is kept in liquid form by heating it in a large central "mother pot," the temperature of which can exceed 400°F. Contact with this liquid form of asphalt invariably results in deep burns.

A second form of asphalt burn occurs from contact with asphalt after it has been removed from the mother pot and placed in a bucket for transport to the work site. At this point, the asphalt has usually cooled significantly, and burns from this type of exposure are typically not as deep as those caused by exposure to liquid asphalt from the mother pot.

Asphalt burns are complicated by the tenacious nature of the material, which makes the asphalt difficult to remove from the skin, thereby prolonging contact with the hot substance and worsening the burn. Removal of asphalt without causing the patient undo pain requires use of a medical adhesive solvent such as Medisol or, if that is unavailable, a petroleum-based ointment such as polysporin or vaseline. The solvent is applied and the patient's burn covered in moist dressings; this is repeated every 2 hours until the asphalt is completely removed. The true depth of the burn is not assessable until the underlying tissue is exposed.

Electrical Burns

There are three kinds of injuries associated with electricity. The first is a true electrical current injury, in which current flows through the body. The second is flash burns, in which no current actually passes through the body, but the electric discharge heats up the air enough to cause (usually very deep) flash burns. The third type is flame burns, in which the patient's clothes catch fire from the heat of the electricity. Flash and flame burns are like all other burns and are treated the same way. The comments below refer to electrical current injury, with and without tissue destruction.

Low-Voltage (110 to 220 Volts) Current without Tissue Destruction

Patients with no persistent symptoms following an exposure to household electrical current (110 to 220 volts of alternating current), and who have a normal electrocardiogram (ECG), no arrhythmia, and no flash or flame burns that require attention, have no need for further observation or treatment and may go home. If there are any ECG or rhythm abnormalities, however, the patient should be admitted for at least 24 hours of ECG monitoring.

In general, electrical current causes little tissue destruction, and usually at the time of exposure the heart either goes into ventricular fibrillation or remains in sinus rhythm. Ventricular fibrillation is relatively uncommon—for example, only about four deaths per year occur from electrical current burns among the 3 million inhabitants of King County (Seattle), Washington. Delayed problems are also very uncommon—probably nonexistent—following electrical current injury.

On the other hand, children who experience electrical current injury after sucking on an extension-cord plug may have serious tissue damage to the mouth and should be admitted to a burn center as they may require splinting of their mouth and possibly reconstructive surgery. Fortunately, such injuries rarely recur as children generally will not put extension cords or similar objects deep into their mouths after the initial contact.

HIGH-VOLTAGE (1000+ VOLTS) CURRENT WITHOUT TISSUE DESTRUCTION

Individuals exposed to high-voltage electrical current are at risk for cardiac arrhythmias even if no ECG or other abnormalities are present at the

Figure 9-5

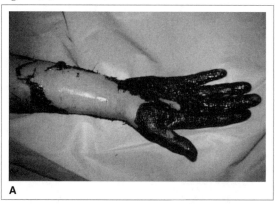

A

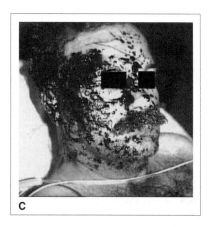

C

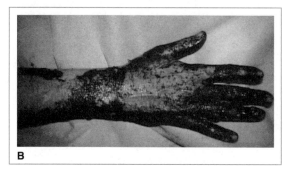

B

Asphalt burn. Photo illustrates typical asphalt burn on **(A)** palmar surface of hand, **(B)** dorsum of hand, and **(C)** face. Note the sticky appearance of the asphalt, which is difficult to remove from the skin. (See also color plate.)

time of initial evaluation. These individuals should be admitted for 24 hours of ECG monitoring.

ELECTRICAL CURRENT INJURY WITH TISSUE DESTRUCTION

The extent of tissue damage in patients with electrical current injuries often bears no relationship to the size of any visible cutaneous burn, because the deep-tissue destruction that occurs in such patients is not visible on the surface skin. The deep-tissue destruction can be extensive, resulting in myoglobinuria from muscle necrosis, and often requiring debridement and even fasciotomy.

The patient's fluid requirements cannot be estimated by the rule of nines and must instead be determined by monitoring vital signs, urine output, and other parameters. Patients with an electrical current injury commonly require large amounts of fluid for resuscitation.

MYOGLOBINURIA   Deep-tissue destruction is often manifest clinically by the presence of myoglobin in the urine, which makes the urine appear brown or red—often the color of a claret or cabernet wine (Fig. 9-6). If inspection of the urine indicates the presence of myoglobinuria, treatment should

Figure 9-6

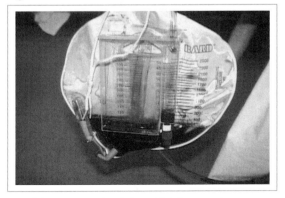

Myoglobinuria. Note the dark, reddish-brown color of the urine in the collection bag. This color is typical of myoglobinuria. (See also color plate.)

Figure 9-7

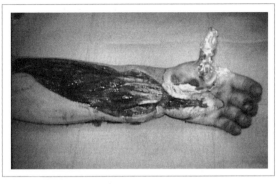

Fasciotomy. This patient has undergone fasciotomy and carpal tunnel release following swelling that occurred as a result of an electrical injury. (See also color plate.)

be instituted to prevent renal damage. Treatment involves maintaining a urine output of about 100 cc/hour. Alkalinizing the urine may also help. Three ampules of bicarbonate in a liter of D5W will produce an isotonic solution of 150 mEq of sodium per liter. Often, simply increasing fluid infusion rates will achieve the desired urine output; however, if increasing fluids does not achieve a sufficient urine output, intravenous mannitol should be administered (12.5 g, followed by another 12.5 g in 30 to 45 minutes). Once mannitol is given, it is no longer possible to assess volume and perfusion status by monitoring urine output; therefore, if there is no evidence of myoglobinuria (i.e., if the urine is clear or light yellow), mannitol should not be used.

SURGICAL DEBRIDEMENT AND FASCIOTOMY   There are two indications for early surgical treatment of patients with electrical current injury. First, if the burn results in persistent gross myoglobinuria or metabolic acidosis, the necrotic tissue load causing these problems can be decreased by operative debridement. Second, if swelling from the burn is compromising vascular flow to an extremity, vascular compromise can be relieved by fasciotomy (Fig. 9-7). Similarly, swelling from electrical burns of the hand may result in progressive median or ulnar nerve symptoms that can be relieved by carpal tunnel release. If these indications for surgery are absent during the first 24 hours after the burn, then operation is usually delayed for 3 to 5 days, a time at which tissue viability can best be assessed, but before necrotic tissue develops invasive infection.

Tissue pressure monitoring to assess need for fasciotomy is widely used in orthopedic surgery, but is used less often in burn management. The reason is that, among burn patients, capillary leakage and associated edema result in elevated tissue pressures, even in totally unburned extremities. Thus, it is necessary to base the need for surgical intervention on clinical parameters such as pulses, pain, and capillary refill, in addition to or instead of tissue pressures alone.

Associated Injuries

Because electrical current injuries result in tetanic muscle contractions and falls, many patients have additional traumatic injuries. In particular, it is important to assess the possibility of spinal cord injury by obtaining appropriate x-rays when patients complain of back or neck pain.

Patients with electrical current injuries often have delayed, persistent, and/or recurrent neurologic symptoms, and subsequent development of premature cataracts is common. Because many electrical burns are work-related and involve insurance claims, it is important to have a baseline examination of both the neurologic system and the eye to establish whether there are any preexisting abnormalities. Therefore, consultation with a neurologist and ophthalmologist, including a slit-lamp evaluation, is often helpful.

Escharotomy

Deep, cutaneous burns decrease the elastic nature of the skin. This, coupled with the burn-related edema, can result in increased compartmental pressures and a burn-related compartmental syndrome. Unlike classic compartmental syndromes,

those that occur in burns can generally be relieved by escharotomy, rather than fasciotomy.

In general, only circumferential full-thickness burns require escharotomy and then only when the distal circulation is compromised. This most often occurs in extremities (Fig. 9-8). Burns on the trunks need escharotomy only very rarely, and fingers almost never do.

Escharotomies are rarely required on an emergency basis. Therefore, if the patient can be transported to a burn center within a few hours of injury, personnel at the burn center can assess the need for escharotomy. Should escharotomy be necessary in a situation in which transport is impossible, consultation with burn center personnel is desirable before performing the procedure.

The procedure of escharotomy involves an incision that should go only through the eschar that is constricting tissue—generally, just under

Figure 9-8

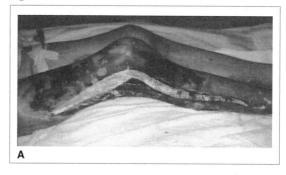

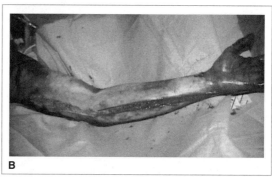

Escharotomy. Escharotomy is most often required in circumferential full-thickness burns of the extremities, shown here on the **(A)** leg and **(B)** arm. (See also color plate.)

the skin and slightly into the fat. The incision should not extend to the muscle fascia. At times, heavy bleeding can occur from incision of the subcutaneous blood vessels. This bleeding can be controlled by coagulating major blood vessels with electrocautery, but it is essential to provide the patient with adequate narcotic analgesia before doing so because, although the eschar itself is insensitive to pain, coagulating subcutaneous tissue is very painful. Rubbing Avitene in the wound and gently wrapping the extremity with Kerlix can often stop oozing, thereby obviating the need for electrocauterization.

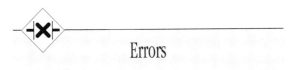

Errors

Several common errors in burn management have been mentioned already, but are worthy of emphasis. These include errors in the management of pain, in the administration of fluids, and in airway management.

Pain Management

The mistakes made in managing pain are giving too little analgesic initially, weaning off analgesic too soon, and failing to place the patient on a weaning schedule. Failure to provide adequate analgesia causes patients to experience pain during dressing changes and physical therapy, resulting in fear and lack of cooperation during these activities. Such patients will generally require increased analgesia later in their course of treatment, will take narcotics more out of fear than out of need, and will often be unwilling to stop taking narcotics after the burn has healed.

Fluid Administration

As discussed earlier, many clinicians administer excessive amounts of intravenous fluids to burn victims in an attempt to maintain a higher-than-necessary urine output. Fluid administration that results in urine output above 50 cc/hour increases the risk of fluid overload, with its complications of tissue edema and pulmonary congestion.

Airway Management

Withholding endotracheal intubation until a burn victim manifests overt signs of respiratory distress is a potentially life-threatening error. Instead, as reviewed earlier in this chapter, prophylactic intubation should be performed early for patients at risk of developing airway edema. This will avoid the subsequent need to intubate an airway that is compromised by laryngeal edema.

Tetanus Prophylaxis

During the flurry of activity that occurs during acute management of burns, clinicians sometimes forget to inquire about the patient's tetanus immunization status. This error occurs infrequently in burn centers, where inpatients are monitored daily and burn-management protocols are used. In the office setting, however, omission of indicated tetanus immunization at the initial visit creates a lost opportunity to immunize the patient, who may or may not return for follow-up care. This is a particular concern for older individuals, who lack sufficient protection against tetanus; most cases of tetanus in the United States occur in geriatric-aged individuals.

A related error is reliance on tetanus toxoid immunization alone, that is, failure to administer tetanus immune globulin when indicated. This error can be avoided by providing tetanus prophylaxis according to standard protocols.

References

Ahrns KS, Harkins DR: Initial resuscitation after burn injuries: therapies, strategies, and controversies. *AACN Clin Issues* 10:46, 1999.

Brigham PA, McLoughlin E: Burn incidence and medical care use in the United States: estimates, trends, and data sources. *J Burn Care Rehabil* 17:95, 1996.

Crawford ME, Rask H: Prehospital care of the burned patient. *Eur J Emerg Med* 3:247, 1996.

Erdmann D, Hussman J, Kucan JO: Treatment of a severe alkali burn. *Burns* 22:141, 1996.

Hadkiiski OG, Lesseva MI: Comparison of four drugs for local treatment of burn wounds. *Eur J Emerg Med* 6:41, 1999.

Hussman J, Kucan JO, Russel RC, et al: Electrical injuries—morbidity, outcome and treatment rationale. *Burns* 21:530, 1995.

Lee RC: Injury by electrical forces: pathophysiology, manifestations, and therapy. *Curr Probl Surg* 34:677, 1997.

Monafo WW: Initial management of burns. *N Engl J Med* 335:1581, 1996.

Parson L: Office management of minor burns. *Prim Care Pract* 1:40, 1997.

Pruitt BA Jr, Cioffi WG, Shimazu T, et al: Evaluation and management of patients with inhalation injury. *J Trauma* 30:S63, 1990.

Pruitt BA Jr, McManus AT, Kim SH, Goodwin CW: Burn wound infections: current status. *World J Surg* 22:135, 1998.

Rabban JT, Blair JA, Rosen CL, et al: Mechanisms of pediatric electrical injury. New implications for product safety and injury prevention. *Arch Pediatr Adolesc Med* 151:696, 1997.

Ratnayake B, Emmanuel ER, Walker CC: Neurological sequelae following a high-voltage electrical burn. *Burns* 22:578, 1996.

Robinson L, Miller RH: Smoke inhalation injuries. *Am J Otolaryngol* 7:375, 1986.

Ryan CM, Schoenfeld DA, Thorpe WP, et al: Objective estimates of the probability of death from burn injuries. *N Engl J Med* 338:362, 1998.

Sheridan RL, Hinson M, Nackel A, et al: Development of a pediatric burn pain and anxiety management program. *J Burn Care Rehabil* 18:455, 1997.

Wallace BH, Cone JB, Vanderpool RD, et al: Retrospective evaluation of admission criteria for paediatric electrical injuries. *Burns* 21:590, 1995.

Williams WG, Phillips LG: Pathophysiology of the burn wound, in Herndon DN (ed): *Total Burn Care*. Philadelphia, WB Saunders, 1996.

Sarvesh Logsetty

Chapter

10

Lacerations

Introduction

Of all surgical injuries seen by primary-care and emergency-room clinicians, lacerations are the most common. Fortunately, when lacerations are evaluated and treated correctly, both the clinician and patient leave the office or emergency room pleased with the results.

In evaluating a laceration, several basic issues must be considered. Clinicians must always check for associated injuries and should not simply assume that the visible laceration represents the full extent of trauma. It is important to clean the wound thoroughly and debride it as needed to remove devitalized tissue. Before repairing a laceration, the clinician must also consider the size, location, and characteristics of the wound, as these parameters will provide a guide for wound closure. It is also necessary to consider what suture materials to use, whether there is sufficient time to perform an adequate repair, whether sufficient support services are available, and whether the wound should be repaired by a surgeon. Finally, it is important to consider the general health of the patient, any underlying medical problems, and the need for tetanus prophylaxis.

This chapter will review the issues described above, thereby providing readers with the general principles that must be considered in evaluating and repairing lacerations. Additional information pertinent to the repair of lacerations is also contained in Chapter 2 (Suturing Techniques and Materials) and Chapter 15 (Skin Lesions), and the reader is referred to those chapters for more detailed information.

Epidemiology

Each year, approximately 11 million lacerations are treated in emergency departments of hospitals in the United States. A large but unknown additional number of lacerations are treated in clinicians' offices and urgent-care centers. Other, usually minor lacerations, are self-treated by patients using adhesive strips or, occasionally, commercially available "super-glues" (cyanoacrylate adhesives).

In the vast majority of cases, when patients seek medical care for a laceration, repair is performed either by an emergency-room clinician or an office-based primary-care clinician. Complicated lacerations requiring management by a surgeon are the exception and are most often seen in the setting of major or multisystem trauma.

Key History

When evaluating a patient who has a laceration, it is important to question the patient about the mechanism and timing of the injury, medical history, and the status of tetanus prophylaxis.

Mechanism and Timing of Injury

The mechanism of injury often determines the treatment and techniques used for laceration repair. For example, clean lacerations sustained from a sharp object can usually be repaired primarily with little need for debridement. Lacerations resulting from irregularly shaped or greasy or dirty objects often require considerable cleansing and debridement to remove devitalized tissue and foreign matter. Lacerations caused by animal or human bites may require antibiotic therapy; in some cases it may not be appropriate to close a bite wound.

Timing of injury also influences treatment. Lacerations on the torso and extremities can be closed up to 8 hours following the injury; when patients with such injuries present more than 8 hours after the injury, the lacerations generally should not be closed. Rather, it is usually preferable to dress the wound daily with sterile, wet-to-dry dressings and either perform a delayed closure 3 to 4 days later or permit the wound to heal by secondary intention. When delayed closure is performed, it is usually necessary to debride the wound to create fresh surgical edges prior to closure. Facial lacerations can generally be closed up to 24 hours after injury, although in some cases they can be closed later, especially if they were cleaned and dressed at the time of injury.

Medical History

Patients should be asked about current and past medical illnesses, medication use, drug allergies, and whether they have undergone laceration repairs in the past. Medical illnesses that affect immunologic function or wound healing may indicate the need for specialized care in laceration repair or the use of antibiotics. Similarly, patients who have developed a keloid or hypertrophic scar after a past laceration repair might be considered for referral to a plastic surgeon instead of having the repair done by a primary-care clin-

Table 10-1

Recommendations for Tetanus Prophylaxis in Patients with Lacerations

CASE SCENARIO	RECOMMENDED TETANUS PROPHYLAXIS	
	TIG	TD
Clean minor wounds		
Unknown immunization status	No	Yes
Received <3 prior doses of Td	No	Yes
Received ≥3 prior doses Td, but last dose >10 yrs ago	No	Yes
Severe wounds		
Unknown immunization status	Yes	Yes
Received <3 prior doses of Td	Yes	Yes
Received ≥3 prior doses Td, but last dose >5 yrs ago	No	Yes

Td, tetanus toxoid—diphtheria toxoid; TIG, tetanus immune globulin.

ician. The clinician should also note whether the patient has allergies to local anesthetics that might be used in the laceration repair or to antibiotics that might be used for treatment or prophylaxis of infection.

Tetanus Prophylaxis

The patient's tetanus immunization status should be determined. If necessary, tetanus toxoid and immune globulin should be administered according to the recommendations in Table 10-1.

Key Physical Examination

A thorough examination must be performed before repairing any laceration. Usually, an initial perfunctory examination will take place on presentation to provide a general idea about the severity of the wound and the instruments and materials that might be required for repair.

Then, as time permits, a more detailed examination can take place. A neurologic and musculoskeletal examination should be performed to detect nerve and tendon injuries, and this examination should always be performed before infiltrating the wound with any anesthetic. Neurologic examinations are especially important for lacerations of the upper extremity, where tendon and nerve injuries are particularly common.

Sensation to light touch, followed by pinprick and two-point discrimination, should be tested and mapped out on a diagram in the medical record if any abnormalities are noted. Also, if any abnormalities are noted, a comparison should be made with the contralateral limb or side. It is important to consider that diminished sensation may or may not indicate nerve injury from the laceration, as a perceived decrease in sensation may in actuality be a preexisting state that is the patient's norm.

After testing sensation, the clinician should systematically test all muscles present in and around the area of the laceration to ensure that they function properly. Any defects may indicate injury to the muscle or tendon itself, or to the innervation of the muscle.

Additional examination involves exploration of the wound for foreign material such as dirt and glass. Such foreign material will need to be removed as part of the wound-repair process.

Treatment

Most lacerations are repaired in the office or emergency department setting. However, for some patients a laceration(s) is part of a multisystem traumatic injury for which emergency surgical treatment of associated injuries is required. Such patients often can have their lacerations explored and repaired in the operating room, concomitantly with other surgical treatments, taking advantage of the general anesthesia used for surgical procedures.

Administration of Local Anesthesia

LIDOCAINE

Assuming the laceration is suitable for repair in an office or emergency-room setting, and once a neurologic examination has been completed and documented, local anesthetic can be administered in preparation for a detailed wound examination and laceration repair. Lidocaine is the usual agent used for local anesthesia, and, in the absence of allergy to the drug, it may be used in any location in the body with little risk. Lidocaine should be injected from within a laceration, rather than through intact skin, because injection from within the laceration is less painful.

EPINEPHRINE   The addition of 1:100,000 epinephrine to lidocaine prolongs anesthetic activity by reducing circulatory removal of lidocaine from the wound site, thereby reducing the need for large amounts of infiltrated lidocaine. The vasoconstrictive action of epinephrine also decreases bleeding, which improves visibility during laceration repair.

The vasoconstrictive action of epinephrine precludes its use, however, in body parts with blood supplies provided by terminal branches of a local circulation such as the tips of fingers, toes, and penis. Ischemia may result if epinephrine is injected into these areas. Similarly, epinephrine should not be injected into cutaneous laceration flaps that have questionable circulatory viability.

SIDE EFFECTS   While lidocaine is generally safe, there are limits to how much can be injected. One limiting factor is lidocaine's physical volume. The other is its toxicity.

Volume Limits   Volume limits on the injection of lidocaine are based on the fact that infiltration of large amounts of lidocaine into the skin results in increased interstitial fluid that can greatly alter the appearance of the wound. This effect can distort anatomic landmarks and make it difficult to repair the laceration properly. When the size or site of a laceration requires quantities of local infiltration that will obscure anatomic landmarks, a good alternative is to use a regional nerve block such as digital, mental, or ulnar nerve blocks. These regional anesthetic techniques are discussed in Chapter 1. A regional block has the advantages of requiring a decreased amount of infiltrated lidocaine, a potentially wider and better-defined area of anesthetic effect, and it does not alter the local topography.

Toxicity   The toxicity of lidocaine also limits the amount that can be injected. While injection of toxic quantities of lidocaine rarely occurs under normal circumstances, lidocaine used for laceration repair is absorbed systemically, and injection of too much lidocaine can result in seizures and cardiac arrhythmias. To avoid toxicity, the amount of lidocaine injected subcutaneously should not exceed 4.5 mg/kg. If epinephrine is present in the lidocaine solution, this amount increases to 6 to 7 mg/kg because of the slower absorption of lidocaine from the skin.

ALTERNATIVES TO LIDOCAINE

BUPIVICAINE   In addition to or instead of lidocaine, small amounts of bupivicaine (marcaine) can be used as a local anesthetic. Bupivicaine is a longer-lasting anesthetic that may provide comfort to the patient when laceration repair will require an extensive amount of time. Bupivicaine is also used if it will be some time before the laceration will be repaired, or if the patient will be unable to quickly obtain oral analgesics at home immediately after the repair.

EUTECTIC MIXTURE OF LOCAL ANESTHETICS   Eutectic mixture of local anesthetics (EMLA) is a pastelike substance containing a 5% mixture of lidocaine and prilocaine. It can be applied to the skin 30 to 90 minutes before anesthetic effect is needed. EMLA often provides sufficient anesthesia for laceration repair without the use of injectable lidocaine or will permit injection of lidocaine with minimal discomfort to the patient. EMLA is widely used for laceration repair in children because of the nonthreatening nature of a paste in comparison with an injection.

TOPICAL ANESTHETIC SOLUTIONS   Several studies have evaluated the effect of topical applications of anesthetic solutions for pain relief during anesthetic repair in children. A variety of solutions are in clinical use, including tetracaine-adrenaline-cocaine (TAC), prilocaine-phenylephrine, bupivacaine-phenylephrine, and lidocaine-epinephrine-tetracaine (LET). These solutions are best used for relatively small (<5 cm in length) lacerations. All of these solutions are applied directly to the laceration, and they achieve reasonable pain relief. However, these solutions must remain in contact with the skin for up to 20 to 30 minutes before

pain relief beings to occur, and pain relief from EMLA and from injectable lidocaine is generally superior to that achieved with these topical anesthetic solutions.

It is important to note that the positive results from topical application of local anesthetics do not pertain to plain lidocaine applied to the skin. Topical application of liquid lidocaine solution, even when the skin is soaked in the lidocaine solution, offers no clinically significant anesthetic effect.

DIPHENHYDRAMINE   Diphenhydramine can be injected subcutaneously and will provide satisfactory anesthesia for repair of many small lacerations. The usual concentration is 0.5% diphenhydramine in a solution that may contain epinephrine if appropriate for the location of the laceration. Higher concentrations of diphenhydramine provide slightly more anesthetic effect, but they are painful to inject. Although not as effective as lidocaine for providing anesthesia, diphenhydramine is a useful alternative for patients allergic to lidocaine and similar agents. If desired, additional anesthesia can be provided by "freezing" the skin with fluoromethane spray prior to injection of diphenhydramine.

Cleaning and Debriding the Wound

Once anesthetized, the injury needs to be cleaned and decontaminated. All wounds should be irrigated with copious amounts of sterile saline and all foreign material meticulously removed—either by irrigation or manually. It should be noted, however, that for a clean, noncontaminated laceration of the face and scalp, research indicates that wound irrigation does not reduce the rate of infection (around 1%) or influence the subsequent cosmetic appearance of the wound.

It is important to avoid instilling substances into the wound that might retard wound healing or cause tissue damage. Hydrogen peroxide and iodine solutions (e.g., Betadine) are two such substances.

If a wound is large or thought to be significantly contaminated, it is appropriate to scrub the wound with a surgical scrub brush. If it is impossible to adequately clean the wound, or if there is doubt about the cleanliness of the wound, it is better to leave it open with a plan to seek surgical consultation, close the wound later, or permit it to heal by secondary intention.

If there is concern that foreign matter remains in a wound even after irrigation and scrubbing, one can consider the possibility of obtaining radiographs to aid in identification of foreign material. The benefit of using radiographs for this purpose is highly dependent on the history, as many foreign materials, including unleaded glass, will not be visible on x-ray.

After the wound has been cleaned, the next step is to remove all nonviable tissue. Not only will dead tissue not heal, but it also serves as a nidus for infection. Debridement should be done sharply (i.e., with a scalpel and/or scissors). If extensive debridement is necessary, it should be performed in the operating room with the proper instruments and lighting.

Closing the Wound

While the wound is being cleaned and debrided, the closure needs to be planned. The primary goal is a cosmetic repair without any tension at the superficial layer. In the simplest form, a shallow linear laceration can be closed with only one layer of interrupted sutures. A running, subcuticular stitch using Monocryl suture is also a nice closure for long, linear lacerations; again, however, the wound edges cannot be under tension. If the wound is deeper or more complicated, sutures in the deeper tissue layers are usually required.

For wounds that are under tension, several maneuvers are used to reduce tension at the skin surface. One common method is to divert the tension in the skin away from the suture line by placing horizontal mattress sutures along the wound edge, thereby allowing the edges of the laceration to be tension-free. The problem with this approach is that the time interval during which

tension reduction is required during wound healing is often longer than the time it takes for the sutures to leave permanent scars. Furthermore, if too much force is transmitted to the mattress sutures, they can cut through the skin.

A better alternative to mattress sutures for relieving tension at the wound edges is to undermine the edges of the laceration slightly. This technique is especially useful in large areas of the skin such as the back and thigh and is applicable to lacerations of up to 1 to 2 cm across the wound. After undermining the wound edges, the surface skin of the remaining "advancement flap" is no longer tethered to the underlying tissue and is therefore more pliable and stretches more easily to the opposite end of the wound. When undermining wound edges to create an advancement flap, it is important to leave some subcutaneous tissue attached to the skin; otherwise, the blood supply to the flap will be compromised.

SUTURE MATERIALS

Choice of suture material is driven by personal experience and the availability of sutures. It is easiest to conceptualize suture material by grouping them as either absorbable or nonabsorbable and then subdividing the absorbable sutures into fast-absorbing and slow-absorbing types. The discussion that follows highlights suture material that is often used for laceration repair; a more detailed review of suture materials is provided in Chapter 2.

Examples of nonabsorbable sutures are monofilaments such as nylon and prolene and braided sutures such as silk. In general, silk sutures should be avoided because they can provoke an aggressive, local, inflammatory response that often results in more scarring. Nylon sutures, on the other hand, are excellent for opposing skin edges; nylon slides smoothly, thereby facilitating removal and minimizing scarring.

A fast-absorbing suture is plain catgut, which absorbs in 7 to 10 days. It can sometimes be used instead of monofilament nonabsorbable sutures for skin closure in areas where suture removal might be difficult or undesirable. The sutures absorb within a few days, and there is no need to remove them.

Long-lasting absorbable sutures include products such as Vicryl (55 to 70 days) and PDS (120 to 180 days). These sutures are used in the deeper layers and are composed of polyglactin, poliglecaprone, and polydioxanone, respectively. Approximately 60% to 70% of the tensile strength of these sutures is still present 2 weeks after laceration repair.

ALTERNATIVES TO SUTURES

SURGICAL STAPLES   Surgical staples are an alternative to sutures for skin closure in noncosmetic areas. Subcutaneous tissues must be approximated and free of tension before using staples. To minimize scarring, staples should be removed 5 to 7 days after laceration repair.

ADHESIVE STRIPS   In cosmetically important areas, the epidermal skin can be closed with adhesive strips (Steri-Strips) instead of sutures. Prior to placing the Steri-Strips, it is important to ensure that the skin is dry and that there is no tension on the approximated edges of the laceration. This can be accomplished by placing intradermal sutures in an inverted (i.e., knot buried) fashion. Dexon or Vicryl absorbable sutures should be used for the intradermal closure to eliminate the need for removal.

TISSUE ADHESIVES   Skin closure can also be achieved with cyanoacrylate adhesives (so-called "super-glues"). These substances have been used for skin closure of lacerations with cosmetic results indistinguishable from those achieved with sutures.

Tissue adhesives are particularly useful in several situations. These include repair of simple lacerations in children, closure of incisions and lacerations that will be covered by a cast, and closure of lacerations for which follow-up visits and suture removal will not be feasible. The use of adhesives for wound closure is not recommended for lacerations of highly mobile areas such as joints, or on areas such as the hands and feet, where heavy use and friction are likely to occur. Adhesives are also not recommended for eyelids and mucous membranes or for when detailed alignment of the wound edges is required, as might occur for some facial lacerations. Adhesives have been used extensively, however, for closing simple, nonjagged facial and extremity lacerations in children, and the cosmetic results are excellent—generally identical to those achieved with sutures.

Several forms of cyanoacrylate are available, including butylcyanoacrylate and octylcyanoacrylate. Although it is easier to work with octylcyanoacrylate because of its physical properties, there is no difference in the cosmetic appearance of wounds, including facial lacerations, repaired with the two substances.

The adhesive forms a pliable waterproof closure of the wound. It is left in place until it disintegrates. Disintegration usually occurs within 7 to 14 days.

Lacerations Requiring Special Considerations

For a variety of anatomic reasons, lacerations in certain areas require special considerations. These include lacerations of the scalp, lips, nose, ear, eyelids, and eyebrows, as well as injuries to muscle, tendon, and vascular structures.

SCALP

Because they bleed heavily and involve multiple tissue layers, scalp lacerations sometimes appear daunting. However, repair of scalp lacerations is actually quite simple if approached systematically with focus on three key points.

The first point is that the scalp is highly vascular; therefore, attention must be focused on control of bleeding. It is not unheard of for a patient to exsanguinate from a scalp laceration. Use of lidocaine with epinephrine, combined with manual pressure, is usually sufficient to stop bleeding from the wound edges. Larger vessels often need to be clamped and tied. If bleeding is not quickly controlled, an intravenous infusion should be instituted and preparation made for transfusion. On occasion, surgical clips (Raney clips) can be used to stop refractory bleeding, but these devices should be used cautiously because they apply a great deal of pressure that can result in hair loss.

Even if a scalp laceration is not actively bleeding at the time of presentation, clinicians should be cognizant of the fact that considerable blood loss may already have occurred, and the patient should be assessed for tachycardia, orthostatic hypotension, or other signs of severe blood loss.

The second point is that the excellent vascular supply of the scalp provides some protection from infection. Therefore, extensive emphasis on creating a clean surgical field often is not necessary. Thus, once the wound is scrubbed clean, it is not necessary to spend a lot of time and effort in shaving the patient's head. A small rim clear of hair should be sufficient to permit suturing without the frustration of grabbing stray strands of hair with the needle holder or having to pull hairs out of the wound.

The third point is that, although the scalp is well organized into layers, it is not always necessary to close the individual layers with subcutaneous sutures. Whenever possible, a single-layer closure of the scalp is best, as it avoids the hair loss that sometimes occurs with subcutaneous sutures. When subcutaneous sutures are required, long-lasting absorbable suture should be used, and the individual layers of the scalp should be accurately approximated to avoid a cosmetic defect. While many surgeons recommend specifically closing the galea aponeurosis, it is probably not necessary to do so if the wound has been adequately debrided.

The skin can then be closed with either staples or vertical mattress sutures. If sutures are used for skin closure, they should either be absorbable sutures, or else a nonabsorbable suture of a different color than the patient's hair. If the sutures are the same color as the patient's hair, it may be difficult to distinguish them from hair at the time of suture removal.

EAR

Ear lacerations must be repaired carefully, especially if the cartilage is injured. When possible, one or two stitches should be placed in the cartilage to approximate its cut edges, using a longer-lasting absorbable suture such as chromic catgut, Monocryl, Vicryl, or Dexon. The skin should then be closed with interrupted 5-0 nylon or plain gut.

Hematomas, if present, need to be aspirated because they apply pressure to the adjacent ear cartilage. Cartilage has a tenuous vascular supply and may undergo necrosis in the presence of pressure from a hematoma. In addition, hematomas on the ear serve as growth media for bacteria and therefore predispose to infection, which can also damage the underlying cartilage. Thus, the ear should be closely observed for signs of infection following laceration repair. If there is any question of infection, with or without the presence of a hematoma, antibiotic therapy should be administered. Ciprofloxacin is commonly used because it has excellent, soft-tissue penetration and reasonable activity against staphylococcal and streptococcal organisms.

EYEBROW

Lacerations of the eyebrow must also be repaired carefully because improper technique can result in a cosmetic defect. A key point is not to shave or trim the eyebrow, as eyebrow hairs may not grow back fully after shaving or trimming. In addition, single-layer closures are preferred to multilayered closures because the subcutaneous sutures used in multilayered closures also increase the risk of hair loss in the eyebrow.

It is also important to be judicious in debriding an eyebrow laceration because removal of tissue may leave a cosmetic defect. While other areas of the body are amenable to skin grafting if debridement involves removal of significant amounts of tissue, a skin graft on the eyebrow or forehead is neither cosmetically nor functionally acceptable. If it appears that jagged edges of an eyebrow laceration preclude accurate approximation of the wound edges, it is still better to repair the laceration without extensive debridement of irreplaceable tissues. If the cosmetic result is unacceptable, the scar can be revised at a later date.

The technique for repairing an eyebrow laceration depends on the exact location of the laceration. If the laceration is totally within the eyebrow, the likelihood of a cosmetically unacceptable scar is minimal because the scar will be hidden by eyebrow hair. If, on the other hand, the laceration crosses the hair-bearing and non–hair-bearing border of the eyebrow, it is essential that these borders are carefully approximated across the laceration. To achieve this approximation, it is best to first line up both the superior and inferior junctions between hair-bearing and non–hair-bearing areas and to tack them together with a small suture before closing the deeper layers of the laceration. If the muscle under the eyebrow is damaged, a single, loose Dexon or chromic gut suture should be placed to approximate the muscle edges; the aim is to gently align the muscle edges without putting tension on the friable muscle. The deeper subcutaneous layers are then repaired with a long-lasting absorbable suture, but, as noted above, a single-layered closure is preferred when possible. Skin repair is accomplished with a fast-absorbing synthetic suture or plain gut; use of these sutures will minimize scarring and eliminate the need for suture removal.

If an eyebrow laceration involves the eyelid, the skin of the eyelid can be closed with plain catgut. However, if the underlying eyelid muscle is traumatized, it is advisable not to undertake the repair and, instead, to refer the patient to an ophthalmologist for exploration and closure of the laceration.

NOSE

Lacerations of the nose can be divided into simple lacerations and complex lacerations; com-

plex lacerations are those involving the nasal ala. For both simple and complex nose lacerations, the skin can be closed with either plain catgut or nylon. No sutures should be placed in the cartilage. The inner nasal mucosa should be closed with either plain or chromic gut. As with ears, follow-up care is important, and it is essential to aspirate any hematomas that develop and to start antibiotics if there is any indication of infection.

LIP

Repair of lip lacerations requires careful attention to the junction between the perioral skin and the pigmented portion of the lip—known as the vermilion border of the lip, which is an important landmark on the face. Therefore, when a lip laceration involves the vermilion border, great care must be exercised to achieve perfect alignment of this border when the laceration is closed. Failure to do this will result in a steplike deformity of the border of the lip, which can mar an otherwise satisfactory repair.

The vermilion border is not a simple line but actually a thin strip, and both the superior and inferior edges of the strip must be approximated properly to prevent a cosmetic defect. It is often helpful to mark out the edges of the vermilion border before injecting local anesthetic because the tissue swelling caused by infiltrated lidocaine can alter topography, making cosmetic closure difficult. Similarly, if epinephrine is used in the lidocaine (which it usually is to diminish bleeding in the highly vascular lip area), the epinephrine-induced vasoconstriction will diminish redness of the lip, making accurate identification of the vermilion border an impossible task. When repairing lacerations of the lower lip, an alternative to marking the vermilion border and using lidocaine is to anesthetize the lower lip with a mental nerve block (see Chapter 1).

Sutures commonly used for repairing lip lacerations are 4-0 Vicryl, Dexon, or Monocryl for the deeper layers; 4-0 or 5-0 chromic for the lip itself; and a 5-0 plain catgut or 5-0 nylon for the adjacent skin. With patience, it is possible to perform a nearly invisible repair. All skin sutures should be removed by day 3 to 5 to minimize noticeable scarring.

Through-and-through lacerations of the lip must be approached in stages. The first stage involves closing the inner mucosa with 4-0 chromic gut or Vicryl in a watertight fashion; horizontal mattress sutures give good results. Next, the deep layer of the lip can be closed from the outside with 4-0 or 3-0 Vicryl, Dexon, or Monocryl sutures. Care should be taken to bring muscle ends together gently ("approximate, don't strangulate!"). The outer layer of skin can be closed with 4-0 plain gut or 4-0 nylon, and these skin sutures should be removed 5 days later.

MUSCLE

In general, it is not necessary to repair a lacerated muscle unless the laceration results in complete or near-complete transection of the muscle. If suture is required, the goal is to gently bring together the muscle tissue without tension and without tearing through the delicate muscle tissue. This is usually achieved with a long-lasting absorbable horizontal mattress suture, or even a simple suture, which incorporates the investing fascia.

TENDON

Both extensor tendons and flexor tendons can be injured. Lacerations of flexor tendons should be referred to an appropriately trained surgeon, because the anatomy involved in flexor-tendon repair is complicated, and accurate repair is essential for return to function.

Extensor-tendon lacerations, on the other hand, sometimes can be repaired by nonsurgeons. Lacerations of extensor tendons are classified as either partial or complete. A clean, partial tendon injury is amenable to a single horizontal mattress stitch of a nonabsorbable braided suture such as braided polyester (e.g., Ethibond, Ticron).

Complete transections of extensor tendons are further classified as either isolated or associated with other injuries. Those associated with other injuries should be referred to a surgeon for exploration. To repair an isolated complete transection of an extensor tendon, the transected edges of the tendon should be positioned together with the least amount of tension on the tendons, and a vertical mattress suture should be placed on either edge of the tendon to secure it together. If there is any tension on the ends, it is best that a surgeon be consulted to perform the repair.

Often, the most important part of treating a lacerated tendon is not the repair itself, but the splinting and the therapy program that follow the repair. Without appropriate splinting, the repair is at high risk to tear apart. Without appropriate physical and occupational therapy, there is a risk that the repair will scar in such a way as to reduce movement of the joint. Thus, once repaired, the tendon should be splinted in the position of least stretch. Patients should be advised against any activity involving the injured extremity, and they should be referred for commencement of a physical and occupational therapy program.

BLOOD VESSELS

It is rarely possible to repair a vascular injury in an office or emergency-department setting. However, while definitive repair may not be achievable, it is often necessary to carefully identify the bleeding vessel and ligate it to prevent exsanguination.

Even if severe hemorrhage precludes visualization of the bleeding blood vessel, it is never appropriate to blindly clamp a structure in an attempt to stop bleeding. Blind clamping can result in damage to the nerves, tendons, and other vessels running in association with the injured vessel. Instead, one should use a temporary tourniquet to stop bleeding and to allow for better visualization.

For extremity lacerations, the best method for creating a tourniquet is to apply a blood-pressure cuff proximal to the wound and inflate it to above systolic blood pressure. The use of a Penrose drain (or other piece of surgical tubing) as a makeshift tourniquet is not recommended because such tourniquets only occlude venous return; thus they do not improve visibility from arterial bleeding, and they potentially worsen edema through venous congestion.

The blood-pressure-cuff tourniquet should not be left in place for longer than 15 to 30 minutes. Once control of significant hemorrhage has been accomplished, the cuff should be deflated and any further minor bleeding managed by local pressure. Although it is tempting to place a tourniquet to prevent bleeding during long transports, this is ill-advised because prolonged hypoperfusion created by the tourniquet can cause ischemic tissue necrosis distal to the tourniquet or an ischemia-reperfusion injury that can result in a severe systemic response once the tourniquet is removed.

The above admonishments aside, it should be noted that tourniquets do have a role in the treatment of lacerations. They can be used on a temporary basis to diminish minor bleeding and improve tissue visibility during the repair of upper extremity lacerations. They are also helpful to maintain visibility when repairing uncomplicated tendon lacerations.

Postoperative Care

After the laceration is repaired, two important issues must be considered. The first is the timing of suture removal. The second is the use of antibiotics.

Suture Removal

As explained in Chapter 2, timely removal of sutures is essential to obtaining the best cosmetic result after laceration repair. General guidelines for timing of suture removal are shown in Table 10-2.

Table 10-2

Timing of Suture Removal

SITE OF LACERATION	USUAL TIMING OF SUTURE REMOVAL (DAYS)
Scalp	7–10
Face	3–5
Outer lip	5
Ear	3–5
Arms and legs	10–14
Hand	10–14
Torso	7–10

Antibiotics

Aftercare of most lacerations involves daily dressing changes and application of antibiotic ointment. Bacitracin ointment is most commonly used.

Systemic antibiotics, on the other hand, are generally appropriate only for obviously contaminated or infected wounds. There is no evidence that routine antibiotics are of benefit for patients with minor lacerations of the arms, legs, face, scalp, or trunk. Similarly, while past practice involved routine prophylactic antibiotic therapy for simple hand lacerations, there is no evidence that this practice reduces the incidence of infection (approximately 1%).

Most dog-bite lacerations can be safely closed after debridement and monitored without prophylactic antibiotics, but cat bites commonly introduce *Pasteurella multocida* into the lacerated tissue and generally should be treated with antibiotics. Penicillin or amoxicillin are the antibiotics of choice for cat-bite lacerations. Doxycycline is the recommended alternative for individuals who are allergic to penicillins.

References

Adler AJ, Dubinisky I, Eisen J: Does the use of topical lidocaine, epinephrine, and tetracaine solution provide sufficient anesthesia for laceration repair? *Acad Emerg Med* 5:108, 1998.

Avner JR, Baker MD: Lacerations involving glass. The role of routine roentgenograms. *Am J Dis Child* 146:600, 1992.

Barnett P, Jarman FC, Goodge J, et al: Randomized trial of histoacryl blue tissue adhesive glue versus suturing in the repair of paediatric lacerations. *J Paediatr Child Health* 34:548, 1998.

Bartfield JM, Sokaris SJ, Raccio-Robak N: Local anesthesia for lacerations: pain of infiltration inside vs outside the wound. *Acad Emerg Med* 5:100, 1998.

Ernst AA, Marvez-Valls E, Mall G, Patterson J, et al: 1% lidocaine versus 0.5% diphenhydramine for local anesthesia in minor laceration repair. *Ann Emerg Med* 23:1328, 1994.

Hollander JE, Richman PB, Werblud M: Irrigation of facial and scalp lacerations: does it alter outcomes? *Ann Emerg Med* 31:73, 1998.

Hollander JE, Singer AJ: Laceration management. *Ann Emerg Med* 34:356, 1999.

Liebelt EL: Current concepts in laceration repair. *Curr Opin Pediatr* 9:459, 1997.

Osmond MH, Quinn JV, Sutcliffe T, et al: A randomized, clinical trail comparing butylcyanoacrylate with octylcyanoacrylate in the management of selected pediatric facial lacerations. *Acad Emerg Med* 6:171, 1999.

Paller AS: A new tissue adhesive for laceration repair in children. *J Am Acad Dermatol* 41:767, 1999.

Penoff J: Skin closures using cyanoacrylate tissue adhesives. Plastic Surgery Educational Foundation DATA Committee. Device and Technique Assessment. *Past Reconstr Surg* 103:730, 1999.

Quinn J, Wells G, Sutcliffe T, et al: A randomized trial comparing octylcyanoacrylate tissue adhesive and sutures in the management of lacerations. *JAMA* 277:1527, 1997.

Quinn J, Wells G, Sutcliffe T, et al: Tissue adhesive versus wound repair at 1 year: randomized clinical trial correlating early, 3-month, and 1-year cosmetic outcome. *Ann Emerg Med* 32:645, 1998.

Romfh RF, Cramer FS: *Technique in the Use of Surgical Tools.* Norwalk, CT, Appleton & Lange, 1992.

Smith GA, Strausbaugh SD, Harbeck-Weber C, et al: Comparison of topical anesthetics with lidocaine infiltration during laceration repair in children. *Clin Pediatr* 36:17, 1997.

Stamou SC, Maltzou HC, Psaltopoulou T, et al: Wound infections after minor limb lacerations: risk factors and the role of antimicrobial agents. *J Trauma* 46:1078, 1999.

Stewart GM, Simpson P, Rosenberg NM: Use of topical lidocaine in pediatric laceration repair: a review of topical anesthetics. *Pediatr Emerg Care* 14:419, 1998.

Sykes LN Jr, Cogwill F: Management of hemorrhage from severe scalp lacerations with Raney clips. *Ann Emerg Med* 18:995, 1989.

Zempsky WT, Karasic RB: EMLA versus TAC for topical anesthesia of extremity wounds in children. *Ann Emerg Med* 30:163, 1997.

Zempsky WT: Use of topical lidocaine in pediatric laceration repair. *Pediatr Emerg Care* 15:239, 1999.

John W. O'Kane and
Peter T. Simonian

Chapter
11

Fractures

Introduction

This chapter will first discuss definitions and general principles of fracture management. Subsequently, the chapter will focus on the evaluation and treatment of specific common fractures.

Definitions

A fracture generally results from the loading of bone beyond its capacity to accommodate the load, causing a disruption of the bony architecture. Fractures can be partial or complete. Partial fractures such as greenstick fractures of immature bone involve only one aspect of the bony cortex. Complete fractures involve both aspects of the cortex and are defined as intra-articular if the fracture line crosses the articular cartilage of a joint surface. Fracture displacement measured in millimeters describes separation of the fracture components, while angulation measured in degrees describes the amount of angular deformity. In an open fracture the fracture site is exposed through a break in the skin. Additional terms to describe fracture configuration include transverse, oblique, spiral, and comminuted (Fig. 11-1).

General Principles of Evaluation

Certain principles are common to evaluation and treatment of any fracture. The initial assessment of a suspected fracture should include a complete neurovascular assessment to ensure that the fracture has not compromised innervation or vascular supply. It is also essential to carefully assess the skin and surrounding tissue; any open fracture should be immediately referred to an orthopedist for surgical treatment.

General Principles of Treatment

Fracture treatment generally consists of a period of immobilization followed by a gradual increase in activity and then rehabilitation to restore normal function. Immobilization of acute injuries decreases pain and allows healing to begin, but must allow space into which predictable swelling can occur. Therefore, splints with soft compression that will accommodate swelling should be employed initially, followed by application of a cast or other prefabricated immobilization device after swelling has diminished (usually by about 5 days after the injury).

Early evidence of neurovascular compromise from compression in a splint or cast includes increasing pain, numbness, skin color change, or

Figure 11-1

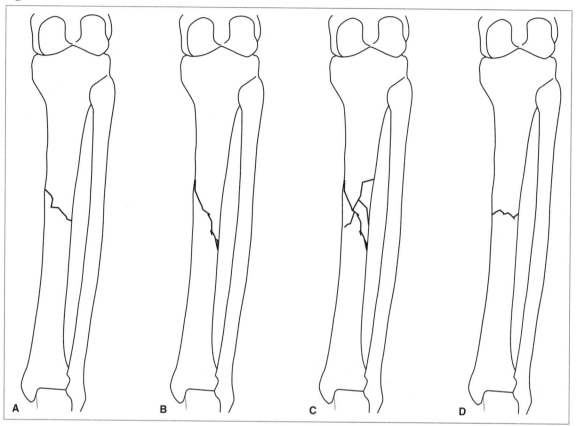

Fracture nomenclature. The four parts of this figure illustrate the principle types of fractures: oblique **(A)**, spiral **(B)**, comminuted **(C)**, transverse **(D)**. The term comminuted refers to a fracture resulting in multiple bone fragments.

impaired motor function. If neurovascular compromise occurs or is suspected, the splint or cast must be removed and the involved limb monitored for normalization of neurovascular function. Cast loosening from limb atrophy is a late complication of cast immobilization, in which case the cast should be refit to ensure adequate immobilization until the end of treatment.

General Principles of Follow-Up

In most cases fractures should be followed radiographically for evidence of bony union. Normal fracture healing involves osteoblast activity result-

ing in the formation of an osteoid callus, followed by remodeling of the callus into normal bone. Fracture healing correlates clinically with resolution of pain and tenderness and is defined by the ossification of the callous osteoid, the disappearance of fracture lines on radiographs, and the stabilization of the fracture fragments. Normal healing time varies between 2 to 6 months, depending on the blood supply of the fractured bone and other variables that affect the rate of healing.

Delayed union is defined as a failure to heal over the normal time course. Nonunion is a failure to heal over 6 to 8 months with radiographic evidence of persistent fracture lines, sclerosed ends of the fracture components with a visible gap, and either hypertrophic or absent callous formation. Clinically, nonunions continue to be painful and tender with an absence of normal bony stability and, possibly, palpable crepitus at the fracture site. The primary risk factors for delayed union and nonunion include the inability to achieve adequate immobilization or fixation and a poor vascular supply. In general, it is advisable to refer nonunions and delayed unions for treatment by an orthopedic surgeon. Electrical stimulation has been advocated for delayed unions, but at this time has not been definitively demonstrated to be effective.

Specific Fractures

Clavicle

INTRODUCTION

Clavicle fractures are among the most common of fractures. They are generally treated nonoperatively and heal with good results. With high-energy injuries to the clavicle, however, nonunion may occur in 0.1% to 5% of cases.

PATHOPHYSIOLOGY

The clavicle is a bony strut connecting the shoulder girdle to the thorax. It is susceptible to injury from a direct blow or a fall onto the shoulder such as occurs with a fall from a bicycle. The clavicle is located superficially, and, as a result, injury to the overlying skin can result if the fracture is displaced superiorly. Because of the clavicle's proximity to the lung and major vascular structures, fractures with inferior or posterior displacement can injure those structures, and careful evaluation should be undertaken to exclude such injuries.

EPIDEMIOLOGY

Clavicle fractures generally occur in the middle third of the bone (Fig. 11-2), with the proximal seg-

Figure 11-2

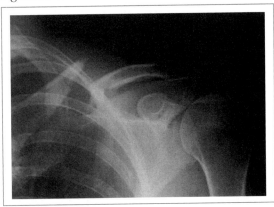

Clavicle fracture. The fracture is through the middle third of the clavicle and shows typical upward displacement of the proximal segment.

ment drawn upward by the sternocleidomastoid and the distal segment anchored by the coracoclavicular (CC) ligaments. Fractures of the proximal (medial) third of the bone are rare in adults, but may occur in individuals under the age of 25 and can involve the sternoclavicular joint. Distal clavicle fractures can be intra-articular, involving the acromioclavicular (AC) joint, which can result in posttraumatic arthritis. Fractures just proximal to the CC ligaments, or those involving disruption of the ligaments, often result in significant displacement of the fracture segments (Fig. 11-3).

TYPICAL PRESENTATION

Patients generally present with a history of a fall onto the shoulder or outstretched hand and complain of pain localized over the clavicle. An obvious deformity may be present. Supporting the weight of the arm, any movement of the arm, and deep breathing are often painful.

KEY HISTORY

When evaluating patients with a clavicle fracture, it is important to seek a history or evidence of associated injuries, particularly injuries of the head or neck. As with all upper extremity injuries, it is also critical to obtain information on handed-

Figure 11-3

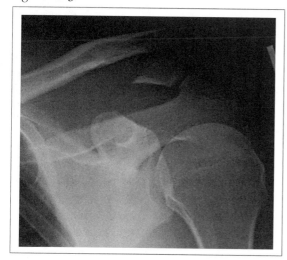

Distal clavicle fracture. Fractures of the distal clavicle often disrupt ligaments, leading to superior displacement of the fracture segments.

ness, occupation, athletic participation, age, and time elapsed since the injury.

Complaints of pain, numbness, weakness, and/or tingling of the arm or hand should alert the clinician to the possibility of a brachial plexus injury. Complaints of significant pain in the upper back could indicate an associated scapular fracture, which can occur in a high-energy injury.

KEY PHYSICAL EXAMINATION

Examination should include a thorough inspection of the skin, to exclude an open fracture or tenting from a displaced fracture segment, and a distal neurovascular examination including pulses and sensory and motor function of the brachial plexus. A pale extremity suggests an axillary artery injury. Finally, the examination should include evaluation of the scapula and glenohumeral joint to rule out associated injury to those structures.

ANCILLARY TESTS

Anterior-posterior (AP) and lateral radiographs are sufficient to confirm the diagnosis of clavicle

fracture. For medial fractures that might involve the sternoclavicular joint, computerized tomography (CT) scanning provides improved visualization.

TREATMENT

The majority of clavicle fractures are treated without surgery. Even those at an increased risk of nonunion (midshaft fractures with significant displacement or distal fractures with disrupted CC ligaments and significant displacement) can initially be treated conservatively, as delayed surgical repair is an acceptable treatment if nonunion occurs.

There are, however, indications for acute surgical treatment in specific situations. These include skin injury or compromise from displaced fracture fragments; associated pulmonary or vascular injury; and, according to some experts, distal fractures with significant displacement (Fig. 11-4). Injuries with associated brachial plexus injury are probably best referred to an orthopedist, although acute surgical intervention may not always be warranted because, in over half the cases, spontaneous recovery of neurologic function occurs.

While traditional conservative treatment consists of a figure-of-eight strap, a sling with a swathe over the injured clavicle is the current recommended treatment. There is no difference in healing and a lower incidence of arm numbness

Figure 11-4

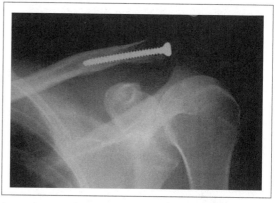

Surgical repair of distal clavicle fracture. Open reduction–internal fixation of distal clavicle fracture shown in Figure 11-3 has corrected displacement.

with the sling, and most patients find the sling more comfortable than a figure-of-eight strap. For initial management of midshaft fractures with overlapping segments and shortening, some authorities recommend a figure-of-eight strap and sleeping in the supine position with a towel roll between the scapulae.

The sling is normally used for 4 to 6 weeks with early, shoulder range-of-motion as tolerated, particularly for older patients at increased risk for developing glenohumeral stiffness as a complication of prolonged immobilization. Follow-up radiographs should be taken at 6-week intervals to document union of the fracture fragments.

ERRORS

The most important error in management of clavicle fractures is failure to identify associated neurovascular, pulmonary, musculoskeletal, or skin injury at the time of presentation. This error can be avoided with a systematic evaluation of the patient that focuses on the history and examination components outlined earlier.

CONTROVERSIES

Current controversy in the management of clavicle fractures relates to treatment of displaced fractures that occur as a result of high-energy injury. Some experts advocate that, because such fractures have up to a 5% chance of nonunion, they should undergo acute surgical repair.

Proximal Humerus

INTRODUCTION

Fractures of the proximal humerus comprise about 5% of all fractures. Most often, these fractures can be managed nonoperatively, but an understanding of fracture patterns and the degree of acceptable displacement and angulation is important in determining when conservative treatment is not appropriate.

PATHOPHYSIOLOGY

The proximal humerus is composed of four parts: the proximal humeral shaft; the greater tuberosity; the lesser tuberosity; and the head, which articulates with glenoid fossa of the scapula. The lesser tuberosity, greater tuberosity, and head each represent a separate ossification center, and either tuberosity can be fractured off the head of the humerus (Fig. 11-5). The surgical neck describes the junction of the head and the shaft. The major blood supply to the humeral head comes through the tuberosities, which also serve as the bony insertions for the rotator-cuff tendons.

Fractures of the proximal humerus tend to occur along the epiphysial lines (see Fig. 11-5)

Figure 11-5

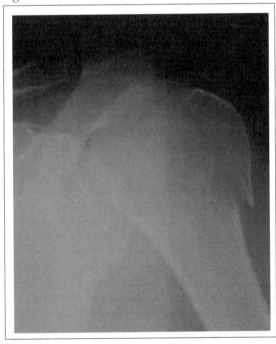

Fracture of greater tuberosity of the humerus. The greater tuberosity of the humerus forms from a separate ossification center from the head of the humerus. This AP radiograph shows a one-part fracture of the greater tuberosity that is displaced from its normal position on the head of the humerus.

and are divided into one-part, two-part, three-part, and four-part fractures, depending on the number of parts displaced. Injury usually occurs from a direct blow to the shoulder or a fall on an outstretched arm.

EPIDEMIOLOGY

Proximal humerus fractures can occur from birth to old age, with most occurring in the elderly, particularly those with osteoporosis. Three-quarters of the total number of proximal humerus fractures occur in women. Two-part fractures of the surgical neck are the most common.

In the elderly minimal trauma is necessary to fracture the proximal humerus, while in younger adults a higher-energy mechanism is necessary. Because the elderly also have a higher incidence of atherosclerosis with brittle arteries, vascular injuries in association with proximal humerus fractures are more common in this age group.

TYPICAL PRESENTATION

Patients normally present following trauma, complaining of pain, swelling, and ecchymosis localized to the proximal arm. Pain is increased with motion of the shoulder.

KEY HISTORY

Key elements of the history include those discussed earlier for clavicle fractures. In addition, a history of a prior osteoporotic fracture should increase suspicion of a proximal humerus fractures, and any complaints of numbness in the axillary dermatome or of distal extremity pain, pallor, numbness, weakness, or tingling indicate the possibility of neurovascular injury. A history of shoulder dislocation may accompany fractures of the greater tuberosity.

KEY PHYSICAL EXAMINATION

Before examining the humerus, examination should focus on associated regional injury such as injury to the cervical spine when the patient has been involved in a high-energy traumatic injury. Examination of the humerus should focus on skin integrity, shortening of the humerus, regional muscle integrity (especially the deltoid and rotator cuff), and a detailed neurovascular examination of the extremity. Overlying crepitus and rotational incongruity between the humeral head and the distal arm suggest a fracture. A dislocation should be suspected if the shoulder appears "squared off" or if the coracoid process is prominent, but fracture-dislocations may not have this characteristic.

ANCILLARY TESTS

Plain radiographs are generally sufficient for diagnosing fractures of the proximal humerus. At minimum, radiographs should include an AP view with the arm in internal and external rotation and an axillary view (Fig. 11-6) to visualize the glenoid fossa to confirm normal articulation with the humeral head. The axillary view is obtained by abducting the arm 25° to 50° and then directing the x-ray beam through the axilla with the film plate placed above the shoulder. A lateral or scapular Y view (Fig. 11-7) assists in visualizing

Figure 11-6

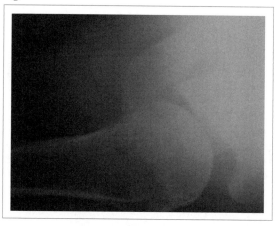

Axillary view of the head of the humerus. The axillary view permits visualization of the head of the humerus within with the glenoid fossa.

Figure 11-7

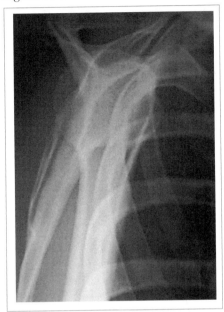

Lateral or scapular Y view of the shoulder. This
view facilitates visualization of the head of
the humerus within the glenoid fossa, as well
as visualization of the tuberosities.

the humeral head to determine its position in the
glenoid, and this view also facilitates visualization
of tuberosity fracture or displacement. CT is useful to determine the extent of fracture displacement, and MRI or ultrasound is useful to visualize
an associated rotator-cuff tear.

TREATMENT

The majority of proximal humerus fractures
will be minimally displaced (less than 5 mm),
angulated less than 20°, and occur in elderly individuals. Under these circumstances, management
consists of a sling and swathe for support, with
early pendulum range of motion to the extent tolerated, beginning at 1 to 2 weeks after the injury.
From 2 to 6 weeks after the injury, range-of-
motion and gentle strengthening is emphasized,
and then the sling is discontinued.

Because shoulder stiffness is common following fractures of the proximal humerus, physical
therapy is important for achieving maximal range
and strength. Common physical therapy exercises
used to facilitate shoulder motion include "churning" and "wall walking." Churning involves the
patient holding a broomstick or similar object in
a vertical position and moving it in a circular
motion, similar to churning butter. In wall walking, the patient faces a wall and places both
hands overhead on the wall and uses the fingers
to "walk" the hands as high as possible on the
wall to facilitate elevation of the arm.

Referral to an orthopedist is recommended for
one-part fractures with greater than 5 mm of displacement or 20° of angulation and for all two- to
four-part fractures, open fractures, intra-articular
fractures, and fractures involving compression of
the humeral head. In addition, referral is recommended when fractures of the proximal humerus
occur in younger individuals, because such fractures in younger persons typically involve higher
energy and the articular surface of the humerus is
often injured.

Generally, two-part fractures with stable reduction are treated nonoperatively, although displacement of a tuberosity greater than 5 mm requires
fixation. Internal fixation is necessary for two- and
three-part fractures, and the humeral head is replaced with a prosthesis in four-part fractures.

ERRORS

Errors in the diagnosis of proximal humerus
fractures include failure to recognize fracture displacement or concomitant posterior or occult dislocation. Other important diagnostic errors include
failure to recognize concomitant rotator-cuff tears
or associated neurovascular injury. All of these
errors can be avoided with careful physical examination and appropriate radiographic views.

The most important management error is prolonged immobilization, which can result in shoulder stiffness from secondary adhesive capsulitis.
The risk of this complication can be minimized
with early mobilization and physical therapy.

CONTROVERSIES

Controversies in the management of proximal humerus fractures relate to selection of appropriate surgical techniques. Specifically, there is controversy regarding the best technique for internal fixation of different fracture patterns and regarding the indications for internal fixation versus insertion of a prosthesis in patients with fractures of the humeral head.

Hip Fractures

INTRODUCTION

Hip fractures are divided into intracapsular femoral neck fractures (Fig. 11-8) and extracapsular intertrochanteric fractures (Fig. 11-9). These

Figure 11-8

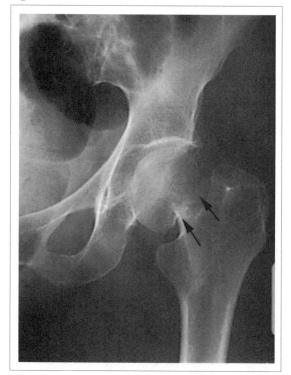

Femoral neck (impacted hip) fracture. The head of the femur is impacted onto the neck of the femur. The arrows indicate the distal margin of the femoral head.

Figure 11-9

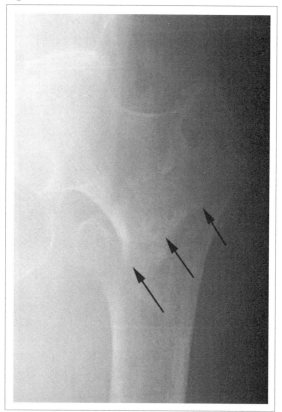

Intertrochanteric hip fracture. The fracture line, indicated by the arrows, extends from the greater trochanter to the lesser trochanter.

fractures generally occur following a fall by an elderly woman who has osteopenia or osteoporosis. In older patients hip fractures generally involve a twisting mechanism, whereas those in younger persons often involve high-energy trauma.

PATHOPHYSIOLOGY

The proximal femur consists of the femoral head, neck, and shaft and the greater and lesser trochanters. The trochanters are found where the neck meets the shaft, with the greater trochanter located superior and laterally and the lesser trochanter located inferior and medially.

The femoral head articulates with the acetabulum to form the hip joint. The hip joint capsule encloses the acetabulum, femoral head, and femoral neck. The major blood supply to the femoral head comes by way of the femoral circumflex arteries, which perforate the joint capsule along the femoral neck. The arterial supply can be compromised by an intracapsular fracture, resulting in avascular necrosis of the femoral head.

EPIDEMIOLOGY

As noted, most hip fractures occur in older women who have decreased bone density. In addition to age and osteopenia, other risk factors for hip fracture include environmental factors that increase the likelihood of falls (e.g., slippery floors or loose throw rugs), Caucasian race, heavy alcohol use, and sedentary life-style.

Hip fractures increase the likelihood of death. Morbidity associated with hip fracture includes loss of the ability to live independently and complications associated with prolonged hospitalization.

TYPICAL PRESENTATION

Patients normally present following a fall, and any elderly person with a history of a fall and pain around the hip should be considered to have a hip fracture until proven otherwise. Persons with a hip fracture are usually unable to walk, and they complain of pain in the hip, groin, or proximal anterior thigh. Normally the affected leg appears shortened and externally rotated. However, patients with impacted, stable fractures, particularly of the femoral neck, may be ambulatory with surprisingly little pain.

It sometimes cannot be determined if the fracture occurred as a result of the fall or if the fracture occurred in the absence of trauma and resulted in the fall. In most cases the former scenario (i.e., fracture resulted from the fall) is thought to apply.

KEY HISTORY

Key historic elements include injury mechanism, general health, prior fractures, malignancy

with a predilection for bony metastasis, and medications. Medications include those that affect bone metabolism (e.g., corticosteroids or thyroid hormone) or that predispose to falls (e.g., benzodiazepines). If the fracture resulted from a fall, potentially inciting medical events such as a cardiac arrhythmia or cerebral vascular accident, as well as other associated fractures (occurring up to 15% of the time), should be considered. A social history inquiring about living situation, physical abuse, substance abuse, and social support network is essential, because rehabilitation from a hip fracture is often prolonged and requires a stable and functional social situation.

KEY PHYSICAL EXAMINATION

The typical presentation may be diagnostic if obvious deformity is present. Hip rotation is most often limited and painful. Neurovascular assessment of the extremity is mandatory. Evidence of significant comorbidity should be noted, as concomitant medical conditions may influence the selection of anesthesia and may affect the methods of and potential for rehabilitation.

ANCILLARY TESTS

AP pelvis and lateral hip radiographs are often diagnostic. If the fracture is subtly impacted or minimally displaced, CT or MRI is helpful in defining the nature of the fracture.

TREATMENT

Treatment varies based on the age of the patient and the type of fracture. In nonelderly patients, a femoral neck fracture is an orthopedic emergency requiring urgent open reduction and internal fixation. If left unreduced for more than 6 hours, the likelihood of femoral head necrosis rises significantly. Intertrochanteric fractures are also treated with internal fixation.

In the elderly, treatment goals are to alleviate pain, to minimize immobilization or bed rest to prevent morbidity associated with inactivity, and to restore ambulation as quickly as possible. These goals are generally met through operative inter-

Figure 11-10

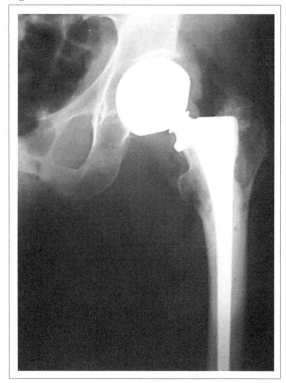

Femoral neck fracture treated with hemiarthroplasty.

patients have extensive medical comorbidity that makes the risk of surgery too great or when patients have preexisting dementia or a nonambulatory status that creates the potential for extremely high morbidity and mortality rates with surgery. Even in bed-bound or demented patients, however, surgery may still be indicated for pain control, and early mobilization is still a goal if feasible for the patient.

ERRORS

One common error is failure to diagnose a fracture in elderly patients who have a stable impacted hip fracture on which they are able to bear weight and walk. As noted earlier, hip fracture should be suspected in any older patient who has fallen down and complains of hip pain, regardless of their ability to bear weight. A second error is failure to rapidly refer patients with femoral neck fractures for surgical repair; failure to do so risks avascular necrosis of the femoral head.

Figure 11-11

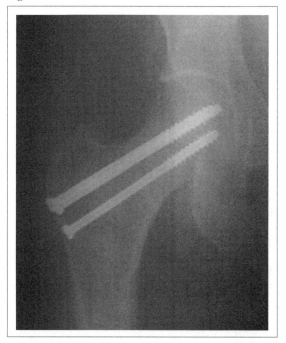

Nondisplaced femoral neck fracture treated by internal fixation.

vention that stabilizes the fracture and permits early mobilization. Prior to surgery, some form of traction (e.g., Buck's traction) can provide some pain relief.

Femoral neck fractures with displacement are generally treated with hemiarthroplasty (Fig. 11-10), while internal fixation is used for nondisplaced or impacted fractures (Fig. 11-11). Intertrochanteric fractures are generally treated with a dynamic hip screw and side plate (Fig. 11-12).

Prophylaxis for deep venous thrombosis is recommended and continued until the patient is ambulatory. Ambulation is encouraged as quickly as tolerated following the procedure.

Nonoperative treatment is appropriate in two situations. The first is for patients with impacted stable fractures without significant pain, who are capable of resuming early ambulation and other physical activity. The second situation is when

Figure 11-12

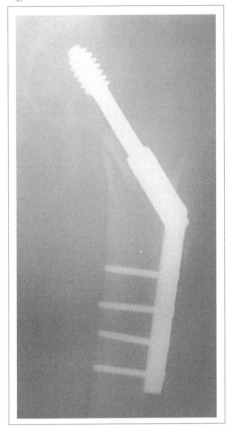

Intertrochanteric hip fracture treated with
dynamic hip screw and side plate.

CONTROVERSIES

Controversies include the method and time
course of prophylaxis for deep venous thrombosis,
which may vary significantly from surgeon to surgeon.
Options include mechanical devices employing
intermittent, lower-extremity compression and
various methods of pharmacologic anticoagulation.

Fifth-Metatarsal Fracture

INTRODUCTION

There are three main types of fifth-metatarsal
(MT) fractures. The most frequent is an avulsion
of the proximal apophysis, otherwise known as
the base of the fifth MT. The second is a fracture
of the diaphysis or metaphysis; fractures of the
proximal diaphysis are often stress fractures. The
third type of fifth-metatarsal fractures is the Jones'
fracture (Fig. 11-13), which refers to a fracture of
the proximal metadiaphyseal junction; Jones' fractures
have a reputation for poor healing.

PATHOPHYSIOLOGY

The peroneus brevis tendon and the lateral
plantar aponeurosis attach to the base of the fifth
MT. Because of the attachment of these structures,
ankle inversion injuries can result in avulsion of
the proximal apophysis. Overuse, particularly in a
supinated foot, can result in a stress fracture of
the proximal diaphysis.

EPIDEMIOLOGY

As noted, fractures at the base of the fifth
metatarsal are the most common. Military recruits,

Figure 11-13

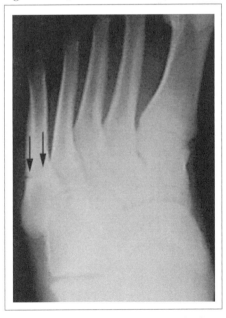

Jones' fracture. A Jones' fracture, shown by the
arrows, is a fracture through the proximal
metaphyseal-diaphyseal junction of the fifth
metatarsal.

hikers, dancers, and athletes in repetitive, weight-bearing sports are at increased risk for stress fractures. Additional risk factors include biomechanical factors (supination, varus knees, tight heel cords) that increase stresses through the lateral foot, medications and illnesses affecting bone metabolism, amenorrhea, and training errors.

TYPICAL PRESENTATION

Patients will present with acute, lateral foot pain that is worse with ambulation, following a direct blow or inversion/plantar flexion injury. In stress fractures the pain presentation may be more insidious, eventually limiting and preventing activity. Local swelling or ecchymosis may or may not be present.

KEY HISTORY

History should include information about the mechanism of injury, regional symptoms predating the acute injury that might signal an acute fracture through a preexisting stress injury, and questions about the risk factors noted above.

KEY PHYSICAL EXAMINATION

Physical examination will reveal local tenderness and possibly swelling at the site of the fracture. If the fracture occurred from an inversion ankle injury, point tenderness over the base of the fifth MT signals the possibility of an avulsion fracture. Lateral ankle tenderness, swelling, and ligamentous laxity may be present, signaling the possibility of a soft-tissue or bony injury of the ankle.

ANCILLARY TESTS

AP, lateral, and oblique radiographs of the foot are sufficient for diagnosis of fifth-metatarsal fractures caused by acute injury. Radionuclide bone scan or magnetic resonance imaging are useful when a stress fracture is suspected but plain radiographs are normal. If initial radiographs show evidence of nonunion (described at the beginning of this chapter), it is likely that the injury represents a chronic overuse mechanism with an associated stress fracture.

TREATMENT

Nondisplaced or minimally displaced avulsion fractures at the base of the fifth MT can be treated with a walking cast, boot, or a hard-soled shoe for about 6 weeks. Weight bearing is permissible to the extent permitted by the patient's pain. Follow-up radiographs are necessary because radiographic non-union occasionally occurs. However, if non-union is asymptomatic, further treatment is not needed.

Acute nondisplaced fractures of the MT diaphysis can be treated similarly, although a cast or boot may be more comfortable than a hard-soled shoe. Displaced fractures should be referred to an orthopedist for internal fixation.

Metadiaphyseal (Jones') fractures with a clear history of acute injury, typical acute radiographic appearance, and no antecedent history consistent with a stress injury can be treated in a non–weight-bearing, short-leg cast for 6 weeks, followed by an additional 2 weeks in a weight-bearing cast.

Metadiaphyseal fractures with a history of chronic symptoms or radiographic changes consistent with a stress fracture should be referred to an orthopedist. Treatment with non–weight-bearing immobilization may be successful, but requires close follow-up and may take many months. Many authors suggest intramedullary screw fixation (Fig. 11-14) with bone grafting for these fractures because of the high likelihood of delayed union or non-union. High-performance athletes are also best referred early following an acute or chronic injury, because many will elect internal fixation to facilitate a shorter rehabilitation.

ERRORS

The most important error in diagnosis and management of fifth-metatarsal fractures is failure to recognize that a Jones' fracture is susceptible to poor healing, especially when it is associated with chronic symptoms or is a stress fracture. If the

Figure 11-14

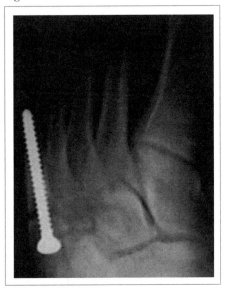

Intramedullary screw fixation for Jones' fracture.
Nonunion of a Jones' fracture can be treated
with intramedullary screw fixation. Some experts
recommend screw fixation as initial treatment.

nature of this fracture is not recognized, it may be treated as a simple displaced fracture of the base of the fifth metatarsal. Jones' fractures with chronic symptoms or stress fractures may require surgical repair and should generally be referred to an orthopedist.

CONTROVERSIES

Some experts recommend surgical treatment for all metaphyseal fractures of the fifth MT, but this recommendation is not universally accepted. The management of fifth-MT stress fractures is also controversial. Many authorities treat these fractures with intramedullary screw fixation, but this often must be removed in the future when it creates a prominence in the skin, placing the bone at risk for refracture. Therefore, some question the wisdom of internal fixation unless evidence of a chronic stress component is clear. Other authorities recommend bone grafting for stress fractures of the fifth metatarsal.

Ankle Fractures

INTRODUCTION

Ankle fractures are among the most common fractures seen in an orthopedic practice. They include fractures of the talar dome and the medial, lateral, or posterior malleolus. Stability of the ankle mortise is the primary variable for determining whether operative versus conservative treatment is appropriate. High-energy fractures of the distal articular surface of the tibia (pilon fractures) should always be referred for orthopedic management and will not be discussed here.

PATHOPHYSIOLOGY

The ankle joint is formed by the articulation of the ankle mortise with the talus. The mortise is formed by the tibia and fibula, which are held together by the tibiofibular ligaments and syndesmosis. The talus is secured within the mortise by the medial deltoid ligament complex and three lateral ligaments: the anterior talofibular ligament, posterior talofibular ligament, and the calcaneofibular ligament. There is a symmetric relationship between the talus and the mortise. Disruption of this symmetry indicates an unstable ankle injury.

The talus is wider anteriorly, and as a result the ankle joint has greater bony stability with a neutral to dorsiflexed foot and less bony stability as the foot moves into plantar flexion. With the foot in plantar flexion, therefore, the ankle is most vulnerable to injury, and stress generally results in ligamentous sprain. Stress applied to the ankle with the foot in dorsiflexion, on the other hand, is more likely to cause a malleolar fracture or tear of the mortise stabilizing syndesmosis (Fig. 11-15). Occasionally in adults but most often in children, a stressed ligament will not tear, but will result in an avulsion fracture of the distal malleolus or through the epiphysis. For most ankle fractures, the injury mechanism is usually a combination of inversion or eversion of the foot with a component of rotation, usually external.

EPIDEMIOLOGY

Ankle fractures are seen in all age groups. The most common injury is a lateral sprain of the anterior talofibular ligament, and the most common fracture is of the lateral malleolus. The Ottawa criteria have been established and successfully employed in emergency departments to identify patients who require radiographs. These criteria are appropriately applied to adults with acute injuries (<10 days) at initial presentation. According to the Ottawa criteria, ankle radiographs are indicated if the patient has tenderness along the posterior aspect or distal tip of either malleolus, or if the patient cannot take four steps immediately following injury *and* during evaluation by a clinician.

Figure 11-15

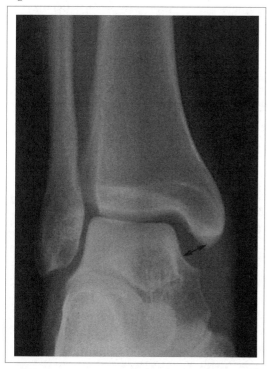

Mortise view of the ankle. The mortise view demonstrates the relationship of tibia, fibula, and talus. The mortise in this radiograph shows widening between the medial malleolus and talus, indicating disruption of the syndesmosis between the tibia and fibula.

TYPICAL PRESENTATION

Patients normally present with a history of a fall or twisting injury with ankle swelling. Weight bearing may not be possible because of pain or may be tolerated with pain.

KEY HISTORY

The history should include questions about prior injury, time since the acute injury, mechanism of injury, ability to bear weight, and overall health status.

KEY PHYSICAL EXAMINATION

Examination should include inspection for swelling, ecchymosis, skin integrity, and gross deformity. On palpation regional tenderness over the foot, both malleoli, the Achilles tendon, and along the lower leg should be noted, as well as symptoms of compartmental syndrome. The entire fibula should be palpated to rule out a Maissoneuve fracture, a rotational ankle injury resulting in proximal fibular fracture, deltoid ligament sprain, and a syndesmosis tear (Fig. 11-16).

Examination should also document neurovascular status (pedal pulses, distal capillary refill and sensation), ankle ligamentous stability (anterior drawer, tilt test), and the integrity of the peroneal tendons, anterior and posterior tibialis tendons, and Achilles' tendon.

ANCILLARY TESTS

Ankle radiographs include AP, lateral, and mortise views. A mortise view is an AP radiograph with the ankle in about 10° of internal rotation. The mortise view is critical; it must demonstrate symmetry of the articulation with the talus and show less than 4 mm of space between the talus and the medial malleolus. If these parameters are not present, surgical repair may be required.

CT is useful to demonstrate osteochondral injury to the talus. MRI is helpful for demonstrating ligamentous disruption or injury to the articular cartilage.

Figure 11-16

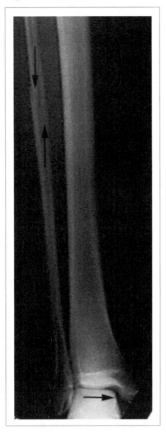

Maissioneuve fracture. The Mais-sioneuve fracture involves a mid-shaft fibular fracture *(arrows in the upper-left portion of the radiograph)* in combination with mortise widen-ing *(arrow in lower-right)*, the latter indicating injury to the deltoid liga-ment and tibiofibular syndesmosis.

TREATMENT

The treatment of ankle fractures is complicated and controversial, but the critical factor determining initial management is the stability of the ankle mortise. Avulsion fractures of the tip of either malleolus can be treated as sprains with early mobilization, weight bearing as tolerated, and then functional rehabilitation. Nondisplaced, dis-tal fibular fractures with a normal mortise can be treated in a non–weight-bearing cast for 6 weeks, followed by functional rehabilitation. Follow-up radiographs in the cast at 2 weeks are necessary to ensure that there is no displacement.

Bimalleolar or trimalleolar fractures, injuries with mortise disruption, Maissoneuve fractures, osteochondral fractures of the talus, isolated fibu-lar fractures above the level of the talus, or fibular fractures with significant tenderness over the me-dial ankle/deltoid ligament complex should be referred to an orthopedist. Surgical treatments vary, but the goal is to restore the normal mortise anatomy and to augment medial and lateral sta-bility if necessary.

ERRORS

Errors include failure to recognize ankle mortise instability and failure to refer such fractures for appropriate (usually surgical) treatment. It is always best to refer a fracture or syndesmosis injury if there is any question of mortise instability.

Scaphoid (Navicular) Fractures

INTRODUCTION

The scaphoid bone, also known as the navicu-lar bone, is the most frequently fractured carpal bone. It is also the second most commonly frac-tured bone in the upper extremity.

PATHOPHYSIOLOGY

The scaphoid is the radialmost bone in the proximal carpal row and functions as a stabilizer between the proximal and distal rows. As a re-sult, it is prone to injury from a fall onto the out-stretched hand when the proximal carpal row is fixed with the wrist in extension.

The scaphoid is anatomically divided into three parts: the proximal pole (tuberosity), the distal pole, and the middle waist. Its blood supply is from branches of the radial artery entering distally and then moving proximally through the bone. As a result, the more proximal the fracture, the greater the likelihood of avascular necrosis or nonunion.

EPIDEMIOLOGY

Scaphoid fractures are common following a fall onto the outstretched extended wrist. About 60% of the fractures occur in the "waist" of the bone (Fig. 11-17), with the remaining 40% divided evenly between fractures of the proximal and distal poles. Between 90% and 95% of scaphoid fractures will heal correctly with appropriate conservative treatment.

TYPICAL PRESENTATION

Patients typically complain of radial wrist pain with swelling. Making a fist and using the wrist against resistance is usually painful.

Figure 11-17

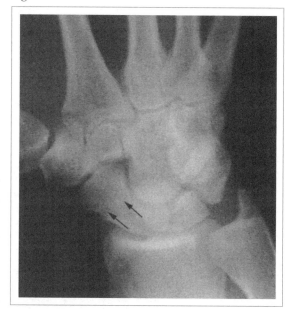

Fracture through scaphoid waist. Typical radiographic appearance of a fracture through the midsection of the scaphoid bone.

KEY HISTORY

As with all upper extremity injuries, it is critical to obtain the following information: handedness, occupation, athletic activity, age, and time elapsed since injury. History of prior injury is also important because of the potential that an injury to the scaphoid bone actually represents a preexisting nonunion.

A history of shoulder, elbow, or arm pain should alert the examiner to the possibility of concomitant injury more proximally. Weakness or loss of sensation in the hand could indicate a nerve injury. A high-energy injury mechanism should alert the examiner to the possibility of an associated wrist ligamentous injury.

KEY PHYSICAL EXAMINATION

Key points in the physical examination include skin integrity, neurovascular assessment, assessment of wrist stability, and identification of regional tenderness indicating the possibility of an arm, wrist, or hand fracture. Radial wrist pain with grip should raise suspicion of a scaphoid fracture, as should tenderness over the scaphoid tubercle (located distal to the volar wrist crease just radial to the long axis of the middle finger).

The most important physical finding, however, is the presence of point tenderness in the "anatomic snuffbox." The snuffbox, visible with the thumb in extension, is located distal to the radial styloid, between the extensor pollicis longus and abductor pollicis longus tendons (Fig. 11-18). Patients with snuffbox tenderness are presumed to have scaphoid fractures regardless of the radiographic findings.

ANCILLARY TESTS

Posterior-anterior (PA), lateral, and oblique wrist radiographs should be obtained. Ulnar deviation of the wrist may increase the sensitivity of the PA radiograph for detecting scaphoid fracture. A PA view with the hand in a fist may demonstrate

Figure 11-18

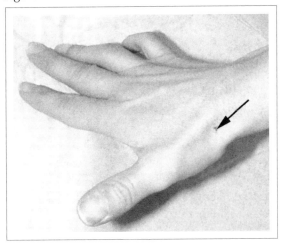

Anatomic snuffbox. The anatomic snuffbox *(arrow)* is the
hollow between the tendons of the extensor pollicus longus
and abductor pollicis muscles. Tenderness in the snuffbox
indicates the possibility of a scaphoid fracture, even if initial
x-rays are negative for fracture.

scapholunate widening, consistent with a scapholunate ligament disruption.

The use of special imaging studies (e.g., CT,
MRI, radionuclide bone scan) for diagnosis of acute
scaphoid fractures is controversial, as discussed
later. CT is the method of choice for identifying
subtle fracture displacement and for visualizing the
fracture in three dimensions. Provided the injury is
at least 72 hours old, a radionuclide bone scan will
identify occult fractures not visible on plain radiographs. Limited MRI of the scaphoid is being used
in a similar fashion in some institutions and seems
to have sensitivity similar to that of CT.

TREATMENT

Treatment of scaphoid fractures requires consideration of many factors. If the fracture is identified on plain radiographs and has more than 1
mm of displacement, any angulation, scapholunate dissociation, or delayed union (>4 months),
the patient should be referred to an orthopedist.
Similarly, fractures identified late (>3 weeks after
injury) or occurring in the proximal pole are best

referred. They may not require surgery, but are
much more likely to heal poorly.

Nondisplaced fractures can be treated conservatively in a long-arm thumb spica cast with the
wrist in a neutral position for 6 weeks. If necessary, the cast should be changed after swelling
subsides to prevent loosening. If repeat radiographs at 6 weeks demonstrate healing, a short-
arm cast should be applied for an additional
6 weeks. Provided interval healing continues and
snuffbox tenderness resolves, mobilization and rehabilitation can start at 12 weeks. Healing may
take up to 3 to 5 months, in which case an extended period of casting is needed. If interval
radiographs demonstrate signs of delayed union
with widening, sclerosis, or displacement, referral
is indicated as some would favor internal fixation
at that point.

If a scaphoid fracture is suspected clinically but
the fracture is not apparent on initial radiographs,
treatment with a long-arm thumb spica splint or
cast is recommended for 2 weeks, with follow-up
radiographs at that time. Treatment proceeds as
outlined above if the fracture is seen in the follow-
up radiographs. If no fracture is apparent and
snuffbox tenderness has resolved, no further
immobilization is required and the patient can
be presumed not to have a scaphoid fracture. If
the patient still has tenderness after removal of the
cast, a fracture should be suspected, and a bone
scan or an MRI is indicated to better delineate the
presence or absence of fracture.

ERRORS

Errors in the management of scaphoid fractures
are common and often result in malpractice litigation. The most important error is failure to recognize that a fracture may be present even in the
presence of a normal radiograph and, thereby,
failing to immobilize an occult fracture. The results of this error may not be noted for years, as
the complication of scaphoid nonunion is wrist
arthritis, which often develops over 5 to 10 years.

Another common error is failure to recognize
associated ligamentous instability of the wrist.

Patients with suspected ligamentous wrist injuries may require surgery and should be referred to an orthopedist.

CONTROVERSIES

Some recommend bone scan or MRI following the initial assessment of a suspected scaphoid fracture if an occult fracture is suspected in the presence of normal-appearing radiographs (for bone scanning, the injury must be >72 hours old). The controversy relates to the relative cost and inconvenience of 2 weeks of immobilization versus the costs and availability of obtaining MRI or bone scans in all cases of suspected scaphoid fractures.

There is also controversy about optimal positioning of the arm for casting and whether the elbow and thumb must included in the cast. While these issues are debated, the recommendations outlined in this chapter reflect current consensus and standard of care. Other controversies relate to the role of surgery for asymptomatic nonunion, to electrical stimulation therapy and timing of surgical intervention for delayed union, and to the role of acute surgery for treating minimally displaced fractures.

Distal-Radius Fractures

INTRODUCTION

Distal-radius fractures are the most common upper extremity fractures. There are two basic types of distal-radius fractures. The more common is known as a Colles' fracture, in which the distal fragment of the fractured radius in angulated dorsally. Smith's fractures, in which the distal fragment undergoes volar angulation, are less common.

PATHOPHYSIOLOGY

The distal radius articulates with the proximal carpal row and the distal ulna at the distal radial-ulnar joint. It assumes about 80% of the axial load across the forearm and is subject to fracture when an individual falls onto the outstretched hand.

Maintenance of the normal anatomic relationships of the wrist joint is critical to normal function. The radius has a normal palmar tilt of 11° to 12°, an inclination of 22° to 23°, and a radial length of 11 to 12 mm (Fig. 11-19). The inclination is the angle between a line drawn perpendicular to the long axis of the radius and a line drawn across the distal radial articular surface. The radial length is the distance in the longitudinal axis between the distal ulna and the radial styloid.

EPIDEMIOLOGY

The fractures generally occur from a fall onto an outstretched hand. Children aged 6 to 12 and the elderly are the most frequently affected. Osteoporosis is a risk factor. Higher energy is required for a younger adult to sustain a distal-radius fracture, and, as a result, significant articular cartilage damage and fracture comminution and displacement are much more likely when distal-radius fractures occur in young adults.

TYPICAL PRESENTATION

Patients present generally following a fall, complaining of distal-arm pain, swelling, and often a deformity. The characteristic deformity in a Colles' fracture is the "silver-fork deformity," in which the orientation of the hand to the wrist resembles the curvature of an upside-down fork.

KEY HISTORY

History must include age, handedness, occupation, life-style considerations, and general medical assessment. Distal weakness or loss of sensation signals a possible nerve injury. Symptoms of possible forearm compartmental syndrome should be sought.

KEY PHYSICAL EXAMINATION

Physical examination includes assessment of skin integrity, deformity, evidence of carpal fracture or instability, finger flexor and extensor function, and distal neurovascular function.

Figure 11-19

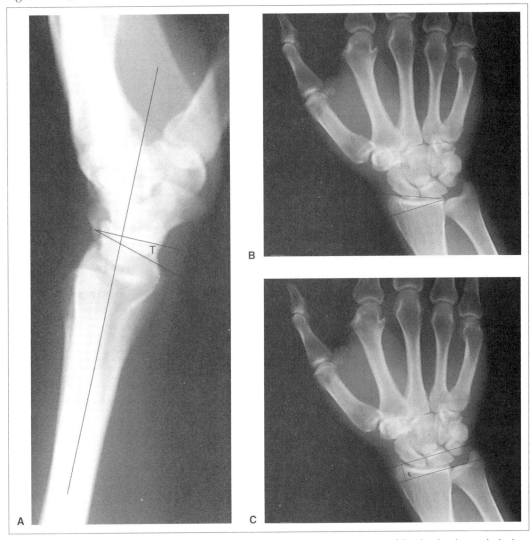

Normal anatomic relationships of the distal radius. The normal anatomic relationships of the distal radius include the following: palmar tilt *(T)* 11–12° **(A)**, inclination *(I)* 22–23° **(B)**, radial length *(L)* 11–12 mm **(C)**.

ANCILLARY TESTS

AP and lateral radiographs are diagnostic and must be carefully evaluated for evidence of comminution, displacement, angulation, intra-articular involvement, and the anatomic relationship discussed above. If there is any question about intra-articular involvement or the extent of the fracture, CT is useful to clarify the anatomic limits of the fracture.

TREATMENT

Fractures with more than 15° of angulation or in which the ulna is also involved should be reduced as described below. Open fractures, intra-articular fractures, and fractures in which appropriate anatomic alignment cannot be achieved with closed reduction should be referred to an orthopedist for consideration of open surgical repair. Fractures in young adults that occurred as a result of a high-energy injury should also be referred.

Conservative treatment (i.e., immobilization without reduction) for a fracture of the distal radius is appropriate if no deformity is present and the fracture is not open or intra-articular. It may sometimes also be appropriate in frail elderly patients in whom deformity is not severe, because the immobilization following reduction in such patients will almost invariably lead to loss of motion at the elbow and wrist joints.

Conservative treatment is indicated for children who have nondisplaced greenstick or torus (buckle) fractures of the distal radius. The bones of children have excellent remodeling potential, and treatment without reduction using 3 to 6 weeks of cast immobilization usually results in a satisfactory outcome.

TECHNIQUE OF CLOSED REDUCTION The first step in performing a closed reduction is administration of anesthesia, which is generally accomplished with a hematoma block. Using sterile technique, a needle is introduced through the dorsum of the fracture into the hematoma between the fracture fragments. Aspiration of blood into the syringe indicates correct placement of the needle, after which about 5 mL of 1% lidocaine (without epinephrine) is introduced.

Reduction is accomplished by applying traction along the axis of the forearm to achieve distraction of the bone fragments and by then reproducing the injury mechanism (i.e., dorsal angulation for a dorsally displaced fracture and ventral angulation for a ventrally displaced fracture). Traction can be applied manually by pulling on the hand while an assistant immobilizes the forearm. It can also be applied by suspending the patient's fingers in finger traps, with the forearm flexed to 90° at the elbow and weights (e.g., sandbags) applied to the upper arm to provide traction.

After the above measures, the fracture is reduced by bringing the wrist into a position of slight flexion and ulnar deviation. The arm is placed in a long-arm splint and postreduction radiographs are taken to ensure satisfactory realignment. Any rotational deformity is unacceptable.

At 1 week following reduction, follow-up radiographs should be obtained to document maintenance of reduction. Of note, a reduced Colles' fracture is more stable than a reduced Smith's fracture and, therefore, more likely to have maintained reduction. If reduction is satisfactory at the 1-week examination, a short-arm cast ending at the metacarpals is applied for 6 to 8 weeks. An interval radiograph should be taken at 3 to 4 weeks to again ensure maintenance of reduction. If reduction is lost at any point, orthopedic consultation is recommended.

ERRORS

Three common errors are worthy of note. One is underestimating the severity of the injury in young adults. While a low-energy fracture in a young adult that is easily reduced, minimally comminuted, and nonarticular can be treated as described above, there should be a low threshold for referral because of the risk of articular involvement.

The second common error is maintaining long-arm immobilization for prolonged periods following the fracture. For older patients, this can result in permanent loss of mobility of casted or splinted joints. In general, it is appropriate to convert long-arm immobilization to short-arm immobilization within about 2 weeks. For some frail elderly patients, long-arm immobilization should be avoided completely.

A third error is applying a circumferential cast as treatment for the acute fracture, a practice that can result in neurovascular compromise when swelling occurs within the cast. Even if reduction is difficult to achieve or maintain, immobilization of acute, distal-radius fractures should be accomplished with a splint, not a circumferential cast.

CONTROVERSIES

The threshold for internal fixation and the methods are controversial. Fractures with any malalignment of the articular surface or any significant angulation are generally repaired. The spectrum of surgical options for fixation include percutaneous fixation, external fixation, internal fixation, and a combination of these approaches with or without bone grafting. The choice depends both on a surgeon's preference and the particular injury.

Hand Fractures: Metacarpal and Phalangeal Fractures

INTRODUCTION

Fractures of the hand are common both from falls and from reaching into a hazardous environment. In this section concepts applicable to all hand fractures will be reviewed, and then principles that make fractures suitable for conservative versus open treatment will be discussed. Finally, one particularly common hand fracture will be discussed—dorsally angulated fracture of the fifth metacarpal, the so-called "boxer's fracture."

PATHOPHYSIOLOGY

Anatomically, metacarpal bones consist of a base, shaft, neck, and head. Each finger has a corresponding metacarpal and a proximal, middle, and distal phalanx (with the thumb lacking a middle phalanx).

The metacarpals are stabilized by deep transverse metacarpal ligaments, giving the second and third metacarpal increased stability but less mobility than the fourth and fifth. As a result, reduced fractures of the middle metacarpals will have greater intrinsic stability, but any angulation will be poorly tolerated. Fractures of the fourth or fifth metacarpal, because of the intrinsic mobility of these bones, do not require precise alignment.

The intrinsic and extrinsic hand muscles, and the finger flexor and extensor tendons, provide angulating forces that can complicate fracture reduction. These forces can be used, however, to augment fracture stability by immobilizing the wrist in 20° extension, the metacarpophalangeal (MCP) joints in 70° of flexion, and the fingers in extension (Fig. 11-20).

Figure 11-20

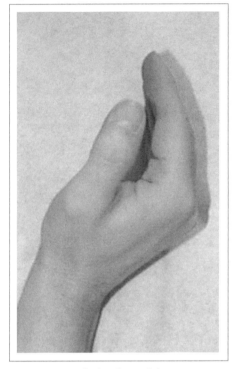

Correct position for hand immobilization. Most hand fractures should be immobilized with the metacarpophalangeal joints in 70° of flexion and the fingers in extension.

EPIDEMIOLOGY

Hand fractures as a group are the most frequent skeletal injuries, with the phalanges fractured more frequently than the metacarpals. Of the metacarpals, the fifth is the most frequently fractured, followed by the first through fourth, respectively. In the United States, about 1.5 million hand fractures occur each year with a cost of 4 billion dollars.

TYPICAL PRESENTATION

Patients normally present following trauma with regional pain, swelling, limited range of motion, and sometimes a gross deformity. Patients may present with open fractures from either protrusion of fractured bone through the skin or when the original injury was a laceration or puncture that directly injured the bone.

KEY HISTORY

Key historic points include age, handedness, occupation, mechanism of injury, any sensory or motor complaints, and assessment of general health.

KEY PHYSICAL EXAMINATION

The skin should be inspected for integrity, swelling, and deformity. Localized tenderness and crepitus, as well as pain over the bone with distal manipulation, are common.

Shortening of a fractured metacarpal may manifest as loss of normal contour of the knuckle dorsally. Assessment for rotational deformity is critical and best performed by having patients flex their fingers while observing for finger overlap, which does not occur in the absence of rotational deformity. A thorough neurovascular examination documenting two-point discrimination is useful for assessing sensory function, and the integrity of the finger extensors and deep and superficial finger flexors should also be confirmed. Wrist, MCP, and interphalangeal joint stability should be documented. A subungual hematoma often accompanies a distal phalanx fracture.

ANCILLARY TESTS

AP, lateral, and oblique radiographs are required to document metacarpal fractures. Two perpendicular views are sufficient for diagnosis of phalanx fractures.

TREATMENT

Fractures that should be referred to an orthopedist include those that are open, multiple, or intra-articular with any displacement. Extra-articular

fractures with significant comminution, displacement, shortening, or rotation also require orthopedic referral.

In general, fractures amenable to conservative treatment are those that are isolated, anatomically aligned, and stable. Fractures likely to be stable include impacted fractures (such as impacted fractures of a metacarpal neck), transverse fractures, and distal phalanx fractures. Nondisplaced oblique or spiral fractures are less stable and require close radiographic follow-up to ensure displacement does not occur. Displaced spiral, oblique, and rotated fractures are very likely to be unstable despite reduction and should be referred for surgical stabilization.

For fractures amenable to conservative treatment, short-arm splinting or casting is recommended for 3 to 4 weeks. Variations on the cast or splint are acceptable provided the hand is immobilized in the correct position (wrist extension, MCP flexion, finger extension, as shown in Figure 11-20), and immobilization includes the joint above and below the fracture.

Potentially unstable fractures should be checked for position at 1 week. After 3 weeks, provided the fracture is clinically stable and healing, range of motion to prevent finger stiffening should begin. Follow-up to document radiographic healing and eventual resumption of full range of motion is recommended. A hand therapist should be consulted for patients having difficulty regaining normal range of motion.

ACCEPTABLE DISPLACEMENT   An additional consideration in fracture management includes the degree of acceptable displacement following reduction. As discussed, neither rotational malalignment nor, in general, any significant angulation or shortening is acceptable.

BOXER'S FRACTURE   One exception to the proscription against malalignment is a dorsally angulated fifth metacarpal fracture or "boxer's fracture" (Fig. 11-21), in which up to 15° of dorsal angulation is acceptable provided the fifth finger can be fully extended. For greater degrees of angulation,

Figure 11-21

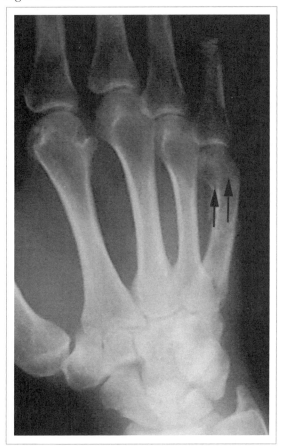

Boxer's fracture. This dorsally angulated fifth metacarpal fracture is known as a "boxer's fracture" or "fighter's fracture."

reduction is attempted using a hematoma block by applying traction to the finger with direct pressure opposing the direction of angulation.

One caveat with this fracture is to beware of the "fight bite," a laceration over the fifth knuckle inflicted by a tooth. Because of the risk of tendon injury and infection, these wounds should be surgically debrided and the extensor tendon inspected with the hand in a closed fist. Intravenous antibiotics covering oral flora are also recommended for these open fractures.

ERRORS

Errors include failure to recognize neurovascular injury, failure to identify loss of anatomic reduction, prolonged immobilization or incorrect hand positioning leading to finger stiffness, and failure to recognize and aggressively treat a "fight bite" complicating a boxer's fracture.

References

Clavicle
Eiff MP: Management of clavicle fractures. *Am Fam Physician* 55:121, 1997.
Gossard JM: Closed treatment of displaced middle-third fractures of the clavicle gives poor results. *J Bone Joint Surg [Br]* 80:558, 1998.
Nordqvist A, Petersson CJ, Redlund-Johnell I: Mid-clavicle fractures in adults: end result study after conservative treatment. *J Orthop Trauma* 12:572, 1998.
Nordqvist A, Petersson C, and Redlund-Johnell I: The natural course of lateral clavicle fracture: 15 (11–21) year follow-up of 110 cases. *Acta Orthop Scand* 64: 87, 1993.
Robinson CM: Fractures of the clavicle in the adult. Epidemiology and classification. *J Bone Joint Surg [Br]* 80:476, 1998.

Proximal Humerus
Mason BJ, Kier R, Bindleglass DF: Occult fractures of the greater tuberosity of the humerus: radiographic and MR imaging findings. *Am J Roentgenology* 172: 469, 1999.
Rasmussen S, Hvass I, Dalsgaard J, et al: Displaced proximal humeral fractures: results of conservative treatment. *Injury* 23:41, 1992.
Szyszkowitz R, Seggl W, Schleifer P, Cundy PJ: Proximal humeral fractures. Management techniques and expected results. *Clin Orthop* 292:13, 1993.
Zyto K: Non-operative treatment of comminuted fractures of the proximal humerus in elderly patients. *Injury* 29:349, 1998.

Hip
Cuckler JM, Tamarapalli JR: An algorithm for the management of femoral neck fractures. *Orthopedics* 17: 789, 1994.

Kane RL, Chen Q, Finch M, et al: Functional outcomes of posthospital care for stroke and hip fracture patients under Medicare. *J Am Geriatr Soc* 46:1525, 1998.

Koval KJ, Skovron ML, Aharonoff GB, Zuckerman JD: Predictors of functional recovery after hip fracture in the elderly. *Clin Orthop Rel Res* 348:22, 1998.

Kyle RF, Cabanela ME, Russell TA, et al: Fractures of the proximal part of the femur. *Instr Course Lect* 44:227, 1995.

Pandey R, McNally E, Ali A, Bulstrode C: The role of MRI in the diagnosis of occult hip fractures. *Injury* 29:61, 1998.

Resch S, Thorngren KG: Preoperative traction for hip fracture: a randomized comparison between skin and skeletal traction in 78 patients. *Acta Orthop Scand* 69:277, 1998.

Fifth Metatarsal

Clapper MF, O'Brien TJ, Lyons PM: Fractures of the fifth metatarsal. Analysis of a fracture registry. *Clin Orthop* 315:238, 1995.

Glasgow MT, Naranja RJ Jr, Glasgow SG, Torg JS: Analysis of failed surgical management of fractures of the base of the fifth metatarsal distal to the tuberosity: the Jones fracture. *Foot Ankle Int* 17:449, 1996.

Quill GE Jr: Fractures of the proximal fifth metatarsal. *Orthop Clin North Am*, 26:353, 1995.

Wiener BD, Linder JF, and Giattini JF: Treatment of fractures of the fifth metatarsal: a prospective study. *Foot Ankle Int* 18:267, 1997.

Ankle

Brage ME, Rockett M, Vraney R, et al: Ankle fracture classification: a comparison of reliability of three x-ray views versus two. *Foot Ankle Int* 19:555, 1998.

Calderone DR, Loder BG, Denny D, et al: Retrospective analysis of operative ankle fractures. *J Foot Ankle Surg* 35:230, 1996.

Ebraheim NA, Mekhail AO, Gargasz SS: Ankle fractures involving the fibula proximal to the distal tibiofibular syndesmosis. *Foot Ankle Int* 18:513, 1997.

Michelson JD: Fractures about the ankle. *J Bone Joint Surg [Am]* 77:142, 1995.

Michelson J, Curtis M, Magid D: Controversies in ankle fractures. *Foot Ankle* 14:170, 1993.

Verma S, Hamilton K, Hawkins HH, et al: Clinical application of the Ottawa ankle rules for the use of radiography in acute ankle injuries: an independent site assessment. *AJR Am J Roentgenol* 169:825, 1997.

Scaphoid

Berna JD, Abaledejo F, Sanchez-Canizares MA, et al: Scaphoid fractures and nonunions: a comparison between panoramic radiography and plain x-rays. *J Hand Surg [Br]* 23:328, 1998.

Grover R: Clinical assessment of scaphoid injuries and the detection of fractures. *J Hand Surg [Br]* 21:341, 1996.

Parvizi J, Wayman J, Kelly P, Moran CG: Combining the clinical signs improves diagnosis of scaphoid fractures. A prospective study with follow-up. *J Hand Surg [Br]* 23:324, 1998.

Rajagopalan BM, Squire DS, Samuels LO: Results of Herbert-screw fixation with bone-grafting for the treatment of nonunion of the scaphoid. *J Bone Joint Surg [Am]* 81:48, 1999.

Tiel-van Buul MM, Roolker W, Broekhuizen AH, Van Beek EJ: The diagnostic management of suspected scaphoid fracture. *Injury* 28:1, 1997.

Distal Radius

Collins DC: Management and rehabilitation of distal radius fractures. *Orthop Clin North Am* 24:365, 1993.

Hastings HD, Leibovic SJ: Indications and techniques of open reduction. Internal fixation of distal radius fractures. *Orthop Clin North Am* 24:309, 1993.

Rodriguez-Merchan EC: Management of comminuted fractures of the distal radius in the adult. Conservative or surgical? *Clin Orthop Rel Res* 353:53, 1998.

Hand

Bowman SH, Simon RR: Metacarpal and phalangeal fractures. *Emerg Med Clin North Am* 11:671, 1993.

Schaffer TC: Common hand fractures in family practice. *Arch Fam Med* 3:982, 1994.

Peter T. Simonian and
John W. O'Kane

Chapter

12

Dislocations

Introduction

Definitions

A dislocation is the movement of a bone's articular surface out of its proper location within a joint. Dislocations are usually described in terms of the relationship of the distal portion of the dislocated joint with the proximal portion.

The vast majority of dislocations are closed (i.e., the skin overlying the joint remains intact). However, open dislocations do occur and require urgent operative irrigation and debridement, along with tetanus prophylaxis and broad-spectrum intravenous antibiotics to minimize the chance of infection.

General Principles of Evaluation

NEUROVASCULAR STATUS

Because dislocations can cause injury to neurovascular structures surrounding the dislocated joint, it is essential to assess and monitor neurovascular status of any patient with a known or suspected dislocation. Neurovascular function can be compromised by a direct injury to blood vessels and nerves or by tissue swelling that occurs in the absence of a direct neurovascular injury. A careful neurologic and vascular examination should therefore be completed and documented before and after any treatment is rendered.

If vascular status has been compromised, it is important to be aware that restoration of circulation, following reduction of the dislocated joint or surgical revascularization, can be associated with elevated pressures in the soft-tissue compartments distal to the point of vascular compromise, resulting in the need for emergent surgical decompression. Elevated compartmental pressures can also result from the soft-tissue trauma of a dislocation without direct vascular injury.

RADIOGRAPHS

Radiographs generally should be obtained for two purposes. The first is to diagnose the dislocation, although, as described later, radiographs are not always needed for diagnosis. The second is to determine the presence or absence of concomitant fractures. In most cases an orthopedic surgeon should be consulted if a fracture is present in conjunction with a dislocation.

General Principles of Treatment

In general, reduction of the dislocated joint should be performed as soon as possible and with as little manipulation of the joint as possible. Typically, the sooner a joint is reduced, the easier and less traumatically the reduction can be accomplished. This has important implications for the joint's blood supply and nerve supply and the condition of the cartilage.

With some dislocations described later, reduction may be performed without first obtaining radiographs. However, if there is suspicion of a concomitant fracture near the dislocation, it may be important to document its existence prior to the reduction to demonstrate that the fracture was

not iatrogenic—that is, that it was not caused during the reduction of the joint.

Several types of dislocations require open surgical reduction. Indications for open reduction include irreducible dislocations, open dislocations, nonconcentric reductions (meaning something is interposed in the joint), loose osteochondral fragments in the joint, and instability after reduction.

General Principles of Follow-Up

IMMEDIATE POSTREDUCTION FOLLOW-UP

After reducing a dislocation, it is important to repeat a detailed neurovascular examination and evaluation of compartmental pressures to ensure that the reduction has not compromised neurovascular status. If compromised, urgent surgical referral is in order.

Similarly, joint stability should be assessed after reduction, as should the range of motion through which the joint should remain stable. If gross instability is detected, the patient should be referred to an orthopedic surgeon.

Radiographs of the joint should also be obtained to ensure that the reduction has been successful. If neurovascular status is normal and the dislocation has been successfully reduced, the joint should be immobilized in a stable position with a splint.

LONGER-TERM FOLLOW-UP

The treatment goals after reduction of a dislocation are often opposing. One goal is to maintain joint stability, while the other is to maintain the joint's range of motion. Joint stability is often improved with immobilization, while early range of motion can decrease posttraumatic stiffness. Thus, treatment of a dislocation requires a careful balance to maximize function by instituting careful range-of-motion exercises to the extent that joint stability will permit.

Although return to preinjury function is the goal after all dislocations, it is often not attainable, especially with high-energy dislocations. Despite appropriate treatment, after some joint dislocations a patient may develop stiffness, arthritis, and/or chronic joint instability.

Specific Dislocations

Interphalangeal and Metacarpophalangeal Dislocations

INTRODUCTION

Dislocations of the fingers at either the interphalangeal or the metacarpophalangeal joints are very common. The most common finger dislocations involve the proximal interphalangeal joints.

PATHOPHYSIOLOGY

Most finger dislocations are a result of combined axial and angular forces exerted on the joint. Dislocations of the interphalangeal joints can occur in the dorsal, volar, radial, or ulnar directions.

EPIDEMIOLOGY

Dislocations of the proximal interphalangeal joints are common and typically occur in the dorsal direction (Fig. 12-1). Dislocations of the distal interphalangeal joint are rare, but when they occur the dislocation is typically in the dorsal direction. Metacarpophalangeal dislocations are somewhat uncommon in the fingers, but more common in the thumb.

TYPICAL PRESENTATION

Patients typically present after an obvious traumatic event—usually one that involves axial loading. The patient often can sense the dislocation when it occurs, and there usually is an obvious deformity.

Figure 12-1

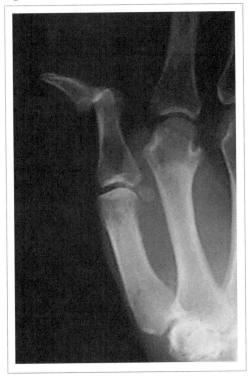

Interphalangeal joint dislocation. Radiograph illustrates a dislocation of the interphalangeal (IP) joint of the thumb. As is typical of IP dislocations, the distal bone is displaced dorsally.

KEY HISTORY

With all hand injuries, it is important to obtain the following information: handedness, occupation, age, and time elapsed since injury. Handedness and occupation may be helpful in determining whether surgical versus conservative treatment is appropriate and in determining the degree, if any, of residual disability that can be accepted. The patient's age should be noted, as increasing age is directly associated with development of joint stiffness after immobilization. The time elapsed since injury may influence the choice of surgical versus closed reduction and the likelihood that closed reduction will be successful.

KEY PHYSICAL EXAMINATION

A meticulous neurologic examination before and after reduction should be performed. One of the most useful tests of neurologic function is measurement of two-point discrimination distance, which can be measured with a simple paper clip (Fig. 12-2). The two ends of the paper clip are applied to the patient's skin, and the patient's goal is to determine the smallest distance between the two points that can be discriminated (without looking) as two separate points rather than one.

Circulatory examination involves measuring the rate of capillary refill of the involved finger in comparison with the others. Capillary refill should be measured before and after reduction.

It is also important to examine the skin for puckering on the palmar crease adjacent to the dislocated digit. If present, it may indicate interposition of the volar plate between the two involved joint surfaces. Interposition of a volar plate often signifies a dislocation that cannot be reduced by simple closed manipulation, and patients with this finding should be referred to an orthopedist.

ANCILLARY TESTS

It is helpful to obtain radiographs prior to reduction to make certain that a fracture is not present. If there is concern that an osteochondral fragment may be present within the joint, further radiographic imaging with special views or computerized tomography (CT) may be needed.

TREATMENT

ANESTHESIA Distal interphalangeal dislocations can often be reduced without anesthesia, while anesthesia is usually needed for dislocations of the proximal interphalangeal joints. If anesthesia is required, the usual technique is a digital (Fig. 12-3), metacarpal, or wrist block using lidocaine without epinephrine

Figure 12-2

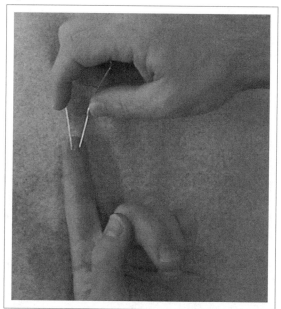

Two-point discrimination test. A simple paper clip can be used to compare two-point discrimination. The width of the ends of the paper clip can be varied. The two-point discrimination distance can be compared between the same fingers on opposite hands.

Figure 12-3

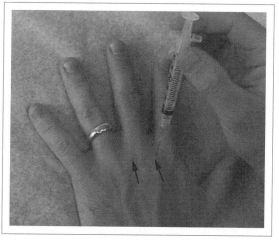

Digital nerve block. Digital nerve block can provide anesthesia for reducing dislocations of the fingers. Approximately 3 cc of lidocaine, with or without bupivicaine, is injected into the sites indicated by the arrows. The solution should contain no epinephrine.

TECHNIQUE OF CLOSED REDUCTION   Distal interphalangeal and proximal phalangeal dislocations can usually be treated by closed reduction. Metacarpophalangeal dislocations, on the other hand, may be difficult to reduce closed because of soft-tissue interposition and often require surgical treatment.

Closed reduction is generally performed with a combination of axial traction on the dislocated joint followed by re-creation of the movement of injury while traction is continued and then by reduction of the joint.

If closed reduction cannot be accomplished, open reduction should be carried out as soon as possible. Similarly, if closed reduction appears to be successful but post-reduction radiographs reveal an asymmetric reduction, soft-tissue interposition is likely and the joint will require operative intervention.

Finally, after reduction the stability of the joint should be evaluated passively and actively. If the patient is unable to extend the joint, the joint may require surgical intervention for repair of a disrupted ligament or tendon.

LONG-TERM MONITORING, TREATMENT, AND PROGNOSIS

Postreduction management varies depending on the particular joint involved, the direction of the dislocation, and the stability after reduction. In general, a splint placed in a direction opposing the deforming force with the interphalangeal joints in nearly full extension, and the metacarpophalangeal joints near 90° of flexion, is initially recommended (Fig. 12-4). Referral to an orthopedist or hand surgeon is recommended within a week to determine if further immobilization, early motion, or surgery is needed. This decision depends on many factors, including the degree of postreduction joint instability and the particular joint of the hand, as well as the occupation, handedness, and age of the patient.

ERRORS

The most common error in managing finger dislocations is failure to identify other injuries associated with a dislocation. The injuries most

Figure 12-4

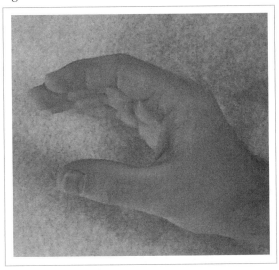

Position for immobilizing the hand after reduction of a finger dislocation. The hand should generally be immobilized with the MP joints near 90° of flexion and the IP joints near full extension.

often missed are associated fractures, tendon injuries, and neurovascular injuries.

A second important error is failure to identify asymmetry of the joint after closed reduction. This error can be avoided by careful inspection of post-reduction x-rays.

Elbow Dislocations

INTRODUCTION

Elbow dislocations—dislocations of the radius and ulna from the humerus—are relatively common. In fact, dislocation of the elbow is the third most common dislocation, exceeded in frequency only by dislocations of the glenohumeral and finger joints. Elbow dislocations are often associated with neurovascular injuries and fractures of the bones surrounding the elbow joint.

PATHOPHYSIOLOGY

The elbow is comprised of three bones—the distal humerus, proximal ulna, and proximal radius.

Any of these bones can be fractured when the elbow is dislocated.

EPIDEMIOLOGY

Elbow dislocations most commonly occur in younger individuals between the ages of 5 and 25 years. Typically, the radius and ulna dislocate as a unit from the humerus, with posterior or postero-lateral dislocations being the most common. Nerve injuries can occur with elbow dislocations and most often involve the ulnar or, occasionally, the median nerve.

TYPICAL PRESENTATION

The mechanism of injury in elbow dislocations is often hyperextension. In some patients, dislocations occur when an axial load is applied to the elbow that is positioned in slight flexion. Patients present with obvious deformity and the inability to flex or extend the elbow.

KEY HISTORY

As with other upper-extremity injuries, it is important to obtain information about the patient's handedness, occupation, age, and the time elapsed since injury. These factors will influence choice of open versus closed reduction and the length of time the joint is immobilized after reduction.

KEY PHYSICAL EXAMINATION

Because elbow dislocations are associated with neurovascular injuries, it is essential to perform a careful neurovascular examination before and after the reduction. The vascular examination should document brachial, radial, and ulnar pulses. Function of the motor and sensory components of the ulnar, median, and radial nerves should also be documented before and after reduction.

The degree of swelling should be noted, because soft-tissue swelling can compromise the circulation distal to the dislocation, even in the absence of direct injury to blood vessels.

ANCILLARY TESTS

AP and lateral radiographs should always be obtained before (Fig. 12-5) and after reduction. Postreduction radiographs must confirm a concentric reduction of all articulations of the elbow.

If there is a question of vascular injury, angiography and consultation with a vascular surgeon should immediately be obtained. Measurement of compartmental pressures should be performed if compartmental pressure elevation is suspected in the forearm; elevated compartmental pressures are most often seen following postreduction revascularization.

TREATMENT

The goal of treatment is to reduce the elbow dislocation as quickly and with as little manipulation as possible. Reduction is typically performed by applying constant, gentle traction on the forearm (distally and slightly downward) with counter-traction applied to the humerus. Reduction will usually occur during application of traction and is often palpable, after which the elbow is brought

Figure 12-5

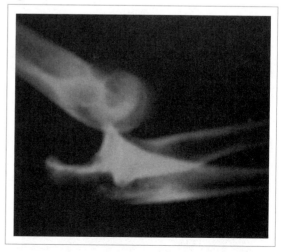

Posterior elbow dislocation. Lateral radiograph demonstrating an elbow dislocation in the most common direction—posterior.

into gentle flexion. During reduction, care should be taken to ensure that medial or lateral displacement has been corrected.

After reduction, the elbow should be gently put through its range of motion to ensure that there is no mechanical block to motion. Because the joint is usually painful, testing range of motion may require local infiltration of lidocaine into the elbow joint. This is done from the lateral side, injecting into the center of a triangle formed by the lateral epicondyle of the distal humerus, the radial head, and the olecranon.

Prior to immobilization, gentle varus and valgus stress should be applied to the joint to assess stability. If stable, the elbow should then be splinted in 90° of flexion for approximately 1 week.

LONG-TERM MONITORING, TREATMENT, AND PROGNOSIS

Contractures of the elbow occur commonly after immobilization, and the degree of contracture has been correlated to the period the elbow was immobilized. Therefore, early range of motion is essential to decrease the incidence and severity of contractures. Sometimes range of motion can be started early within a stable arc of motion, avoiding the extremes of extension or flexion. Then, as the elbow becomes more stable, any contracture-induced blocks or restraints on motion are removed as soon as joint stability permits.

COMPLICATIONS

Important complications at the time of an acute dislocation are neurovascular injury and compartmental syndromes of the forearm. The most common complication in the months following an elbow dislocation is stiffness of the elbow, a complication that is often avoidable with early mobilization. Late complications include heterotopic ossification in the tissues surrounding the elbow and chronic ligamentous instability, which often was present but unrecognized at the time of the reduction. Reconstructive elbow surgery can be performed for chronic liga-

mentous instability and in some cases for elbows with acute instability.

EMERGING CONCEPTS

Early mobilization is essential for an optimal outcome. Therefore, surgeons are recognizing that, if gross ligamentous instability is present after reduction, surgical ligament stabilization should be considered to facilitate early motion, rather than treating the instability with prolonged immobilization, as has been done in the past.

Shoulder Dislocations

INTRODUCTION

Dislocations of the shoulder are relatively common. They can be classified into two broad categories.

The first category is known as "TUBS," which stands for *T*raumatic dislocation, *U*nidirectional laxity, *B*ankart lesion (discussed below), and *S*urgery as a primary treatment. The common, traumatic, anterior-inferior shoulder dislocations usually fall into the TUBS category.

The second category of shoulder dislocations is "AMBRI," which refers to dislocations that are *A*traumatic, *M*ultidirectional (laxity in more than one direction), and *B*ilateral, and that have *R*ehabilitation as the primary treatment and an *I*nferior capsular shift if surgery is performed. AMBRI dislocations are relatively uncommon and will not be discussed in detail in this chapter.

PATHOPHYSIOLOGY

The vast majority of shoulder dislocations are TUBS dislocations that occur in the anterior (actually, anterior-inferior) direction. The arm movement that results in dislocation is typically abduction and external rotation.

Posterior TUBS dislocations are much less common and can be missed on physical examination alone. Posterior dislocations most commonly occur after a generalized tonic-clonic seizure or in association with a fracture.

EPIDEMIOLOGY

Shoulder dislocations represent almost 50% of all major joint dislocations. Nearly all (95%) of these dislocations are in the anterior direction, and about 70% occur among patients less than 30 years of age. Axillary nerve injuries occur in about 10%, and fractures in about 40% of anterior dislocations.

Some patients develop recurrent anterior dislocations. The most important factor determining whether recurrent dislocations will occur is the patient's age at the time of the first traumatic dislocation. Recurrent shoulder dislocations develop in up to 90% of patients who were less than 20 years of age at the time of the first dislocation and who were treated without surgery.

TYPICAL PRESENTATION

The most common presentation is dislocation of the shoulder after a significant traumatic event, in which the patient's arm is forced into an extreme abducted and externally rotated position. Patients who develop recurrent dislocations typically require less and less trauma for each subsequent dislocation. Some of these patients ultimately develop recurrent dislocations that occur with no trauma.

If a patient's first shoulder dislocation occurs without trauma, the patient may have an AMBRI dislocation. This would indicate a problem with ligamentous laxity in the shoulder and, often, in other joints as well.

KEY HISTORY

In addition to the history usually obtained from a patient with upper extremity injuries (age, occupation, handedness, time since injury), it is also important to ask if the patient has experienced previous shoulder dislocations. If so, further questioning should be directed at determining whether

prior dislocations occurred on the same or opposite side as the current dislocation, whether the first dislocation was associated with trauma, and the patient's perception of joint laxity in the dislocated shoulder.

KEY PHYSICAL EXAMINATION

A detailed neurologic and vascular examination before and after reduction is essential to detect neurovascular injuries caused by the dislocation or the reduction. It is also important to perform a careful evaluation of the function of the rotator-cuff muscles and to palpate the greater tuberosity of the humerus to detect fractures at that site.

Palpation and inspection of the shoulder is useful, as patients with anterior dislocations often have a visible or palpable deformity of the shoulder joint resulting from displacement of the head of the humerus. In contrast to anterior dislocations, however, there may be few or no signs on physical examination that indicate a posterior dislocation.

When evaluating patients with a history of shoulder dislocation, the "apprehension test" is useful because it is almost always positive in patients who have had anterior TUBS dislocations. To perform an apprehension test, the clinician externally rotates the patient's arm and, while maintaining external rotation, gradually abducts the arm. A positive test occurs when the patient experiences apprehension and a sensation that the shoulder is about to dislocate, usually when the arm reaches about 90° of abduction.

The final examination that should be performed when evaluating a patient who has a shoulder dislocation is an assessment of laxity in other joints. This is achieved by testing for significant hyperextension in joints such as the elbows, fingers, and knees. If present, an AMBRI dislocation should be suspected, especially if the patient does not report a convincing history of traumatic dislocation.

ANCILLARY TESTS

Radiographs before reduction are not always essential, especially for patients who have had multiple recurrent dislocations and/or when radio-graphs cannot be obtained without a significant time delay. However, x-rays are mandatory after reduction and should include both AP (Fig. 12-6) and lateral views. Typically, a scapular "Y" radiograph is used for the lateral view (Fig. 12-7) because a posterior dislocation may only be seen on this view.

In addition to documenting the presence of a dislocation, x-rays may reveal fractures that are commonly associated with shoulder dislocations—especially with recurrent dislocations. Two common radiographic signs of fractures are the Hill-Sachs defect and the Bankart lesions. The Hill-Sachs defect (Fig. 12-8) occurs on the back of the humeral head and represents an impaction fracture of the humerus into the anteroinferior glenoid fossa. A Bankart lesion (see Fig. 12-9), part of the TUBS syndrome, represents the corresponding fracture on the glenoid, in which the fracture involves the anteroinferior glenoid rather than the head of the humerus. Special radiographic views can

Figure 12-7

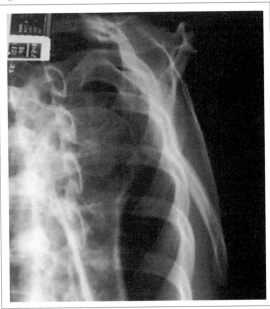

Scapular Y view of a shoulder dislocation. The scapular Y view is typically obtained as the lateral shoulder view in patients with a suspected shoulder dislocation. The x-ray shown here demonstrates an anterior dislocation of the head of the humerus, with its typical displacement anterior and inferior to the glenoid. The scapular Y view may be the only view on which a posterior shoulder dislocation can be visualized.

Figure 12-6

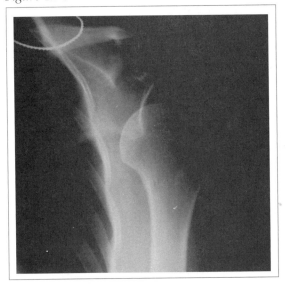

Anteroposterior x-ray of shoulder dislocation. This AP view shows the typical anteroinferior position of the shoulder in a common anterior dislocation.

highlight these lesions. The most common special views for this purpose are the Stryker notch view (see Fig. 12-8), which is basically an AP view of the shoulder with the arm maximally flexed, and the Westpoint view, which is a prone axillary view with the arm hanging over the side of the x-ray table.

Treatment

Reduction of a dislocated shoulder can be done in many settings, but the most favored is an emergency room in which intravenous sedation can be administered with appropriate monitoring. Except in some patients who are heavily intoxicated with alcohol, sedation is almost always necessary for

Figure 12-8

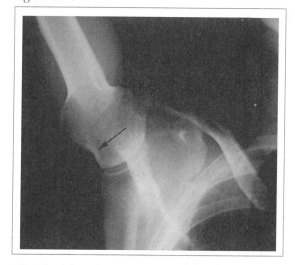

Hill-Sachs defect. The arrow points to a Hill-Sachs defect in the back of the humeral head, which represents an impaction fracture from repetitively impacting the head of the humerus into the anteroinferior glenoid. It typically occurs in shoulders that have been dislocated multiple times. It is best seen with the Stryker notch view used for this radiograph.

reduction of a shoulder dislocation because successful reduction requires relaxation of the muscles surrounding the shoulder joint.

TECHNIQUES FOR REDUCTION Many techniques have been described for reducing a dislocated shoulder. One of the easiest and most commonly used methods involves simple traction on the patient's arm. Two bed sheets are used. One sheet is wrapped around the patient's torso and used by an assistant to apply countertraction. A second sheet is wrapped around the patient's forearm just below the elbow, with the elbow flexed to 90°. This second sheet is also wrapped around the clinician's waist to facilitate application of controlled longitudinal traction, while leaving the clinician's hands free to manipulate the patient's arm (Fig. 12-10). While applying traction to the patient's arm, gentle internal and external rotation, and sometimes adduction, is applied to the patient's arm with the clinician's free hands; reduction will usually occur if traction is sufficient.

A second common method involves having the patient lie in the prone position with the dislocated shoulder hanging off the side of the examination table. Traction is applied to the shoulder by hanging a weight from the patient's forearm or wrist to applying downward pressure (Fig. 12-11). When this technique is used with adequate sedation, reduction is spontaneous, occurring without need for manipulation of the patient's arm.

SURGICAL TREATMENT When younger patients (below age 20) present with a first TUBS dislocation, surgical stabilization of the shoulder joint should be considered to reduce the likelihood of recurrent dislocations. The procedure can often be performed arthroscopically. However, whether performed as an open or arthroscopic procedure,

Figure 12-9

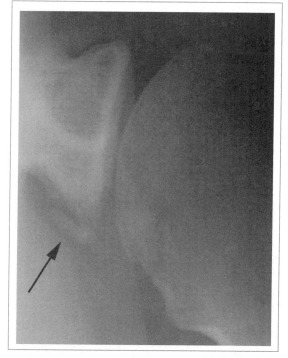

Bankart lesion. The arrow points to a Bankart lesion, which represents an impaction fracture of the anteroinferior glenoid. It occurs in shoulders that have had multiple dislocations.

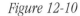

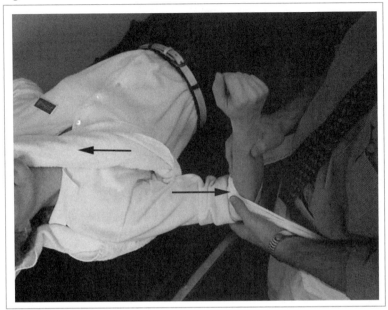

Reducing an anterior shoulder dislocation with two sheets. Reduction of a dislocated shoulder can be done with two sheets or towels. One sheet is wrapped around the torso of the patient to apply countertraction in the direction shown by the left-pointing arrow. A second sheet is wrapped around the forearm just below the elbow with the elbow flexed to 90°. This second sheet is also wrapped around the clinician's waist to assist in application of longitudinal traction in the direction of the right-pointing arrow.

surgical stabilization should be performed within 10 days after reduction, before the injured tissues become friable.

LONG-TERM MONITORING, TREATMENT, AND PROGNOSIS

POSTREDUCTION IMMOBILIZATION AND MOTION As with other dislocations, treatment of shoulder dislocations has two opposing goals: maintaining stability and maintaining range of motion. Initially, the shoulder should be immobilized in a sling with gentle range of motion limited to 90° of flexion (forward elevation) with 0° of external rotation. Elbow range of motion should be started immediately to avoid elbow stiffness, and isometric, rotator-cuff strengthening should also be initiated to maintain muscle strength about the shoulder.

Forward elevation can be increased to 140° and external rotation to 40° at 6 weeks after the injury in younger patients and 3 weeks in older patients. Return to athletic activities can begin once full range of motion and rotator-cuff strength is obtained.

RECURRENT DISLOCATIONS As noted, there is a propensity to experience recurrent dislocations of the shoulder, and each time a patient sustains a dislocation, subsequent dislocations often occur with less force and increased frequency. The goal of long-term management therefore is to minimize the risk that recurrent dislocations will occur. As discussed previously, younger patients should be considered for arthroscopic surgical stabilization procedures following a first dislocation. For patients already experiencing recurrent dislocations, the

Figure 12-11

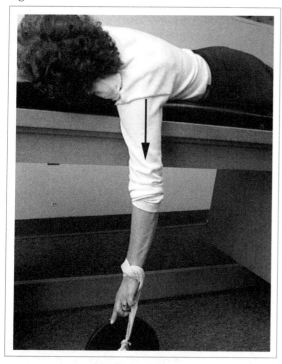

Reducing an anterior shoulder dislocation with the "bucket" method. The shoulder can be reduced with the patient in the prone position with a weight hanging from the wrist applying downward traction. A commonly used weight is a bucket that is gradually filled with sandbags or water.

clinician should educate the patient on how to avoid arm movements that predispose to dislocation of the joint. When patients experience multiple recurrent dislocations with minimal trauma, the best treatment is surgical stabilization of the shoulder joint.

ERRORS

Most of the common errors in management of shoulder dislocations involve failure to recognize injuries associated with the dislocation. These include vascular injuries (more common in elderly patients with less compliant blood vessels), axillary nerve injuries, and rotator-cuff tears. Each of these associated injuries can be detected with a careful physical examination.

Another common error is failure to identify posterior dislocations and/or associated fractures (such as the Bankart or Hill-Sachs fractures mentioned earlier). Posterior dislocations are missed because they are often not apparent on physical examination and cannot be seen on standard AP x-rays. Failure to identify a posterior dislocation can be avoided if appropriate lateral radiographs are obtained. As described above, special views can also identify the Bankart and Hill-Sachs fractures.

Finally, many clinicians make the error of instituting prolonged immobilization in the elderly individuals, leading to stiffness of the shoulder and elbow. Early movement of the upper extremity joints is essential and becomes increasing important with advancing age.

CONTROVERSIES AND EMERGING CONCEPTS

In a departure from traditional management, surgical stabilization for first-time TUBS fractures is now being recommended for younger patients. Considerable evidence exists that such an approach will decrease the rate of recurrent shoulder dislocations.

Acromioclavicular Joint Dislocations

INTRODUCTION

Acromioclavicular (AC) joint separations are very common and typically result from a direct blow on top of the joint or shoulder. As described below, AC joint injuries are classified based on the degree of injury.

PATHOPHYSIOLOGY

AC separation represents an injury to the soft-tissue restraints between the end of the clavicle and the bony prominence of the acromion. These soft-tissue restraints include the joint capsule and the coracoclavicular ligaments. The joint capsule is weaker and fails before the stronger coracoclavicular ligaments. In children, an injury to the epiphysis of the distal clavicle can appear similar to an AC separation.

EPIDEMIOLOGY

AC joint dislocations are categorized into three types. A type I injury represents injury to the joint capsule only, with no apparent displacement of the clavicle and no abnormalities on x-ray. A type II injury represents injury to the joint capsule and partial injury to the coracoclavicular ligaments, resulting in a radiographically evident partial displacement of the clavicle relative to the acromion. The displacement is usually superior.

A type III AC joint injury represents a complete dislocation of the joint with complete disruption of the soft-tissue structures. The clavicle is usually dislocated superiorly, but, rarely, can be dislocated inferiorly or posteriorly to the acromion. These uncommon directions of dislocation are important to recognize because, when they occur, the clavicle can injure neurovascular or thoracic structures and can thus require surgical repair.

TYPICAL PRESENTATION

There is usually a history of a direct blow to the AC joint. Common scenarios for this injury are a fall from a bicycle or motorcycle onto the superior aspect of the shoulder or a similar injury while skiing.

Patients usually complain of pain and tenderness localized over the AC joint. They may have difficulty lifting the arm.

KEY HISTORY

In addition to the usual history required in upper-extremity injuries (handedness, occupation, age, and the time elapsed since injury), the clinician should ask the patient about prior injury to the shoulder or AC joint. Questions should also be directed at detecting other areas of injury (e.g., arm, cervical spine, or thorax).

KEY PHYSICAL EXAMINATION

The most common finding on physical examination is tenderness, and sometimes swelling, directly over the AC joint. In type I injuries, AC-joint tenderness may be the only finding, as x-rays are typically normal (see below). In type II and type III dislocations, deformity may be obvious with the distal clavicle displaced in the superior direction. In addition to examination of the AC joint and clavicle, the examination should include assessment of the upper extremity neurovascular supply, the shoulder joint, and the neck.

ANCILLARY TESTS

X-rays are normal in type I injuries because type I AC joint injury involves no dislocation of the clavicle. In type II or III AC dislocation, x-rays demonstrate superior dislocation of the clavicle (Fig. 12-12). An AP view is typically adequate for this purpose. A view of the normal shoulder is often helpful for comparison; both AC joints can be included on the same radiograph.

If uncertainty exists about the presence of an AC joint injury, x-rays can be repeated while the

Figure 12-12

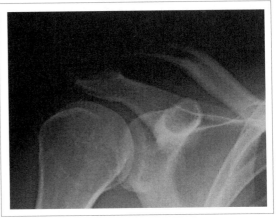

Acromioclavicular dislocation. An AP radiograph of the shoulder demonstrates a type III acromioclavicular (AC) dislocation, with typical upward displacement of the clavicle.

patient holds a 10-lb weight in each hand. Weights may move the scapula (and therefore the acromion of the scapula) inferiorly, making superior dislocation of the clavicle more obvious

TREATMENT

For type I and II injuries, immobilization in a sling is used until comfort allows discontinuation of the sling. To avoid stiffness of the shoulder and other upper extremity joints, range-of-motion exercises should be started as soon as pain subsides.

Treatment of type III injuries is controversial. Currently, there is no consensus about the correct approach to treatment.

There is consensus, however, about the need for surgical repair when the AC dislocation is associated with injuries to adjacent structures. This most commonly occurs in the rare situation in which the distal clavicle is displaced in an inferior or posterior direction.

LONG-TERM MONITORING, TREATMENT, AND PROGNOSIS

Many patients develop a mild, chronic deformity following an AC joint injury, commonly manifest as a bump over the joint. Chronic arthritis and pain may also develop after AC joint injury and can be treated surgically with distal clavicle resection if conservative measures fail to relieve pain. Chronic instability of the distal clavicle may also develop; late surgical stabilization can be performed for this problem.

ERRORS

Perhaps the most common error in management of AC joint injuries is prolonged immobilization leading to shoulder stiffness. Because type I and type II AC joint dislocations are stable injuries, this error can be avoided by instituting early range-of-motion activities as soon as the patient's pain permits movement of the joint.

A second error is failure to diagnose injuries associated with AC joint dislocation. Such injuries include fractures of the end of the clavicle; fractures of the acromion; epiphyseal injuries of the clavicle in persons under 20; and injuries of the rotator cuff, glenohumeral join, and cervical spine. Failure to diagnose these injuries can generally be avoided with a careful physical examination and appropriate x-rays.

CONTROVERSIES

As discussed above, there is controversy about the risks and benefits of surgical repair versus conservative treatment of type III AC joint injuries. Clinicians managing patients with these injuries should seek consultation from a specialist in orthopedic surgery.

Hip Dislocations

INTRODUCTION

Dislocation of the hip represents displacement of the femoral head from the acetabulum. Typically, this occurs in the posterior direction, but it can also occur in the anterior direction. Hip dislocations are emergencies and should be reduced as soon as possible to avoid compromising vascular supply to the area.

Hip dislocations occur more commonly in prosthetic hip joints than in native hip joints because prostheses dislocate with much less force than a normal hip. In addition, suboptimal positioning of a hip prosthesis may contribute to the propensity for dislocation.

PATHOPHYSIOLOGY

Substantial force is required to displace a normal femoral head from the acetabulum. The cause of the hip dislocation therefore is usually high-energy trauma such as a fall from a height or motor vehicle accident. Because of the high energy involved in these injuries, there are often associated fractures of the acetabulum, femoral head and neck, and pelvis, and there may also be other injuries involving the musculoskeletal system and visceral organs.

The mechanism of injury in posterior hip dislocations, the common type of dislocation, is usually axial force applied to a flexed hip such as occurs in an automobile crash in which an individual's knee collides with a car dashboard. Anterior dislocations, which are less common, result from abduction and external rotation forces.

EPIDEMIOLOGY

Posterior hip dislocations account for approximately 90% of all hip dislocations. The remaining 10% of hip dislocations occur in the anterior direction.

As noted, the highest incidence of hip dislocations is in persons who have undergone hip replacement surgery, making them more frequent in older individuals. However, hip dislocations also occur in younger persons, particularly after high-energy trauma.

TYPICAL PRESENTATION

Patients with a posterior hip dislocation will hold their hip in a flexed, adducted, and internally rotated position. Patients with an anterior dislocation will hold their hip more extended, abducted, and externally rotated. In either case, patients usually have significant pain and are unwilling or unable to move the hip.

KEY HISTORY

As with any injury from high-energy trauma, a general trauma history involving all organ systems is required. An attempt should be made to quantify the energy of the injury (i.e., speed of the motor vehicle or height of the fall) and to determine the position of the hip and lower extremity at the time of the dislocation.

KEY PHYSICAL EXAMINATION

In addition to a general trauma survey, the hip area and lower extremity should be examined, focusing attention on the neurovascular status of the lower extremity. Particular emphasis should be placed on evaluating sciatic nerve function, as the sciatic nerve is injured in 10% to 20% of patients who sustain a hip dislocation.

ANCILLARY TESTS

Radiographs should include an AP pelvis and lateral view (Fig. 12-13) and should include both hip joints in the radiographic field. These x-rays should be obtained before reduction. The posterior dislocated femoral head will appear smaller, while the anterior dislocated head will appear larger on

Figure 12-13

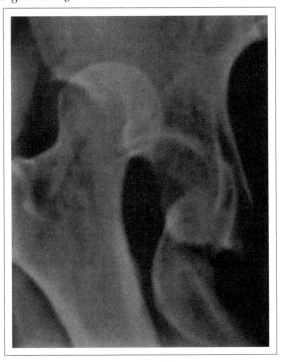

Hip dislocation. An AP radiograph of the hip demonstrates a posterior dislocation of the femur.

Figure 12-14

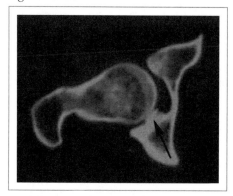

Hip dislocation with intra-articular bone fragment.
CT scan after reduction of the hip is recommended
to rule out an intra-articular bone fragment *(arrow).*

the AP pelvis x-ray when compared with the normal side. It is important to document the presence of associated fractures about the hip and femur prior to manipulation.

AP and lateral x-rays should be repeated after reduction to ensure that reduction has been successful. Postreduction x-rays should demonstrate that the bilateral femoral heads and hip joint spaces appear equal in size. A CT scan of the hip joint after reduction is recommended to detect intra-articular bone fragments (Fig. 12-14).

TREATMENT

Reduction of a dislocated hip can often be performed successfully with intravenous sedation. The patient's cardiopulmonary function must be carefully monitored while sedation is in effect.

The procedure for reducing the dislocation involves application of traction to the extremity. While applying traction, the clinician attempts to recreate the deforming force, following which the femoral head should return to its place in the acetabulum. If the hip is dislocated posteriorly, the traction force is applied with the hip in a flexed and adducted position. In the anterior dislocation, force is applied in extension and internal

rotation. In either case, the force is applied gently to avoid injury to the hip joint. If these maneuvers fail to reduce the dislocation, the procedure should be performed under general or spinal anesthesia.

LONG-TERM MONITORING, TREATMENT, AND PROGNOSIS

After the hip is reduced and found to be stable, patients are allowed to bear weight with crutches to the extent that pain permits. Crutches or a cane are continued until weight bearing causes no pain. This typically takes 4 to 6 weeks. Subsequently, progressive exercises are continued to strengthen the muscles about the hip.

If the hip is unstable after reduction, the extremity can be placed in traction for 4 weeks to allow soft-tissue healing. Deep venous thrombosis prophylaxis should be initiated if the patient is immobilized in traction.

Even with appropriate treatment, several long-term complications can develop in patients who have had a hip dislocation. These include redislocation, posttraumatic arthritis, and avascular necrosis of the femoral head.

ERRORS

Common errors in management of hip dislocation include failure to recognize loose, bony fragments within the joint or associated fractures of the acetabulum, femoral head, or femoral neck. Fractures about the hip can also occur iatrogenically if too much force is used during reduction; such fractures are particularly likely in elderly patients who have an artificial hip.

Patellar Dislocations

INTRODUCTION

Dislocations of the patella often reduce spontaneously, and therefore the dislocation may not be recognized. Instead, dislocations of the patella may be confused with anterior cruciate ligament, medial collateral ligament, or medial or lateral meniscus injuries.

PATHOPHYSIOLOGY

The patella nearly always dislocates in the lateral direction, resulting in tears of the medial retinaculum and vastus medialis. Direct contact between the medial patella and lateral femur often occurs during patellar dislocations, resulting in osteochondral injuries to either of these two bones.

EPIDEMIOLOGY

Patients with hyperlaxity and/or with genu valgus alignment are more prone to patellar dislocations. Patients with recurrent dislocations often require less force for each subsequent dislocation.

TYPICAL PRESENTATION

Typically, patellar dislocations occur following a direct blow to the patella or a pivoting movement of the knee. Patients may present with the patella dislocated (usually in the lateral direction). More commonly, however, the patella has spontaneously reduced, and the patient is left with a painful joint effusion.

The patient typically is unable to bear weight after the injury. Often, patients sense that the knee joint, rather than the patella, has dislocated.

KEY HISTORY

The patient should be questioned about preexisting patellofemoral problems or past knee or patellar surgery, as these factors may influence the choice of treatment. Similarly, when patients have had recurrent patellar dislocations, it is useful to document the number of prior patellar dislocations sustained by the patient and whether the problem occurs unilaterally or bilaterally. Information about the mechanism and level of energy required to dislocate the patella, along with the timing of the injury, may also be helpful.

KEY PHYSICAL EXAMINATION

Patients with a patellar dislocation typically have an effusion, and, if the dislocation has reduced spontaneously, they will have a positive apprehension test. To perform an apprehension test the clinician creates a lateral patellar subluxation (movement of the patella laterally from its normal location) with the knee in about 20° of flexion, and the patient will complain of pain and fear of dislocation.

There will often be pain in the area of the medial retinaculum, medial articular surface of the patella, and/or the lateral femur. Evaluation should also include an assessment of laxity and integrity of the knee ligaments and the extensor mechanism of the knee, along with measurement of the Q-angle.

ANCILLARY TESTS

Appropriate radiographs for evaluating patients with a patellar dislocation include AP, lateral, and bilateral Merchant views. Lateral displacement or tilting can be seen on the Merchant view (Fig. 12-15). A MRI scan can be used to determine if an articular cartilage injury has occurred or if the medial retinaculum has been torn (Fig. 12-16).

TREATMENT

The dislocation has almost always reduced spontaneously, and treatment simply involves immobilization. In the uncommon situation in which reduction is required, it can usually be achieved with gentle manipulation.

The knee is immobilized in extension for about 4 weeks, but vastus medialis strengthening and resisted straight-leg raises are begun immediately. A patellar stabilization brace may be helpful.

For patients with congenital factors that predispose patellar dislocation, surgical repair is preferred at the time of the first dislocation. Such factors include increased Q-angle and/or hyperlaxity of the knee. Surgery for these patients results in better long-term outcomes.

Figure 12-15

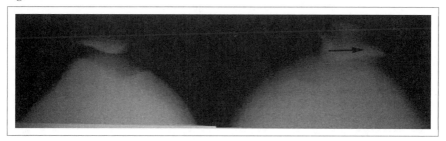

Patellar dislocation: Merchant view. Merchant view of the patella demonstrates persistent lateral subluxation after reduction of an acute patellar dislocation.

LONG-TERM MONITORING, TREATMENT, AND PROGNOSIS

Despite appropriate treatment, whether conservative or surgical, patellofemoral arthrosis may result from damage to the articular cartilage at the time of injury. Patients with recurrent dislocations often have chronic ligamentous instability as a result of the initial injury, and surgical stabilization is indicated for these patients if conservative measures have failed to prevent recurrent dislocations.

ERRORS

The most common errors in diagnosis and management of patellar dislocations are failure to diagnose osteochondral fractures or fragments in the joint and failure to detect injury to knee ligaments or the extensor mechanism. These errors can be avoided with careful physical examination and radiographic studies.

CONTROVERSIES

While surgical repair is often recommended for individuals with recurrent dislocations or those who have congenital conditions predisposing to patellar dislocations, the need for surgery in other situations is controversial. In particular, some experts are now recommending primary surgical repair of complete tears of the medial retinaculum at the time of the first patellar dislocation.

Knee Dislocation

INTRODUCTION

Knee dislocation is defined as a complete disruption in the articulation of the tibia with the femur. These injuries are relatively unusual. Knee

Figure 12-16

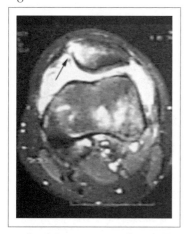

Patellar dislocation: MRI. After patella dislocation, an MRI scan can be used to determine if an articular cartilage injury has occurred *(black arrow)* and also if the medial retinaculum has been completely torn.

dislocations often reduce spontaneously or are reduced by lay or medical personnel at the accident scene, resulting in a relatively benign appearance on presentation for medical care.

While they are uncommon, knee dislocations have potentially devastating outcomes because they generally occur following high-energy trauma and are accompanied by a high incidence of serious neurovascular injuries. Initial management is centered on limb salvage and viability. Stabilization of fractures and management of ligamentous injuries are secondary priorities.

PATHOPHYSIOLOGY

CLASSIFICATION   Knee dislocations are classified by the position of the tibia relative to the femur. Anterior dislocations are the most common (approximately 30%) and are typically the result of a hyperextension force. Posterior dislocation is present about 25% of the time, occurring when posterior force is applied to the anterior tibia with the knee flexed; posterior dislocations require the greatest force.

Lateral and medial dislocations are less common and are the result of valgus and varus forces, respectively, and the combination of rotary and directional forces make possible any number of additional injury patterns. Posterolateral dislocations are worthy of mention because they can be irreducible because of the tendency of the medial femoral condyle to buttonhole through a characteristic vertical tear in the joint capsule, resulting in a trapdoor effect that blocks reduction.

ASSOCIATED INJURIES   The vascular anatomy of the knee plays an important role in determining the sequelae of arterial injury in knee dislocations. The popliteal artery, a direct continuation of the femoral artery, is tethered proximally to the femur in the adductor hiatus and distally to the fibula by the fibrous bands of the soleus fascia. Both of these points serve as tethers and are common sites of injury. While five genicular arteries arise from the artery within the popliteal space, these anastamoses generally do not provide adequate flow to ensure limb survival after popliteal artery injury, and amputation rates in acute knee dislocation with popliteal artery injury approach 75% unless surgical revascularization is performed.

Nerve injuries are also frequent complications of knee dislocation. The common peroneal nerve is most often injured, but damage to the superficial peroneal nerve, deep peroneal nerves, and distal peripheral nerves may also occur.

Knee dislocation can result in injury to the anterior cruciate ligament, posterior cruciate ligament, medial collateral ligament, lateral collateral ligament, the posterolateral complex, the capsule, the extensor mechanism, the menisci, and the articular surface.

EPIDEMIOLOGY

Knee dislocations are usually the result of high-energy trauma. Popliteal artery injury occurs in one-third of patients, and the dislocation is open in 20% to 30% of cases. The amputation rate ranges from zero in low-velocity dislocation, to 85% in high-velocity injuries with prolonged ischemia (>8 hours). Nerve injury and fracture of the ipsilateral extremity is reported in 30% to 40% of patients.

The incidence of associated injuries is linked to the type of dislocation. Anterior and posterior dislocations have a significantly higher incidence of vascular injury; they cause 40% to 50% of vascular injuries associated with knee dislocations. The nature of the vascular injury pattern is usually an intimal tear with anterior dislocations and complete transection in posterior dislocations. The incidence of peroneal nerve injury is highest in lateral and posterolateral dislocations.

KEY PHYSICAL EXAMINATION

NEUROVASCULAR FUNCTION   Careful evaluation of the neurovascular structures is critical before and after reduction of the joint. Physical examination should focus particularly on evaluation of pulses. Normal pulses, however, do not rule out vascular injury, and as discussed later, arteriography or other vascular studies should be considered in all patients with a knee dislocation. In fact, significant injury to the popliteal artery has been reported in 10% to 50% of patients who have palpable distal pulses after knee dislocation.

A warm but pulseless foot should not be "observed," as reperfusion of a compromised popliteal artery must be accomplished within 6 hours of injury. Similarly, absent pulses in a patient with a knee dislocation should not be attributed to spasm, as diminished or absent pulses in knee dislocations are almost always the result of a true injury to the vessel. Even if the skin appears well-perfused, metabolic demands of the underlying muscle are much greater, and muscle necrosis can occur even while superficial tissues seem to have adequate vascular supply.

ANTERIOR CRUCIATE LIGAMENT   Careful examination of the ligaments is also critical because the status of the ligaments influences surgical planning. Physical examination of the anterior cruciate ligament is best done with the Lachman test at 30° of flexion (Fig. 12-17). Both the amount of excursion and the end point of the anterior cruciate ligament are evaluated.

The examiner should also be suspicious of posterior cruciate insufficiency when doing the Lachman test. If one notes significant anterior excursion with a firm end point, this might indicate that the starting point was subluxated posteriorly, incriminating an injury to either or both the posterior cruciate ligament or the posterolateral complex. The pivot shift (Fig. 12-18) and pivot jerk tests may also be used.

POSTERIOR CRUCIATE LIGAMENT   The posterior cruciate ligament is best evaluated with the posterior drawer maneuver (Fig. 12-19) at 90° of flexion, comparing the "drop back"of the tibial tubercle to that of the opposite knee flexed at 90°. The quadriceps active test performed in 70° of flexion and the posterior sag sign can help confirm a posterior cruciate injury. The reverse pivot shift may also be used.

LATERAL LIGAMENTS   The lateral ligaments of the knee include the lateral collateral ligament and the posterolateral complex. The primary restraint to varus stress of the knee is the lateral collateral ligament. The posterolateral complex (i.e., the lateral collateral ligament and popliteus muscle)

Figure 12-17

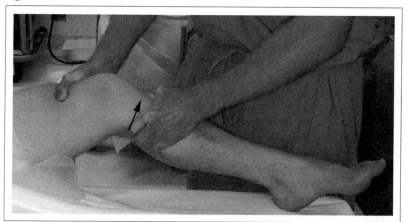

Lachman's test. After dislocation of the knee a Lachman test can be used to determine anterior cruciate ligament (ACL) laxity. Laxity is indicated by a positive Lachman test, in which the upper tibia moves forward relative to the femur when force is applied in the direction of the arrow.

Figure 12-18

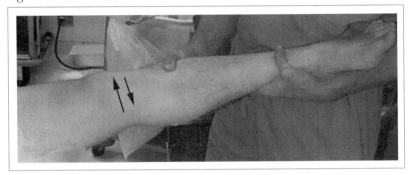

Pivot shift test. A pivot shift can also be used to determine ACL laxity, in which case the lateral tibia will subluxate relative to the femur. However, the pivot shift is difficult to perform after knee dislocation when patients are awake because of pain and guarding.

resists external rotation of the tibia with respect to the femur.

Evaluation of the lateral ligaments and posterolateral complex is performed by stressing the knee into varus with the knee in extension and again in 30° of flexion (Fig. 12-20), as well as sub-

jecting the tibia to external rotation at 30° and 90° of flexion (Fig. 12-21). The posterolateral drawer test (a posterior drawer test with the foot externally rotated), if positive, can also indicate an injury to the posterolateral complex.

The "external rotation recurvatum test" can be also used evaluate posterolateral stability. The test is performed by holding the patient's heels up off the table while the patient is supine on the examining table. A positive test is manifest as varus and hyperextension with internal tibial rotation.

MEDIAL LIGAMENTS   Stability of the medial side is evaluated both in extension and in 30° of flexion. The primary restraint is the superficial medial collateral ligament. Instability in extension, whether to varus or valgus stress, incriminates disruption of the cruciate ligaments.

Figure 12-19

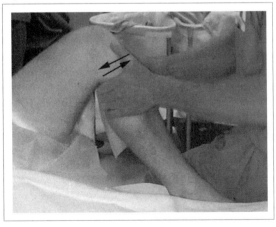

Drawer maneuver. The anterior and posterior drawer can be used, respectively, to evaluate stability of the anterior cruciate ligament (ACL) and posterior cruciate ligaments (PCL). The tibia can be shifted backward relative to the femur in PCL injuries and forward in ACL injuries. Always compare with the contralateral normal knee.

ANCILLARY TESTS

PLAIN RADIOGRAPHS   Although plain radiographs will identify a frank dislocation, it is not desirable to await the results of x-rays before reducing an obviously dislocated knee joint, especially when vascular compromise is suspected. Plain x-rays are useful, however, to detect associated fractures and to confirm dislocation if the presence of dislocation is not certain.

Figure 12-20

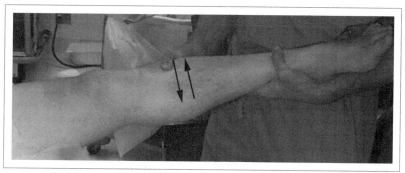

Valgus and varus stress. The examiner is moving the tibia laterally (valgus) and medially (varus) relative to the femur to stress and test the stability of the medial and lateral ligaments of the knee.

VASCULAR STUDIES   The need for evaluation of possible arterial injury beyond simple physical examination is controversial, particularly when the patient has normal pulses. Some experts have advocated serial physical examinations and Doppler evaluation with calculation of ankle-brachial indices and comparisons with the opposite side. Concern with this approach centers around reports of a 16% rate of false-negative results using Doppler ankle-brachial indices as a screening tool.

Others have recommended arteriography in all cases of knee dislocation, even when patients have normal distal pulses, and the high rate of vascular injuries makes this a reasonable approach.

When pulses are absent or diminished following reduction, some surgeons advocate immediate surgical exploration without the delay inherent in obtaining an arteriogram. Communication between the orthopedic surgeon, general surgeon, vascular surgeon, and the radiologist is critical in developing a workable clinical pathway for evaluating patients with knee dislocation.

Figure 12-21

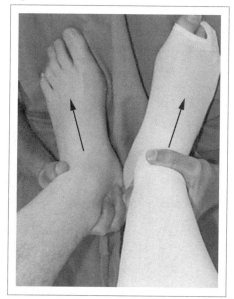

Assessing external rotation. Simply looking at the degree of external rotation of the foot at 30° and 90° of knee flexion can help determine if the patient has damaged structures at the posterolateral corner of the knee.

OTHER TESTS   Magnetic resonance imaging can also be used to help operative planning. MRI has been shown to better predict the extent of soft-tissue injury (including ligamentous injuries) than any other technique.

Compartmental pressures in the leg should be measured if compartmental pressure elevation is suspected. Elevated pressures are particularly likely when revascularization occurs following reduction.

TREATMENT

The majority of experts have concluded that even after reduction of a dislocated knee, operative management is the treatment of choice for the ligament injuries that occur in association with knee dislocations. Prior to surgical repair, a thorough examination under anesthesia is done to evaluate ligamentous stability. Surgical repair permits early motion and mobilization of the knee, which improves long-term outcomes.

Patients who have undergone surgical repair of knee dislocations are at high risk for developing deep venous thrombosis (DVT). Appropriate prophylaxis for DVT prevention should be instituted.

LONG-TERM MONITORING, TREATMENT, AND PROGNOSIS

Following multiligament reconstruction, continuous passive motion is started immediately, beginning at 0° to 30° of motion and advanced as tolerated to include weight bearing. A variety of braces and orthotic devices can be used, with the choice of device dependent on the ligaments involved in the injury. With significant collateral ligament surgery, immediate weight bearing is delayed for 6 weeks. In that setting, hydrotherapy, especially toe-touch weight bearing in a pool or on an underwater treadmill, can be helpful.

Myositis ossificans can develop in some patients, especially on the medial side of the knee, years after treatment of a dislocated knee. Indomethacin is an appropriate therapy for this complication.

ERRORS

The most serious error in management of knee dislocations is failure to realize that popliteal artery injury may be present even if distal pulses are normal. Another important error is failure to be vigilant for the development of compartmental syndrome after revascularization if the vascular supply was compromised for a period before reduction or revascularization of the extremity. Finally, knee dislocations can be associated with injuries of the ipsilateral hip and ankle joint, and

care must be taken to ensure that these other joints are appropriately evaluated.

CONTROVERSIES

As discussed earlier, a principal controversy in management of patients with knee dislocations revolves around selection of the best method for assessing the integrity of the popliteal artery. Until this controversy is resolved, arteriography should at least be considered in all patients with a knee dislocation.

A second controversy surrounds the timing of ligamentous reconstruction. Some have recommended immediate reconstruction of all ligaments, while others have recommended early range of motion with delayed reconstruction. If gross instability is present, the latter approach is not an option.

Dislocations of the Ankle, Talar Joints, and Tibial-Fibular Syndesmosis

INTRODUCTION

Dislocations of the tibiotalar (ankle) joint typically are associated with fractures (Fig. 12-22), and one-third of ankle dislocations are open. Neurovascular and skin injuries are relatively common with ankle dislocations. Closed reduction of closed ankle dislocations is typically successful with limited risk of posttraumatic arthritis.

Combined dislocations of the talus at its other articulations, the subtalar and talonavicular joints, are associated with high rates of avascular necrosis of the talus. Isolated injury to the syndesmosis between the distal tibia and fibula can also occur and easily be overlooked. Osteochondral fractures can occur with any of these dislocations.

PATHOPHYSIOLOGY

The ankle joint is composed of the distal tibia, distal fibula, and the talus. The tibia and fibula are attached to each other through a syndesmosis. Ankle dislocations are usually associated with ankle

Figure 12-22

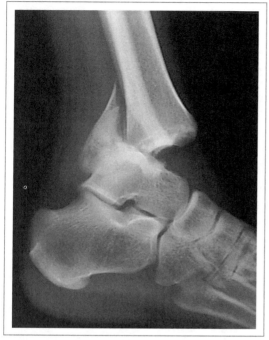

Fracture-dislocation of the ankle. Radiograph shows a dislocation of the talus from the tibia, accompanied by fractures of the tibia and fibula. Ankle dislocations are often associated with fractures.

fractures. Dislocations of the talar joints produce an obvious deformity. Injuries to the tibial-fibular syndesmosis are not always obvious and should be carefully investigated in the appropriate clinical setting.

EPIDEMIOLOGY

Although ankle and talar dislocations are uncommon, they often result in open injuries because of the superficial nature of the bones. The neurovascular structures are also at risk because of their superficial location.

TYPICAL PRESENTATION

Dislocations of the ankle joint and peritalar dislocations produce significant deformity and typi-

cally occur following high-energy trauma. Syndesmosis injuries may appear relatively benign on physical examination.

KEY HISTORY

An understanding of the mechanism and the energy of the injury is helpful in predicting the degree and extent of the injury.

KEY PHYSICAL EXAMINATION

Careful neurovascular examination before and after reduction of the dislocation is essential. Vascular examination should include the posterior tibial and dorsalis pedis pulses. Neurologic examination should focus on the tibial nerve and the deep and superficial peroneal nerves.

The condition of the skin is critical. The skin must be carefully inspected for evidence of an open injury, which may be small and not immediately apparent. If there has been significant skin tenting or deformity for a prolonged period prior to reduction, necrosis of the skin can occur.

Subtalar-talonavicular dislocations show a classic positioning of the foot medially on the leg; there is always significant tenting of the skin with this injury. With a talar dislocation, the talus will usually displace to the lateral side with significant skin tenting.

ANCILLARY TESTS

Radiographs of the ankle should include the mortise, AP, and lateral views. If an osteochondral injury is suspected, MRI or CT scans should be obtained. If there is any suspicion of proximal leg injury, the entire leg must be imaged with plain radiographs.

It is important to carefully study the symmetry of the ankle mortise on radiographs. Any medial widening is indicative of a significant syndesmosis injury. Radiographs of the proximal leg should also be considered to rule out a proximal fibula fracture.

TREATMENT

Reduction of a closed dislocation is typically accomplished with steady longitudinal traction. Reduction can be blocked by an interposed posterior tibial tendon, in which case surgical reduction is required. If closed reduction is successfully accomplished, further management is dictated by the nature of the associated fractures.

Syndesmotic disruptions that result in no widening of the ankle mortise can be treated with casting and non–weight bearing for 4 weeks followed by a weight-bearing cast or boot for an additional 4 weeks or until pain is absent. If there is displacement and/or asymmetry of the ankle mortise on radiograph, then open reduction and internal fixation of the syndesmosis is indicated.

LONG-TERM MONITORING, TREATMENT, AND PROGNOSIS

Posttraumatic arthritis and stiffness can occur following any of these dislocations, as can chronic ligamentous instability. Late surgical stabilization for instability can be performed if conservative treatment fails. The talus is also susceptible to avascular necrosis if the blood supply has been significantly compromised. Progressively disabling arthritis can be treated with fusion of the involved joints.

ERRORS

Skin necrosis and sloughing can occur because of delayed reduction of an ankle or peritalar dislocation. Syndesmosis injuries should not be missed, especially if there is radiographic widening or asymmetry on the ankle mortise radiograph. Finally, it is important to evaluate the proximal leg to determine if the proximal fibula has been injured.

References

Interphalangeal/Metacarpophalangeal
Capo JT, Hastings H 2nd: Metacarpal and phalangeal fractures in athletes. *Clin Sports Med* 17:491, 1998.

Hossfeld GE, Uehara DT: Acute joint injuries of the hand. *Emerg Med Clin North Am* 11:781, 1993.
Kung J, Touliopolis S, Caligiuri D: Irreducible dislocation of the proximal interphalangeal joint of a finger. *J Hand Surg [Br]* 23:252, 1998.
McCue FCD, Meister K: Common sports hand injuries. An overview of aetiology, management and prevention. *Sports Med* 15:281, 1993.
Stiles BM, Drake DB, Gear AJ, et al: Metacarpalphalangeal joint dislocation: indications for open surgical reduction. *J Emerg Med* 15:669, 1997.
Takami H, Takahashi S, Ando M: Complete dorsal dislocation of the metacarpophalangeal joint of the thumb. *Arch Orthop Trauma Surg* 118:21, 1998.

Elbow
Andrews JR, Whiteside JA: Common elbow problems in the athlete. *J Orthop Sports Phys Ther* 17:289, 1993.
Cohen MS, Hastings H 2nd: Acute elbow dislocation: evaluation and management. *J Am Acad Orthop Surg* 6:15, 1998.
Endean ED, Veldenz HC, Schwarcz TH, et al: Recognition of arterial injury in elbow dislocation. *J Vasc Surg* 16:402, 1992.
Slowik GM, Fitzimmons M, Rayhack JM: Closed elbow dislocation and brachial artery damage. *J Orthop Trauma* 7:558, 1993.

Shoulder
Arciero RA, St. Pierre P: Acute shoulder dislocation. Indications and techniques for operative management. *Clin Sports Med* 14:937, 1995.
Cicak N, Bilic R, Delimar D: Hill-Sachs lesion in recurrent shoulder dislocation: sonographic detection. *J Ultrasound Med* 17:557, 1998.
Gates JD, Knox JB: Axillary artery injuries secondary to anterior dislocation of the shoulder. *J Trauma* 39:581, 1995.
Kirkley A, Griffin S, Richards C, et al: Prospective randomized clinical trial comparing the effectiveness of immediate arthroscopic stabilization versus immobilization and rehabilitation in first traumatic anterior dislocations of the shoulder. *Clin J Sports Med* 7:242, 1997.
Pevny T, Hunter RE, Freeman JR: Primary traumatic anterior shoulder dislocation in patients 40 years of age and older. *Arthroscopy* 14:289, 1998.
Riebel GD, McCabe JB: Anterior shoulder dislocation: a review of reduction techniques. *Am J Emerg Med* 9:180, 1991.

Valentin A, Winge S, Engstrom B: Early arthroscopic treatment of primary traumatic anterior shoulder dislocation. A follow-up study. *Scand J Med Sci Sports* 8:405, 1998.

Acromioclavicular

Lemos MJ: The evaluation and treatment of the injured acromioclavicular joint in athletes. *Am J Sports Med* 26:137, 1998.

Phillips AM, Smart C, Groom AF: Acromioclavicular dislocation. Conservative or surgical therapy. *Clin Orthop* 353:10, 1998.

Hip

Dorr LD, Wan Z: Causes of and treatment protocol for instability of total hip replacement. *Clin Orthop* 355:144, 1998.

Frick SL, Sims SH: Is computed tomography useful after simple posterior hip dislocation? *J Orthop Trauma* 9:388, 1995.

Kelley SS, Lachiewicz PF, Hickman JM, et al: Relationship of femoral head and acetabular size to the prevalence of dislocation. *Clin Orthop* 355:163, 1998.

Tennent TD, Chambler AF, Rossouw DJ: Posterior dislocation of the hip while playing basketball. *Br J Sports Med* 32:342, 1998.

Yang RS, Tsuang YH, Hang YS, et al: Traumatic dislocation of the hip. *Clin Orthop* 265:218, 1991.

Patella

Henry JH, Craven PR Jr.: Surgical treatment of patellar instability: indications and results. *Am J Sports Med* 9:82, 1981.

Nikku R, Nietosvaara Y, Kallio PE, et al: Operative versus closed treatment of primary dislocation of the patella. Similar 2-year results in 125 randomized patients. *Acta Orthop Scand* 68:419, 1997.

Knee

Almekinders LC, Logan TC: Results following treatment of traumatic dislocations of the knee joint. *Clin Orthop* 284:203, 1992.

Dennis JW, Jagger C, Butcher JL, et al: Reassessing the role of arteriograms in the management of posterior knee dislocations. *J Trauma* 35:692 1993.

Kwolek CJ, Sundaram S, Schwarcz TH, et al: Popliteal artery thrombosis associated with trampoline injuries and anterior knee dislocations in children. *Am Surg* 64:1183, 1998.

Merrill KD: Knee dislocations with vascular injuries. *Ortho Clin North Am* 25:707, 1994.

Noyes FR, Barber-Westin SD: Reconstruction of the anterior and posterior cruciate ligaments after knee dislocation. Use of early protected postoperative motion to decrease arthrofibrosis. *Am J Sports Med* 25:769, 1997.

Twaddle BC, Hunter JC, Chapman JR, et al: MRI in acute knee dislocation. *J Bone Joint Surg [Br]* 78:573, 1996.

Ankle and Peritalar

Davis AW, Alexander IJ: Problematic fractures and dislocations in the foot and ankle of athletes. *Clin Sports Med* 9:163, 1990.

Frankel MR, Tucker DJ: Ankle dislocation without fracture in a young athlete. *J Foot Ankle Surg* 37:548, 1998.

Merchan EC: Subtalar dislocations: long-term follow-up of 39 cases. *Injury* 23:97, 1992.

T. Al West and
Ronald V. Maier

Resuscitating Victims of Major Trauma

Introduction

The care of the patients with multiple injuries presents an important challenge to primary-care clinicians. Although the ultimate destination of the patient is often the operating room or transfer to another facility, the initial minutes of care after arrival to the hospital are crucial in determining the patient's outcome. The goal of this chapter is to provide primary-care clinicians with a guide to managing those first minutes of care, focusing on the early assessment, resuscitation, and stabilization of trauma patients.

Epidemiology

Trauma accounts for a significant portion of visits to physicians and hospitals. Almost 3 million hospital admissions each year result from injuries,

accounting for 9% of admissions at acute-care hospitals. It is the leading cause of hospitalization for people younger than 45 years, with about 1.6 million admissions per year.

The statistics regarding mortality rates are just as striking. About 150,000 deaths, or one death out of every 14 in the United States, are caused by injury. This makes trauma the third leading cause of death in the country. The incidence of injury-related death (62 per 100,000 population) is surpassed only by the rates for heart disease and cancer. Injury is by far the leading killer in people less than 45. For ages 5 to 34, injuries account for more deaths than all other causes combined.

Males have a higher incidence of hospitalization for trauma than females. Injury death rates vary substantially according to race as well, with Native Americans having the highest mortality from unintentional injuries, African-Americans having the highest homicide rate, and Caucasians and Asians having the highest suicide rate. There is significant evidence that much of the racial differences in injury rates are related to economic status. There are also differences in injury-related death rates in rural and urban settings, with unintentional-injury death rates highest in rural areas and with homicide rates several times as high in urban centers compared with other areas.

Pathophysiology

Shock is usually defined as inadequate oxygen delivery to tissues and is the most important pathophysiologic process that occurs in the multiply injured patient. Shock can be classified by its underlying cause: hypovolemic, cardiogenic, neurogenic, or septic. While septic shock is rarely present in the acute phase of traumatic injury, any of the other causes can contribute to shock in trauma patients. Hypovolemia is by far the most common cause of shock in trauma patients. It must be aggressively treated on a presumptive basis, because only the timely restoration of perfusion and oxygen delivery can reverse the progression of organ damage caused by shock.

Hypovolemic Shock

Hypovolemia is most often a direct result of hemorrhage. Blood loss that is rapid and severe enough to cause hemorrhagic shock is usually obvious when it is external, such as from a scalp laceration or major vascular injury. However, internal hemorrhage can occur into the pleural or peritoneal cavities, the retroperitoneum (usually from a pelvic fracture), or the muscular compartments of the thigh (from a femur fracture). In addition to hemorrhage, direct soft-tissue injury can lead to hypovolemia through sequestration of fluid in muscle, bowel wall, and other tissues (the so-called "third space"). These fluid shifts can be massive and can cause hypovolemia in and of themselves. Soft-tissue injury also initiates the release and activation of inflammatory mediators, which lead to further extravasation and potentiate the effects of hypoxic cellular injury.

A fall in circulating blood volume initiates compensatory mechanisms aimed at restoring homeostasis. Aortic and carotid sinus baroreceptors mediate an increase in sympathetic tone, causing increased systemic vascular resistance and enhancing venous return to the heart. This change in tone is most prominent in skeletal muscle and splanchnic vascular beds; flow to these organs is sacrificed in an effort to maintain perfusion to the brain, heart, and kidneys. Other microvascular mechanisms lead to changes in capillary hydrostatic and oncotic forces, resulting in a net influx of interstitial fluid into the intravascular space and re-expansion of plasma volume. Such mechanisms can compensate for up to a 10% to 15% reduction in circulating blood volume, with maintenance of relatively normal vital signs.

As circulating volume decreases, more mechanisms are called into play in order to maintain perfusion of the vital organs. Further increases in sympathetic vascular tone lead to an increase in diastolic blood pressure; the resulting decrease in pulse pressure is usually the earliest and most subtle shock-related change in the vital signs. Tachycardia ensues in an effort to maintain adequate cardiac output in the face of a lowered stroke volume. Urine output then begins to fall as blood flow to the kidneys is decreased and redistributed instead to the cerebral and coronary circulations. Once losses exceed 25% to 30% of blood volume, compensatory mechanisms ultimately fail to preserve normal blood pressure, and hypotension occurs.

Cardiogenic Shock

Cardiogenic shock in trauma patients can result from either intrinsic or extrinsic causes. Intrinsic causes such as blunt cardiac injury can bring about a decrease in inotropy. A decrease in inotropy can result from direct myocardial bruising, hemodynamically significant arrhythmias, or valvular or septal rupture and their respective hemodynamic changes. Extrinsic compression of the heart from pericardial tamponade or tension pneumothorax leads to obstruction of ventricular filling and results in drastic decreases in cardiac output.

Neurogenic Shock

Spinal cord injury or severe head injury can result in the failure of the sympathetic nervous system to maintain adequate vascular tone. As a result, generalized vasodilation and venodilation ensues, causing a decreased systemic vascular resistance and increased venous capacitance. As the available intravascular space expands, the relative hypovolemia causes hypotension and decreased perfusion. However, in contrast to hypovolemic or cardiogenic shock, there is no tachycardia, diaphoresis, or pallor because of the absence of sympathetic activity.

Effects of Shock

Regardless of the cause of the shock, basic metabolic changes occur at the cellular level. As oxygen delivery to the tissues decreases, anaerobic metabolism ensues, leading to a marked decrease in intracellular energy stores. The cell membrane loses its electrical and chemical gradients, and sodium and water flow into the cell. This intracellular fluid sequestration causes an extracellular volume deficit, which in turn leads to intravascular depletion. This volume deficit is best replaced with a balanced salt solution such as lactated Ringer's solution.

During periods of shock, especially from hypovolemia, a direct ischemic tissue insult occurs. Microvascular sludging and thrombosis produce a subclinical disseminated intravascular coagulopathy, with recurring cycles of ischemia, reperfusion, and capillary injury. As the hypoperfusion phase is reversed, inflammatory cells, especially neutrophils, are activated and begin adhering to endothelial walls. Here they release oxygen radicals, injuring the endothelial lining and leading to extensive capillary leak and massive interstitial edema. This ischemia-reperfusion injury takes place throughout the body, but is especially prominent in the lungs where it may result in severe difficulties with oxygenation, thus leading to further hypoxic insults in a vicious cycle. The longer and more severe the period of ischemia, the worse the reperfusion injury. Therefore, it is important to restore circulating volume and oxygen delivery as soon as possible, to allow intracellular aerobic metabolism and energy stores to recover.

Typical Presentation

There is a wide range in the presentation of patients with major trauma. Most patients, especially in urban settings with well-developed trauma systems, arrive at the emergency department by ambulance directly from the scene of the injury; however, some patients arrive hours or days after the event. Patients may be sedated, pharmacologically paralyzed, and intubated at the injury scene for transport, or they may be fully alert and able to cooperate with a history and physical examination. Some patients have external signs of trauma such as obvious fractures, which, by their impressive appearance, can divert the clinician's attention away from other, more life-threatening injuries. Many patients arrive in extremis, with worrisome or even absent vital signs, prompting a rapid diagnostic and therapeutic response. However, even the most seriously injured patients may have initially normal vital signs, which can lull the unwary clinician into a false sense of security.

Key History and Physical Examination

The role of the initial history and physical examination is distinctly different in the trauma setting than in other diseases. Although a detailed history and a physical examination are important, they must often be delayed because of the immediate need to inspect for life-threatening injuries. The details of the physical examination will be addressed in the sections on initial management and specific injuries, as will certain aspects of the patient history. However, there are several points in the history that are universally applicable and will be discussed here.

Mechanism of Injury

The mechanism of injury influences the trauma patient's condition and outcome and dictates the focus of the clinician's diagnostic and therapeutic mind-set. An understanding of mechanisms of injury and how they relate to specific anatomic patterns of injury is essential to the ability to anticipate the patient's course and to take a proactive approach to resuscitation.

BLUNT TRAUMA

Blunt trauma results from a combination of forces, including acceleration, deceleration, crushing, compression, and shearing. The most common specific cause of blunt trauma that results in multisystem injury is motor vehicle collisions; others include falls, assaults, and other transportation-, recreation-, and occupation-related injuries. Blunt injuries often have a delay in diagnosis because overlying soft tissue and bony structures may show little external sign of injury, while considerable force may have been transmitted to underlying organs.

Specific information should be gathered about the mechanism of blunt traumatic injury as early as possible in the course of the resuscitation. The position in which the patient was found, estimated blood loss at the scene of injury, and the time course of extrication and transport are helpful pieces of information in seriously injured patients and should be asked of prehospital personnel if the information is not volunteered. In automobile collisions, it is important to ask about seat-belt use, direction and presumed speed of impact, position of the patient in the passenger

compartment, damage to the vehicle, and whether the patient was ejected from the vehicle. Motorcycle crashes are associated with increased morbidity and mortality because the vehicle offers no protection for the driver; information on whether the patient was wearing a helmet is vital for raising the index of suspicion regarding occult head injury.

PENETRATING TRAUMA

Penetrating trauma refers to injury produced when a foreign object (usually a missile or knife) passes through tissue. Such injuries are, in the setting of civilian trauma, focal and therefore more anatomically predictable than those from blunt forces. Details about the kind of weapon used, the direction and distance from which the attack came, and how many shots were heard can provide important clues to the location and extent of injury.

Treatment

The overall goal in resuscitating the multiply injured patient is to maintain oxygen delivery to tissues. Such delivery depends on both adequate perfusion and adequate oxygen content of blood. Thus, the maneuvers undertaken in the initial care of the trauma patient are intended to maximize both these factors. A systematic approach focuses first on the ABCDE of resuscitation (a mnemonic in which A is for airway, B for breathing, C for circulation, D for disability, and E for exposure).

Airway

The first priority in any resuscitation is to ensure an adequate airway. Management of the airway is outlined in Figure 13-1.

Any patient who can answer questions in a normal voice can be assumed (at least initially) to have an intact airway. Labored breathing with

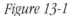

Figure 13-1

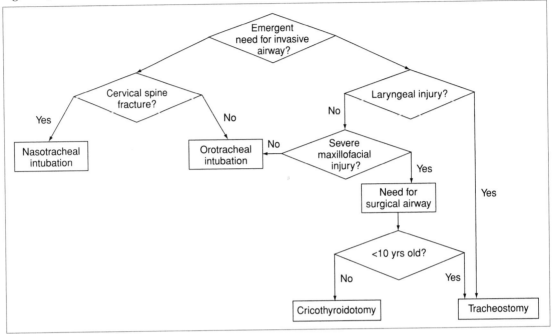

Algorithm for airway management.

retractions or noisy breathing with hoarseness, gurgling, or stridor may be signs of partial pharyngeal or laryngeal obstruction and require attention to the airway. This may be as simple as manual removal of vomitus and blood from the oropharynx or as performing the chin lift or jaw thrust maneuver, or it may involve the use of an oropharyngeal airway or nasal trumpet. Agitation should never be assumed to be caused by intoxication; it is often the earliest sign of hypoxia and can be a clue to impending airway occlusion.

In the setting of obtundation, severe maxillofacial or neck trauma, or profound shock, placement of a definitive artificial airway (defined as a tube in the trachea with an inflated cuff) is necessary. This is usually accomplished by orotracheal intubation. Inline cervical stabilization is mandatory during intubation of the injured patient to protect against cervical spinal-cord injury in the presence of unrecognized spinal fractures. If neuromuscular blockade is required, succinylcholine is

the agent of choice because of its rapid onset and short duration of action. Nasopharyngeal intubation can be accomplished with little neck movement, but requires a spontaneously breathing patient with no evidence of facial or basilar skull fractures. Inability to intubate by either the orotracheal or nasotracheal route is a clear indication for a surgical airway, either through a needle or open cricothyroidotomy, as described later in this chapter.

Breathing

Once a patent airway is secured and supplemental oxygen administered, the adequacy of ventilation must be assessed. Physical examination, including observation, auscultation, and palpation of the chest, are the best ways to evaluate whether a patient is breathing effectively.

Cyanosis, tachypnea, and mental-status changes are indicative of insufficient ventilation. Causes of hypoventilation in the injured patient include hemothorax, pneumothorax, chest-wall instability, cervical spinal-cord injury, and decreased drive resulting from central nervous system depression.

The hemodynamically unstable, injured patient with diminished breath sounds should be presumed to have a tension pneumothorax and should have immediate decompression of the pleural cavity by inserting a 14- to 16-gauge intravenous catheter into the anterior second intercostal space. This is a temporizing method and should be followed by tube thoracostomy.

There are several adjuncts to the physical examination that are helpful in determining a patient's ventilatory status. A pulse oximeter attached to the finger or earlobe can indicate adequacy of oxygen saturation and peripheral perfusion; it does not ensure adequate ventilation. Arterial blood gases are particularly useful and are essential in severely injured patients—not only to assess breathing, but to assess circulatory status as well. A chest x-ray is also mandatory in any multiply injured patient.

Circulation

Key goals in the care of injured patients are to stop bleeding and restore circulating volume and vital organ perfusion. External bleeding can frequently be controlled with manual pressure or a compressive dressing over a blood vessel or open wound. The pneumatic antishock garment (PASG) or other air splints can be placed to assist in control of severe bleeding from pelvic or lower extremity fractures. Operative therapy is usually necessary for control of internal hemorrhage.

Vascular access must be obtained promptly. At least two, large-bore (14 or 16 gauge), peripheral IV lines should be placed. They should not be inserted distal to extremity wounds that have potential vascular injuries. If peripheral access is impossible, saphenous vein cutdown or central venous access with a large (8 French) introducer catheter can provide a route for rapid volume infusion. In children under the age of 3 years, inter-

osseous lines should be used rather than central access.

If the patient is in shock, an infusion of 2 liters (20 mL/kg in children) of warm, lactated Ringer's solution is given as rapidly as possible. Vital signs, urinary output, acid-base balance, and/or central venous pressure are used to monitor the response to this initial fluid challenge. A lack of response, or a transient response, indicates that ongoing hemorrhage is likely.

Blood is administered if there is no response to the initial crystalloid bolus. Type O blood (Rh negative for women of childbearing age) is universally compatible and should be immediately available. A blood sample should be sent to the blood bank as soon as possible to avoid delay in obtaining cross-matched blood.

Disability

Disability refers to assessment of neurologic status, an assessment that requires a brief neurologic examination after airway, breathing, and circulation are ensured. The key points in the examination include level of consciousness, pupillary function, and movement of extremities. The Glasgow Coma Scale (GCS) is an often-used method of assessing the severity and following the progression of neurologic injury (Table 13-1).

Exposure

Once the immediately life-threatening injuries have been addressed, a complete head-to-toe physical examination is performed. It is important to completely expose the patient to avoid overlooking any subtle but important injuries. Additional IV lines, nasogastric tube, and a Foley bladder catheter should be placed at this time. Other monitoring devices such as continuous EKG monitors and pulse oximeters should also be applied if not already in place.

Hypothermia must be prevented and reversed by the use of warm blankets and all intravenous

Table 13-1

The Glasgow Coma Scale

PARAMETER	RESPONSE	SCORE
Eyes open	Never	1
	To pain	2
	To verbal stimuli	3
	Spontaneously	4
Best verbal response	No response	1
	Incomprehensible sounds	2
	Inappropriate words	3
	Disoriented but conversant	4
	Oriented and conversant	5
Best motor response	No response	1
	Extension (decerebrate)	2
	Flexion (decorticate)	3
	Withdraws to pain	4
	Localizes pain	5
	Obeys commands	6
Total		3–15

fluids must be warmed. Blood warmer/infusion devices are essential since administration of refrigerated blood and blood products can rapidly lower body temperature. Crystalloids can be stored in a warmer or heated carefully to 39°C in a microwave before use.

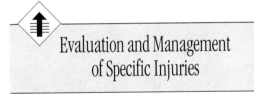

Evaluation and Management of Specific Injuries

Intracranial Injury

Brain injury is very common and is often the main determinant of survival in a multiply injured patient. Treatment of the patient with traumatic brain injury is directed toward rapid assessment of the severity of injury and prevention of secondary neurologic insult. The latter depends mainly on establishment

of adequate ventilation, oxygenation, and perfusion during the initial minutes of resuscitation.

HISTORY

All head-injured or multiply injured patients should be asked about loss of consciousness during the incident that caused their injury. Prograde or retrograde amnesia can indicate mild head injury. Headache and other postconcussive symptoms such as tinnitous, vertigo, and emotional lability are often associated with head injury and can persist for days or sometimes weeks.

Obviously, head-injured patients may not be able to provide information regarding their injury. In this situation the emergency response personnel should be questioned about the patient's level of consciousness at the injury scene, whether movement has been witnessed in all four extremities, the observation of any lateralizing neurologic signs, and the stability or progression of neurologic status during transport. Seizures may occur as a result of brain injury or may be the cause of a fall or vehicular crash.

PHYSICAL EXAMINATION

The level of consciousness is usually described by the Glasgow Coma Scale (GCS), which takes into account eye opening and verbal and motor responses (see Table 13-1). The GCS is scored with a value of 3 to 15, with higher values reflecting better neurologic function. The GCS should be calculated on arrival to the emergency department and reassessed on a frequent basis. A change of three or more points indicates a significant change in neurologic status and requires prompt evaluation and intervention.

Identification of lateralizing signs is critical in the early assessment. Pupillary size and response to light are recorded and compared between eyes. Any difference in size or shape must be assumed to be caused by intracranial injury until proven otherwise. Lateralized extremity weakness can be subtle, but is usually easily detected in patients who can follow commands. Asymmetry of movement in response to a painful stimulus is sometimes the only lateralizing sign in the patient with an altered level of consciousness.

ANCILLARY TESTS

Computed tomography (CT) of the head usually makes a definitive diagnosis of the type and severity of brain injury. Any patient with an altered level of consciousness or lateralizing neurologic signs should undergo a CT as soon as their respiratory and circulatory systems are stabilized. An adequate CT scan can identify mass lesions such as epidural or subdural hematoma, as well as parenchymal contusions, subarachnoid blood, and diffuse brain injury.

TREATMENT

Early neurosurgical consultation is mandatory in the care of the moderately or severely brain-injured patient. Any patient whose GCS is less than 11 or who has abnormalities on CT scan falls

into this category. Operative treatment is frequently required for the treatment of significant mass lesions.

Once the diagnosis of head injury is made, treatment is oriented toward maintaining delivery of oxygen and nutrients to the brain. Supplemental oxygen is mandatory, whether delivered by nasal cannula, face mask, or endotracheal tube. Cerebral perfusion pressure (CPP) is defined as the difference between mean arterial pressure (MAP) and intracranial pressure (ICP); even brief drops in CPP to levels less than 70 mm Hg are associated with decreases in long-term functional outcome. Therefore, the temptation to restrict fluids to reduce cerebral swelling must be tempered by the need to maintain circulating blood volume and MAP.

The patient with evidence of increased ICP and impending herniation (unilateral pupillary dilation or other lateralizing signs) should be treated promptly to reduce the ICP. Raising the head of the bed to 30°, moderate hyperventilation (P_{CO_2} of 30 to 35 mm Hg), and osmotic diuresis (20% mannitol, 30 g IV) all reduce ICP. However, they do so at the expense of cerebral blood flow and should be considered temporizing measures to be instituted prior to potential definitive surgical care.

Spinal Column

Injuries to the vertebrae and spinal cord account for only a small percentage of injury-related hospitalizations, but they often require extensive long-term medical care and rehabilitation. Most spinal-cord injuries are complete by the time the patient arrives at the emergency department, but prompt diagnosis and treatment can still have a beneficial effect on outcome in many patients. Initial care is directed toward maintenance of spine stabilization and prevention of secondary injury, to prevent further neurologic damage to patients whose cord injury is not complete.

All trauma patients should be regarded as having a spinal injury until proven otherwise. Injudicious manipulation or inadequate immobilization of the spine can result in conversion of an incomplete to a complete lesion and can worsen the outcome. Conversely, as long as appropriate protection of the spine is maintained, evaluation of the spinal column can be deferred until respiratory and hemodynamic stability is achieved.

HISTORY

Information regarding the mechanism of injury and the patient's neurologic status at the scene should be gathered from the patient or paramedics. Numbness, tingling, paresthesias, or weakness are subjective complaints that should raise suspicion of spinal injury.

PHYSICAL EXAMINATION

With the patient's head in a neutral position, the cervical collar is removed and the posterior elements of the spine palpated. Any midline tenderness, gap, or step-off is noted, and the collar replaced. The patient should then be log-rolled and the spine palpated along its entire length, again noting any palpable defects or tenderness. A motor and sensory examination of the extremities is performed to detect and document any deficits.

If any deficits are present, careful attention is paid to the level of injury. A complete injury will have no motor or sensory function below a specific anatomic level. However, incomplete lesions will often have mixed sensory and motor findings, with sparing of function at some levels. Documentation of perineal sensation and sphincter contraction and reflexes is important, as sacral sparing can be a subtle indicator of an incomplete lesion.

ANCILLARY TESTS

Any patient who complains of significant neck pain, is tender to palpation, has neurologic findings, or is not reliably evaluable because of distracting injuries, diminished consciousness, or intoxication requires a plain-film radiographic examination of the spine. The cervical spine is evaluated by three views: anteroposterior (AP), lateral, and open-mouth odontoid. All cervical

vertebrae down to the top of T1 must be visible on the film for the examination to be considered adequate. A swimmer's view is often necessary to evaluate the lower cervical spine. Even subtle "chip" fractures or misalignment on these films should be considered evidence of potential spinal instability, and orthopedic or neurosurgical consultation should be obtained.

If the plain films are normal, but the patient still complains of significant pain, flexion-extension films of the cervical spine can be used to detect ligamentous instability. The cervical collar is removed, and the patient is asked to voluntarily flex and extend the neck while x-rays are taken. Flexion-extension films should be taken only if and when a patient is awake, alert, and neurologically normal. Flexion and extension should be under the patient's own power—under no circumstances should the neck be forced into flexion or extension. If no instability is detected on these films, the cervical spinal cord can be considered free of injury.

It is important to realize that 10% of patients with a cervical-spine fracture have a second, noncontiguous vertebral fracture. Therefore, radiographic evaluation of the complete spine is mandatory for patients with a cervical-spine fracture. Comatose patients should also have complete spine–screening films. Two views (AP and lateral) are usually adequate for thoracic and lumbar evaluation. CT scanning is a useful follow-up of suspected fractures.

TREATMENT

IMMOBILIZATION As has been stressed earlier, proper immobilization is the primary initial treatment of spinal fractures. This includes the use of a semirigid cervical collar, backboard, sandbags, straps, and tape. Occasionally, sedatives or paralytic agents are required to achieve adequate immobilization if a patient is agitated. The patient should be removed from the hard backboard as soon as possible to reduce risk of decubitus ulcers. In the meantime, padding should be placed under weight-bearing bony prominences. Reduction of an obvious deformity should not be attempted, as this can increase the severity of injury—rather, a neurologic or orthopedic surgeon should be consulted.

FLUIDS AND VASOPRESSORS Neurogenic shock occurs because of a loss of sympathetic innervation to the heart and peripheral blood vessels, resulting in bradycardia and hypotension, which are caused by vasodilation and relative hypovolemia. However, even if spinal shock is suspected, the injured patient who is hypotensive must be treated for hemorrhagic shock by administering fluids. Treatment for hypovolemic shock must be continued until it is certain that no bleeding is present. Once hemorrhage-induced hypovolemia has been excluded, judicious use of vasopressors (preferably an alpha-adrenergic agent such as phenylephrine) can restore blood pressure and improve perfusion.

STEROIDS Corticosteroids have been shown to improve outcome in patients with blunt spinal cord injury if given within 8 hours after injury. Intravenous methylprednisolone, 30 mg/kg, is given as an initial bolus, followed by an infusion of 5.4 mg/kg/hour over the next 23 hours. Steroids should not be given to victims of penetrating spinal cord trauma or later than 8 hours after the injury; administering steroids to such patients exposes them to an increased risk of infectious complications without any proven beneficial outcome.

Neck

Injury to the neck presents a clinical challenge because of the fact that so many vital structures in the neck—the aerodigestive tract and major blood vessels—are contained within such a small, relatively unprotected space. Since these important structures pass through the anterior part of the neck, penetrating wounds through or anterior to the sternocleidomastoid muscle have the highest potential for injury. Conversely, wounds to the posterior triangle rarely involve these structures. Wounds that do not penetrate the platysma muscle are considered superficial and do not require extensive evaluation of deeper structures. The management of penetrating neck injuries is summarized in Figure 13-2.

The neck is divided into three anatomic zones (Fig. 13-3). Zone I is the base of the neck. Because this zone includes the thoracic outlet, wounds here put the intrathoracic organs and great vessels at

Figure 13-2

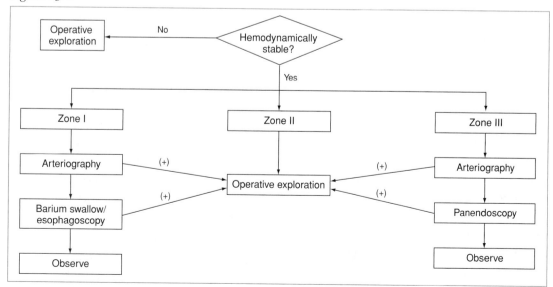

Algorithm for penetrating neck trauma.

Figure 13-3

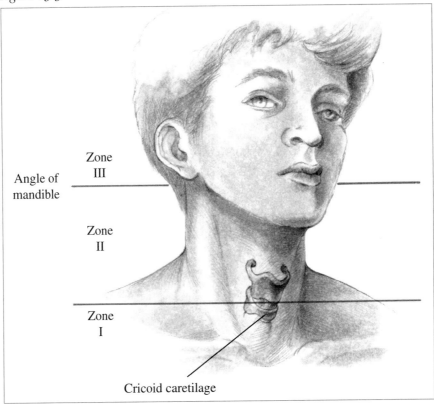

Angle of
mandible

Zone
III

Zone
II

Zone
I

Cricoid caretilage

Zones of the neck. Zone I is the base of the neck, which includes the thoracic outlet. Injuries in this area may involve the lungs and great vessels, leading to pneumothorax and hemothorax, respectively. Zone II is the body of the neck, which is the most commonly injured area and includes the airway, esophagus, and vascular structures. Zone III lies above the angle of the mandible; injuries to this area may involve the upper carotid artery. *(Reproduced by permission from Perry MO: Vascular injuries of the neck, in Carrico CJ, Thal ET, Weigelt DS (eds):* Operative Trauma Management. *New York, McGraw-Hill, 1999, p 221.)*

risk for injury. Zone II, the body of the neck, is the most commonly injured area. Zone III lies above the angle of the mandible, where surgical exposure of injured structures can be particularly difficult.

HISTORY

Aside from the basic information regarding mechanism of injury, patients with neck injuries should be questioned about subjective complaints referable to the aerodigestive tract. Dysphagia or odynophagia can be indicative of pharyngeal or esophageal injury. Hoarseness,

dysphonia, or change in vocal quality can signal injury to the airway.

PHYSICAL EXAMINATION

Attention should be directed first toward identifying injuries that mandate surgical exploration. So-called "hard" signs of vascular injury include shock, external hemorrhage, expanding hematoma, and abnormalities of the carotid pulse. A bruit may be present over an arteriovenous fistula. Stridor, subcutaneous air, hemoptysis, or hematemesis indicate injury to the aerodigestive tract.

In zone I injuries, particular attention should be paid to the possibility of hemothorax or pneumothorax. To evaluate for subclavian or innominate arterial injury, blood pressure should be taken in both arms and compared.

ANCILLARY TESTS

Radiologic evaluation is particularly helpful in the diagnosis of both blunt and penetrating neck trauma. Chest x-ray is indicated for all zone I injuries, as the cupola of the pleural cavity can extend up to the level of the clavicles. Plain films of the neck can show a hematoma that displaces or distorts the airway, subcutaneous or retropharyngeal air, missile fragments, and bony fractures. CT of the neck is useful in the evaluation of blunt trauma, especially when injury to the laryngeal cartilage is suspected. Suspicion of blunt carotid artery injury, either because of neurologic findings not explained by intracranial injury or because of significant contusions and abrasions on the neck, should be evaluated by arteriography after consultation with a surgeon.

TREATMENT

Early surgical consultation is mandatory for any neck wound that penetrates the platysma muscle. Many surgeons prefer immediate exploration regardless of symptoms, especially in isolated zone II injuries; others argue for exploration only in the presence of objective findings of injury, with angiography, esophagography, and panendoscopy as adjunctive diagnostic measures. Angiography is usually pursued for asymptomatic penetrating wounds to zone I (to evaluate for possible great-vessel injury) and zone III (for preoperative planning in difficult-to-expose, high-carotid-artery lesions).

Thorax

Thoracic injury accounts for approximately one-fourth of all trauma deaths, with two-thirds of these deaths occurring after arrival at the hospital. Although injury to the thorax can be life-threatening, operative intervention is usually not required. Rather, attention to the aforementioned principles of airway control, adequate ventilation, and circulatory stability can successfully treat most injuries. The management of penetrating chest trauma is summarized in Figure 13-4.

HISTORY

The mechanism and details of an injury are important factors in evaluating thoracic trauma. Rapid deceleration, whether from a high fall or a motor vehicle collision, is associated with aortic disruption. A bent or broken steering wheel is often associated with a sternal fracture and/or blunt cardiac injury. A gunshot wound should prompt a search for the exit wound or missile to determine the possibility of transmediastinal injury.

PHYSICAL EXAMINATION

Physical examination is directed toward identifying the immediately life-threatening chest injuries. Tension pneumothorax is diagnosed by respiratory distress, diminished breath sounds with a resonant percussion note, tracheal deviation, distended neck veins, and hypotension that is refractory to volume infusion. The findings in pericardial tamponade (almost always a result of penetrating trauma) are similar, but breath sounds are normal and the trachea remains in the midline; distant heart sounds may or may not be present. Flail chest can be detected by observing for paradoxical motion of the chest wall—collapse rather than expansion during inspiration. Absent or diminished breath sounds with a dull percussion note indicate hemothorax. Subcutaneous emphysema should alert the clinician to the potential presence of tracheobronchial or esophageal injury.

ANCILLARY TESTS

CHEST X-RAY An AP chest x-ray can reveal a variety of thoracic injuries and is mandatory early in

Figure 13-4

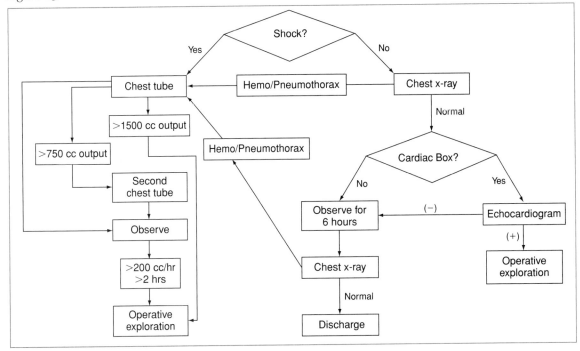

Algorithm for penetrating chest trauma.

the evaluation of any patient with multiple traumatic injuries. It should be performed as soon as the patient's airway is controlled and adequate ventilation is ensured. All penetrating thoracic wounds should be identified and marked with a radiopaque marker before taking a chest x-ray.

In chest x-ray interpretation, just as in resuscitation, attention is turned to the airway first — correct positioning of the endotracheal tube (the tip of the tube 2 to 3 cm above the carina) must be confirmed by a chest x-ray. The trachea is then examined; tracheal deviation on chest x-ray can indicate compression by a mediastinal or neck hematoma. Mediastinal air should alert the clinician to the possibility of tracheobronchial or esophageal injury.

The pleural space and lung parenchyma are assessed next. Hemothorax can be detected by a hazy appearance as the blood layers out posteriorly or by blunting of the costophrenic angle. Deepening of the costophrenic sulcus indicates a

pneumothorax. Parenchymal consolidation immediately after injury suggests a pulmonary contusion or laceration or the aspiration of stomach contents.

The bony structures on the chest x-ray can provide clues to the magnitude and mechanism of injury and can prompt searches for associated injuries. Clavicular fractures are common and often isolated; however, severely displaced clavicular fractures or dislocations can compress or lacerate the airway or great vessels. First and second rib fractures are indicative of a substantial transmitted force and, if present, should raise concern about major intrathoracic vascular injury. Lower rib fractures (ribs 9 through 12) are associated with intra-abdominal injury, most commonly of the spleen, liver, or kidney.

The finding of a nasogastric tube or gastrointestinal gas pattern in the pleural space on chest x-ray is pathognomonic of diaphragmatic rupture. An abnormally elevated hemidiaphragm is a less specific sign of injury, but still suggests diaphragmatic injury. Free air under the diaphragm requires abdominal exploration for hollow-viscus injury.

ANGIOGRAPHY   Arch aortography to rule out great vessel injury should be performed in any patient with chest x-ray signs of mediastinal hematoma (Table 13-2). Any penetrating wound in proximity to the great vessels should also prompt angiography.

ELECTROCARDIOGRAPHY   A electrocardiogram is warranted for patients who have experienced blunt trauma to the chest. Any significant arrhythmia or sign of ischemia should be considered evidence of blunt cardiac injury, and the patient should be admitted to a critical-care or telemetry unit for observation.

ECHOCARDIOGRAPHY   Patients with penetrating trauma to the "cardiac box" (below the sternal notch, above the xiphoid process, and between the nipples) are at high risk for cardiac injury. In the stable patient suspected of penetrating cardiac injury, echocardiography is a useful examination to evaluate for pericardial fluid. The hypotensive patient with penetration in this area is assumed to have a mediastinal injury, and immediate surgery is needed.

Table 13-2

Chest X-Ray Signs of Mediastinal Hematoma

Wide mediastinum (>8 cm on AP view)
Abnormality of aortic knob contour
Opacification of aortopulmonary window
Rightward deviation of trachea
Rightward deviation of nasogastric tube
Abnormal or wide paraspinous stripe
Fracture of first rib
Left apical cap (extrapleural hematoma)
Depression of left main-stem bronchus
Elevation of right main-stem bronchus
Evidence of diaphragmatic rupture

TREATMENT

The initial management of a patient with thoracic trauma follows the same guidelines as stressed previously: airway control, adequate ventilation, and reversal of shock. Tension pneumothorax or massive hemothorax are not diagnoses to be made with a chest x-ray in the unstable patient; rather, a chest tube should be inserted immediately in any patient with diminished breath sounds and respiratory distress or hypotension. Cardiogenic shock can be caused by tension pneumothorax, cardiac tamponade, or blunt cardiac injury; these diagnoses should be entertained whenever shock persists despite adequate oxygenation and volume resuscitation.

Most cases of pneumothorax and hemothorax are definitively treated by tube thoracostomy; thoracotomy is necessary in less than 15% of all patients with thoracic trauma. A chest tube acts to reexpand the collapsed lung, restoring capacity for oxygenation and ventilation. Lung expansion also allows for the tamponade of bleeding from the low-pressure pulmonary circulation in parenchymal injuries. Retained blood in the pleural space acts to promote bleeding by a local fibrinolytic effect and by preventing tamponade. If the initial output from a thoracostomy tube exceeds 500 mL, a second chest tube should be inserted to diminish the likelihood of a retained hemothorax. Indications for thoracotomy are an initial output of 1500 mL from a chest tube or continued bleeding at a rate exceeding 200 mL/hour.

Abdomen

HISTORY

There are several specific patterns of abdominal injury that are each associated with particular mechanisms of trauma. Side-impact blunt trauma is more likely to result in injuries to the solid organs on the side of the impact: the liver and right kidney are often injured together, as are the spleen and left kidney. Rapid deceleration can injure mobile organs at their fixed points: the liver and spleen at their peritoneal attachments, small bowel in the mesentery, and (less often) the small bowel at the ligament of Treitz. Focal frontal forces (commonly from a bicycle handlebar) can crush the pancreas against the spine, and/or the duodenum may have a "blowout" caused by the acute rise in intraluminal pressure. Improperly positioned lap-belts riding above the iliac crests causes a transverse abdominal wall contusion ("lap-belt" sign) and is frequently associated with lumbar-spine flexion-distraction injury and shear-induced intestinal rupture. Figure 13-5 outlines the approach to evaluation and management of blunt abdominal trauma.

PHYSICAL EXAMINATION

Inspection of the abdomen should focus initially on the presence and location of abrasions, contusions, and penetrating wounds to assess likely direction and magnitude of transmitted forces. The contour of the abdomen is important as well; a patient with a distended abdomen and hypoten-sion usually has hemoperitoneum, often from a vascular injury. Evisceration of small bowel or omentum from a stab wound is an indication for immediate laparotomy.

The abdomen should be palpated for guarding or rebound tenderness. These signs of peritonitis, if present, mandate operative exploration. The absence of peritonitis, however, does not rule out intra-abdominal injury, as blood is not a consistent cause of symptomatic peritoneal irritation. Minimal transmural bowel injuries, as well as those in the retroperitoneum, can take hours to cause peritonitis.

The rectal examination cannot be overlooked in the evaluation of the abdomen. A high-riding prostate gland is indicative of urethral transection and is a contraindication to Foley catheter insertion. Gross blood on the examining finger indicates a bowel injury and is an indication for sigmoidoscopy and possible surgical exploration. Diminished sphincter tone is a sign of spinal-cord injury and should prompt a search for a vertebral

Figure 13-5

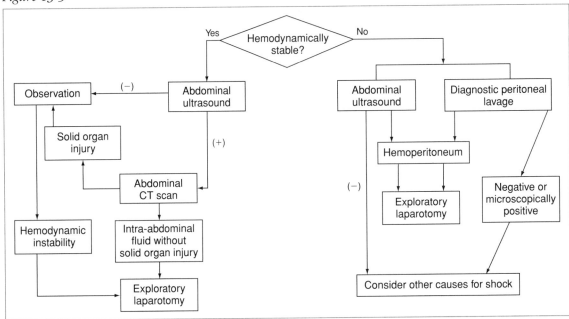

Algorithm for blunt abdominal trauma.

fracture. Fragments from a pelvic fracture can cause a laceration of the rectal wall, which can be noted on digital examination. Likewise, the vagina should be examined for lacerations from penetrating wounds or pelvic fracture fragments.

ANCILLARY TESTS

Patients with abdominal trauma often require adjunctive tests to properly evaluate whether they have sustained a significant injury. The physical examination can be equivocal or the abdomen unevaluable because of intoxication, head injury, or spinal-cord injury. Moreover, some patients require operative procedures such as fracture fixations that preclude serial examinations.

PERITONEAL LAVAGE Diagnostic peritoneal lavage (DPL) has for many years been the major tool for diagnosing intraperitoneal injury. Its advantages include its high sensitivity (95% to 97%) and rapidity. However, it is the most invasive of the abdominal diagnostic procedures, and it cannot determine which organ has been injured, or how severely. Furthermore, the specificity of DPL, cited in many studies as 98% to 99%, is somewhat misleading—as this specificity refers only to whether any injury is present, not whether a laparotomy is necessary to treat that injury. These concerns, combined with a trend toward nonoperative management of solid-organ injuries, have decreased the use of DPL. However, DPL still occupies an important role, especially in the diagnosis of hollow-viscus injuries and in settings where other diagnostic modalities are not accessible. The DPL procedure is described later in this chapter.

COMPUTERIZED TOMOGRAPHY Computed tomography (CT) of the abdomen has become a mainstay in the management of hemodynamically stable patients with abdominal trauma. It is especially useful in its visualization of the retroperitoneum, which is not well evaluated by DPL. Intravenous and, selectively, oral contrast agents are necessary to obtain a good quality study. The use of the newer helical (spiral) CT scanners adds even more to the accuracy of the test (sensitivity 97%, specificity 95% in blunt trauma). It is worthwhile to emphasize that CT should not be performed in an unstable patient, as it only delays definitive treatment and places the patient at significant risk while sequestered in the CT scanner.

ULTRASOUND Ultrasound has been used in Europe for several years in the diagnosis of abdominal injury and has recently gained some acceptance in the United States. In experienced hands, it has a specificity and sensitivity that approaches that of CT and DPL. Its main advantages include its non-invasive nature, as well as its ability to be done serially and at the bedside of unstable patients. Its major limitation is that visualization is often restricted by the presence of obscuring bowel gas or subcutaneous air. Furthermore, ultrasonography has low sensitivity for detection of bowel perforation and should not be used as the test of choice when bowel perforation is suspected (e.g., when a "lap-belt" sign is present).

TREATMENT

Early surgical consultation is important in the management of penetrating abdominal trauma, as many of these patients will require exploratory surgery. Emergent surgical exploration is required when such patients are hypotensive.

GUNSHOT WOUNDS A gunshot wound to the abdomen is associated with an 85% incidence of significant intra-abdominal injury. For this reason, even hemodynamically normal patients require surgical exploration.

STAB WOUNDS If a patient with an anterior abdominal stab wound is hemodynamically normal, with no evisceration or signs of peritonitis, further evaluation is needed to determine the presence of significant intra-abdominal injury. This evaluation often involves local wound exploration, which can be performed in the emergency department under local anesthesia by enlarging the incision as necessary to visualize the wound tract through the layers of the abdominal wall. Probing the wound without visualization is not recommended, as false passages can be created, and the information gained is minimal. If wound exploration reveals that the wound tract clearly ends in the subcutaneous tissue, the exploration is negative, and no further diagnostic workup is needed. If the exploration is positive (i.e., the wound penetrates the posterior fascia) or the end of the tract cannot be visualized, then a DPL can be performed to evaluate for intraperitoneal injury.

Stab wounds to the flank or back have the potential to injure retroperitoneal structures, including the pancreas, duodenum, ascending and descending colon, kidney, and ureter. For this reason, triple (oral, IV, and rectal) contrast CT scan is the test of choice to rule out injury in stable patients suspected of having such injuries. DPL may be performed prior to CT and, if positive, laparotomy is indicated because the positive DPL indicates peritoneal penetration from a posterior stab wound that has traversed the retoperitoneum. Unstable patients require immediate surgery.

BLUNT TRAUMA   The unstable patient with blunt trauma also requires rapid diagnosis of abdominal injury. DPL or ultrasound should be performed during the primary survey, as soon as airway, ventilation, and IV access are established. A positive test is an indication for immediate exploratory laparotomy. CT should be reserved for the hemodynamically normal patient and should never delay a transfer to a definitive-care facility.

Pelvis

Pelvic fractures are common blunt injuries and are indicative of a large, transmitted force. Associated injuries are common and are usually the main source of morbidity and mortality. However, the fracture itself can be the cause of life-threatening hemorrhage resulting from cancellous bone bleeding, tearing of the pelvic venous plexus, and injuries to branches of the internal and external iliac artery. Thus, the diagnosis of pelvic fracture must be made expediently to permit institution of adequate resuscitation and, for severe pelvic fractures, early surgical consultation.

HISTORY AND PHYSICAL EXAMINATION

History yields little information in the diagnosis of a major pelvic fracture. Rather, the only initial sign of such a fracture is often unexplained hypotension (caused by hemorrhage) refractory to fluid administration. Swelling and ecchymosis of the scrotum, perineum, or (less commonly) the flank can be important clues to an unstable pelvic fracture. Blood at the urethral meatus is indicative of an associated urethral injury, as is a high-riding or free-floating prostate on rectal examination. Rectal examination can also reveal bony fragments. Inspection of the patient's lower extremities may show a leg-length discrepancy or rotational deformity. These are caused by the cephalad-directed, unopposed, muscular pull and external rotation of the unstable hemipelvis.

The bony pelvis should be tested for mechanical instability by grasping the anterior and posterior iliac spines and administering anterior-posterior and lateral compression. Cephalad-caudad instability can be determined in this manner as well. This procedure will be painful in the presence of significant pelvic fractures and often not tolerated by patients who are awake and alert.

ANCILLARY TESTS

The AP plain film is the mainstay of diagnosis of pelvic injuries. It should be performed early during the resuscitation of the blunt trauma patient, along with the chest x-ray and lateral cervical-spine film. Interpretation of the pelvis film should focus on identifying disruptions of the pelvic ring, because these fractures are most likely to cause hemorrhage. Single fractures of the pelvic ring rarely occur; if one fracture is identified, a careful search is needed to identify a second fracture. Anteriorly, widening of the symphysis pubis or fractures of the pubic rami are common. Widening of the sacroiliac joint indicates a disruption of the strong posterior ligaments.

Different vectors of transmitted force result in different fracture patterns. Frontal impact causes widening of the symphysis and external rotation of both hemipelves, the so-called AP-compression pattern. The lateral compression pattern consists of internal rotation of the hemipelvis and overlapping of the ramus or symphysis fracture. Other less common patterns result in vertical shear and mixed forces. Although the AP-compression fracture is most commonly associated with bleeding, it is important to stress that *any* pelvic ring fracture (no matter how limited) can cause major hemorrhage.

TREATMENT

Early stabilization is one of the keys to the treatment of an unstable pelvic fracture, especially if hemorrhage is present. Instability of the pelvis allows significant increases in pelvic volume and permits the resulting retroperitoneal hematoma to expand unchecked, leading to further displacement and more bleeding. As much as 4000 mL of blood can accumulate in the retroperitoneal space of a patient who has an unstable pelvic fracture. By stabilizing the fracture, bleeding from veins and cancellous bone is reduced by the tamponade effect of reducing pelvic volume.

There are several temporary means of achieving stabilization, including inflation of the abdominal compartment of the pneumatic antishock garment (PASG). Just as effective, and much simpler, is to snugly wrap and "tourniquet" a folded sheet circumferentially around the patient at the level of the iliac spines. These are temporizing measures only, and the patient should undergo arteriography as soon as possible to diagnose and treat pelvic arterial bleeding.

Although simple pelvic stabilization can reduce venous bleeding, arterial injury can continue to cause severe blood loss. For this reason, early arteriography is essential in the management of the severe pelvic fracture with evidence of ongoing hemorrhage. Selective embolization of arterial bleeding is usually possible, but occasionally it is necessary to embolize the entire internal iliac system on one side to control bleeding. Ongoing

resuscitation with crystalloid, blood, and coagulation components should continue during angiography, as well as efforts to prevent and treat hypothermia. Definitive care of the pelvic fracture(s) will frequently require operative reduction and stabilization by an orthopedic surgeon with expertise in pelvic surgery.

Extremities

Injuries of the extremities are extremely common, especially in blunt trauma. Fortunately, such injuries are rarely life-threatening. It is therefore important to remember that no matter how impressive an extremity injury looks, its care does not take precedence over the expedient resuscitation of the patient and the search for less obvious but more serious injuries. Once the immediate stability of the patient is ensured, priority should be given to finding and treating limb-threatening injuries such as open fractures, occult vascular or neurologic injuries, and compartmental syndrome.

PHYSICAL EXAMINATION

A rapid visual inspection of the extremities will usually identify the most serious injuries. Major external hemorrhage is usually obvious and should be initially treated with pressure at the site of the injury. Most major, long-bone fractures can be identified clinically by the presence of angular deformity and swelling. All open wounds should be documented—an open wound in the same extremity segment as a fracture should be considered an open fracture until proven otherwise. A pale distal extremity may be indicative of a vascular injury causing critical ischemia.

Palpation of the extremities should be carried out as part of the secondary survey. Any areas of tenderness, swelling, or deformity should have further evaluation to rule out a fracture. Joint stability should be determined by cautious application of stress to specific ligaments. Tight swelling in any of the major muscle groups may indicate crush injury or ischemia resulting in compartmental syndrome. A brief neurologic examination should be carried out at this time as well, by testing sensation to pinprick and light touch along the extremities. Motor testing of muscle groups can give clues both to peripheral nerve injuries and to central nervous system lesions.

An important part of the physical examination of the injured extremity is the vascular examination. Brachial blood pressure should be recorded bilaterally, with any differences of 10 mg Hg or greater prompting further evaluation of the upper extremity vascular tree. The presence and character of the distal pulses is assessed by palpation. Auscultation and palpation over a penetrating injury may reveal a bruit or thrill, both considered "hard" signs of vascular injury that require surgical exploration. "Soft" signs of arterial trauma include a small, stable hematoma; apparent injury to a peripheral nerve (most of which lie in close proximity to a major artery); or reduction in Doppler-measured blood indices in an injured extremity.

Hypotension may limit the ability to palpate pulses; in this situation, examination of the pulses with a Doppler device must be performed distal to any penetrating injuries or suspected fractures. The ankle pressure index (API) is determined by taking the systolic blood pressure measured by Doppler at the ankle (posterior tibial and dorsalis pedis arteries) of the injured leg. The highest of these two values is divided by the brachial systolic blood pressure (also measured by Doppler). Any API of less than 0.9 is indicative of abnormal flow to the extremity resulting from arterial injury or preexisting peripheral vascular disease.

ANCILLARY TESTS

PLAIN X-RAYS   Although x-rays are an essential part of the process for diagnosing extremity fractures, as stated before, extremity x-rays should not be performed until other life-threatening injuries have been identified and appropriately treated. Plain x-ray films should, of course, be obtained in hemodynamically normal patients in whom the physical examination raises suspicion of a fracture or dislocation. Abnormalities of joints such as effusions or tenderness also require x-rays. Two

orthogonal views are necessary to fully evaluate a fracture and plan for treatment.

ANGIOGRAPHY   Radiographic evaluation of the vascular system is necessary when there is a question of injury to an artery and should be considered when hard or soft signs (described above) of vascular injury are present. However, proximity of an injury to major peripheral vascular structures is rarely an indication in and of itself for arteriography. Positive signs on arteriography include obstruction, extravasation, false aneurysm, arteriovenous fistula, vessel-wall irregularity, and filling defect or intimal flap. More recently, noninvasive arterial imaging with duplex-mode ultrasound has been used with good results in the detection of arterial injury. As a general rule, a surgeon should be consulted if such studies are being considered.

TREATMENT

The extremities are only rarely involved with immediately life-threatening injuries, and these usually involve exsanguinating hemorrhage from a major artery. Such life-threatening injuries are most often penetrating injuries, but they can also be associated with fractures caused by massive blunt trauma. Direct pressure over the injured artery is usually sufficient to control bleeding; under critical conditions, a proximal tourniquet can be used as a temporizing measure. Early surgical intervention is crucial to definitively treat the hemorrhage and restore flow to the extremity.

IMMOBILIZATION   Early immobilization of fractures is an important part of the care of the injured patient. The goal of such early treatment is to achieve realignment in as close to anatomic position as possible and prevention of further injury by limiting motion at the fracture site. Such immobilization helps reduce pain and control blood loss and further soft-tissue injury at the site of the fracture.

OPEN FRACTURES   If an open wound exists in the same extremity segment as a fracture, it should be assumed to be an open fracture. Such wounds should be covered with a sterile dressing soaked in an iodine-based disinfectant solution. Administration of intravenous antibiotics prior to transport is appropriate if definitive orthopedic care is not readily available.

VASCULAR INJURIES   Vascular compromise of an extremity must be recognized and treated rapidly. Muscle necrosis resulting from decreased blood flow begins within 4 to 6 hours, and nerves are even more sensitive to ischemia. Therefore, early operative intervention is necessary to avoid devastating complications, including amputation. If an extremity is pulseless distal to a displaced fracture or dislocation, reduction of the bony injury may restore flow and provide time to more fully evaluate the vascular injury. Arteriography often serves only to delay definitive treatment and should not be ordered without consulting a surgeon for immediate operative intervention with intraoperative angiography.

COMPARTMENTAL SYNDROME   Compartmental syndrome can occur as a result of vascular compromise, massive soft-tissue trauma, or bony injury with hematoma formation or in situations resulting from a prolonged time until extrication of a "trapped extremity." Any clinical suspicion of a compartmental syndrome should prompt surgical consultation—its presentation is often subtle, and its only definitive treatment is operative fasciotomy. Direct measurement of compartmental pressures is frequently necessary to confirm the diagnosis.

TRAUMATIC AMPUTATION   Traumatic amputation is impressive in appearance and often diverts attention away from other more life-threatening injury. However, the same treatment principles of management—attention to airway, breathing, circulation, and neurologic status—apply in the care of patients with traumatic amputation. Early resuscitation is crucial to ensuring an optimal outcome, regardless of whether that involves replantation of the amputated extremity.

Replantation is usually considered an option only in a patient with a sharp, isolated extremity injury distal to the knee or elbow. Such patients should be transported to an appropriate surgical facility. The amputated part should be washed with saline, wrapped in sterile gauze soaked in an antibiotic solution (usually penicillin G), placed in a plastic bag, and transported in an ice-filled cooler. Multiply injured patients requiring aggressive resuscitation and emergency operations because of torso or head trauma are not replantation candidates.

Procedures

There are a number of relatively simple procedures that can be accomplished in the emergency department, each of which has the potential to be lifesaving. Clinicians managing trauma patients should be familiar with the performance of these procedures. Each is directed toward alleviating problems of airway, breathing, or circulation.

Cricothyroidotomy

While obtaining an airway is the first priority in the multiply injured patient, endotracheal intubation is sometimes impossible because of glottic edema, laryngeal fracture, or severe oropharyngeal hemorrhage obstructing the airway. In these situations, rapid procurement of a surgical airway is necessary. This can be achieved in the form of either a needle cricothyroidotomy, which allows temporary jet insufflation of oxygen directly into the trachea; or a surgical cricothyroidotomy, which is a definitive airway with placement of a cuffed tube into the trachea. For children, only needle cricothyroidotomy can be used, as surgical cricothyroidotomy is contraindicated in children less than 12 years old.

NEEDLE CRICOTHYROIDOTOMY

In preparation for needle cricothyroidotomy, oxygen tubing is assembled, and a Y-connector is placed between a high-flow (15 L/min) oxygen source and the patient end of the tubing. The patient is then placed supine, and the neck is prepared with povidone iodine or similar agent.

To perform the procedure, the cricothyroid membrane is identified by palpation. It is located anteriorly in the neck, between the thyroid cartilage and cricoid cartilage. The cricoid cartilage is best identified by anterior tracheal palpation from caudad to cephalad. After a small skin nick is made with a scalpel in the skin overlying the cricothyroid membrane, a 14-gauge, over-the-needle IV catheter attached to a 10-mL syringe is used to puncture the cricothyroid membrane, directing the needle caudally at a 45° angle. The metal needle is withdrawn, the flexible catheter advanced, and the oxygen tubing connected to the catheter hub.

Intermittent insufflation of oxygen is provided by occluding the Y-connector for 1 second, allowing passive exhalation for 4 seconds. Ventilation by needle cricothyroidotomy is a temporary measure, as adequate oxygenation can only be maintained for about 30 minutes; CO_2 retention will occur even earlier.

Complications of needle cricothyroidotomy include hematoma, aspiration of blood, posterior tracheal-wall perforation, esophageal laceration, and thyroid-gland perforation. These can usually be avoided by careful attention to anatomic landmarks and negative pressure on the syringe during membrane perforation. Aspiration of air verifies position within the tracheal lumen.

SURGICAL CRICOTHYROIDOTOMY

Surgical cricothyroidotomy (Fig. 13-6) is performed using the same anatomic landmarks. A transverse incision is made over the cricothyroid membrane, taking care to avoid the anterior jugular veins. The membrane itself is then incised transversely. The scalpel handle is inserted into the incision and rotated 90° to the vertical position, thereby opening the airway.

A #5 or #6 cuffed endotracheal or tracheostomy tube is inserted through the incision into the trachea and the cuff inflated. The tube is then secured to the patient with tracheostomy tape.

Surgical cricothyroidotomy carries several complications, including hemorrhage and aspiration of blood, laceration of the esophagus or trachea, mediastinal emphysema, and creation of a false passage into the tissues of the neck. Long-term complications include subglottic or laryngeal stenosis and vocal cord paralysis resulting in hoarseness or partial airway obstruction.

Tube Thoracostomy (Chest Tube)

A well-placed chest tube can definitively address many of the life-threatening complications that accompany thoracic trauma. In the trauma setting, a 36-French tube should be used to minimize the chance of the tube becoming obstructed with clot. It should be placed in the fifth intercostal space, just anterior to the midaxillary line, high enough to ensure entry into the pleural space rather than the peritoneal cavity, particularly with abnormal elevation of the diaphragm. This landmark can be found directly lateral to the nipple line (Fig. 13-7).

The ipsilateral upper extremity is abducted and secured, and the chest is surgically prepared and draped. If the patient is conscious, lidocaine (1% with epinephrine) is infiltrated in the skin, subcutaneous tissues, rib periosteum, and parietal pleura.

A 3-cm transverse incision is then made over the sixth intercostal space, and blunt dissection is directed cephalad to create a subcutaneous tunnel to the fifth intercostal space. A curved clamp is used to puncture through the intercostal muscle and pleura just above the sixth rib and is then spread to create an opening to accommodate the tube. A gloved finger is inserted to verify entry into the pleural space and sweep away adhesions and clot. The tube is inserted, directed toward the lung apex, to the desired depth (the last side hole in the tube should be within the pleural space). "Fogging" of the tube and movement of air and fluid within the tube verifies placement in the pleural cavity. The tube is sutured securely to the skin, covered with a sterile dressing, and then connected to an underwater-seal suction device. A chest x-ray should be obtained to verify placement and assess whether the tube has successfully addressed the pneumothorax or hemothorax.

The most serious complications of tube thoracostomy are laceration or puncture of the lung and injury to intraperitoneal organs. Both of these complications can be avoided by using the finger sweep technique, noted above, to ensure proper location of the tube. The intercostal neurovascular bundle can also be injured during this procedure, especially if the clamp is advanced under rather than over the rib. Kinking or clogging of the tube can result in a persistent pneumothorax or hemothorax and necessitates a second tube. Care must be taken to ensure a tight seal in the tubing of the collection system and at the skin around the tube; a pneumothorax can result from air leaks at these sites.

Pericardiocentesis

Cardiac tamponade is a lethal and difficult-to-diagnose complication of cardiac injury. It is almost always associated with a penetrating injury to the heart (blunt rupture of a cardiac chamber is rare). When cardiac tamponade occurs, it is often lethal before arrival at the hospital.

Figure 13-6

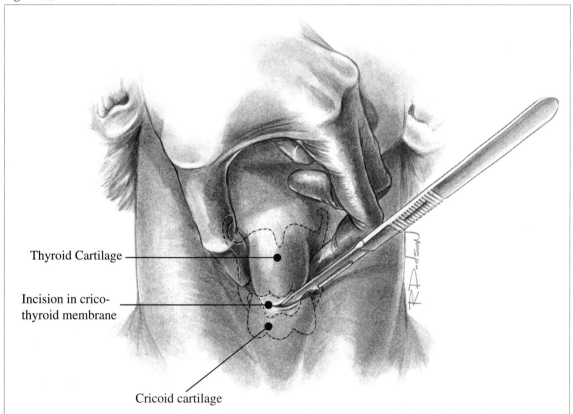

Thyroid Cartilage

Incision in crico-
thyroid membrane

Cricoid cartilage

Anatomic landmarks for cricothyroidotomy. A transverse incision is made over the cricothyroid cartilage. *(Reproduced by permission from Mulder, DS: Airway management, in Carrico CJ, Thal ET, Weigelt DS, (eds): Operative Trauma Management. New York, McGraw-Hill, 1999, p 11.)*

Figure 13-7

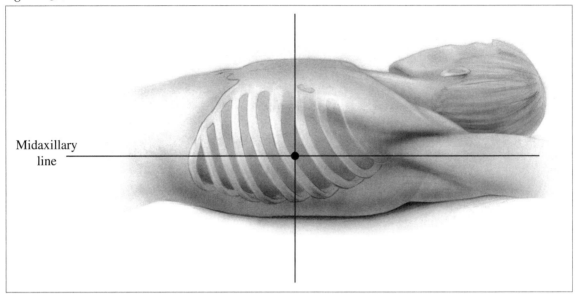

Midaxillary
line

Anatomic landmarks for tube thoracostomy. The correct site for insertion of a thoracostomy tube is the fifth intercostal space, just anterior to the midaxillary line. *(Reproduced by permission from McNeil J, Rozycki GS, Thal ET: Diagnostic procedures used to establish priorities, in Carrico CJ, Thal ET, Weigelt DS (eds):* Operative Trauma Management. *New York, McGraw-Hill, 1999, p 29.)*

Pericardiocentesis is an effective method of decompressing the pericardial sac and temporarily restoring cardiac output, assuming the patient has an adequate circulating blood volume. Cardiac tamponade should be suspected, and pericardiocentesis performed, when a patient has evidence of penetrating trauma in the "cardiac box" or across the mediastinum and when the response to volume administration is absent or transient.

When performing pericardiocentesis, continuous electrocardiographic monitoring should be used throughout the procedure. The subxiphoid area is surgically prepared with an antiseptic solution. A long (1½ to 2 inch) intravenous catheter is attached to a 30-mL syringe. The skin entry site for the needle is just to the left of the xiphoid process, with the needle angled toward the tip of the left scapula (45° in the sagittal, coronal, and transverse planes).

While inserting the needle, mild negative pressure should be maintained on the syringe at all times. Advancement of the needle should stop when an injury pattern is noted on the EKG monitor. If pericardial tamponade is present, 20 to 30 mL of nonclotting blood may be withdrawn, usually with dramatic improvement of the patient's vital signs. The needle should be withdrawn from the catheter, and the catheter left in place within the pericardial space for use if further drainage is needed. If bleeding is rapid, tamponade may occur quickly, prior to initiation of spontaneous thrombolysis, and pericardiocentesis may fail because of the presence of clot within the pericardial sac.

Pericardiocentesis is only a temporizing method to be used if the patient requires transport, and it should not delay definitive surgical repair of a cardiac injury if a surgeon and operating room are immediately available. Complications of the procedure include pneumothorax and laceration of the heart or coronary arteries.

Saphenous Vein Cutdown

The greater saphenous vein is an ideal choice for vascular access by the cutdown technique because of its subcutaneous course, constant position, and large size. This route should be used whenever peripheral upper-extremity access is unobtainable because of either upper extremity trauma or a history of intravenous drug abuse.

The ankle area is surgically prepared and draped. Lidocaine (1% with epinephrine) is infiltrated into the skin and subcutaneous tissue. A transverse incision is made 1.5 cm anterior and superior to the medial malleolus (Fig. 13-8). The subcutaneous tissues tend to be very thin and are dissected bluntly in an inferior-superior direction to expose and mobilize the vein without causing injury. Approximately 3 cm of vein should be exposed and mobilized for cannulation. A 3-0 silk suture is then passed around the proximal portion of the vein and elevated gently for traction.

A transverse venotomy is made and gently dilated with the tip of a hemostat. A 14-gauge intravenous cannula or 7-Fr introducer sheath is inserted through the venotomy and secured in place with the silk suture. Intravenous tubing can then be attached to the cannula for fluid administration. The incision is closed with interrupted sutures and the cannula sutured to the skin. The wound should be dressed sterilely with a topical antibiotic ointment.

Diagnostic Peritoneal Lavage (DPL)

As discussed earlier, DPL has limitations and has been somewhat supplanted by CT and ultrasound in recent years. Nonetheless, DPL is a rapid and sensitive method of detecting intraperitoneal injury and may still be preferable in the situations mentioned previously.

Before beginning the procedure, a nasogastric tube and Foley catheter are placed to decompress the stomach and urinary bladder. The periumbilical area is prepared and draped in sterile fashion, and

Figure 13-8

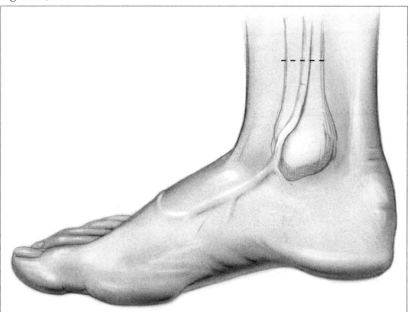

Anatomic landmarks for saphenous vein cutdown. The incision is made 1.5 cm anterior and superior to the medial malleolus. *(Reproduced by permission from Borgstrom DC: Intravenous access and emergency thoracotomy, in Carrico CJ, Thal ET, Weigelt DS (eds): Operative Trauma Management. New York, McGraw-Hill, 1999, p 13.)*

the skin and subcutaneous tissue are infiltrated with 1% lidocaine with epinephrine.

An 18-gauge introducer needle attached to a 10-mL syringe is inserted perpendicularly through the skin and subcutaneous tissue just below the umbilicus and is advanced until resistance from the fascia is encountered. Countertraction using a penetrating towel clamp placed in the umbilicus is useful to avoid iatrogenic injury to internal organs. Gentle pressure will result in first fascial and then peritoneal penetration (accompanied by a small tactile "pop"). The needle is directed toward the pelvis, and the flexible guidewire is advanced through the needle until resistance is felt. The needle is then withdrawn over the wire. A small skin nick is made for the catheter, and the catheter introduced over the guidewire into the peritoneal cavity.

The wire is then removed, and a syringe is used to aspirate through the catheter. If no gross blood is obtained, the syringe is removed and 1 liter of warm lactated Ringer's solution is instilled through the IV tubing connected to the catheter. The IV bag containing the solution is placed on the floor, and the intraperitoneal fluid is drained. A sample of the fluid is sent to the laboratory for analysis. The indications of a positive test are listed in Table 13-3.

Inadequate return of instilled fluid is the most common difficulty encountered during DPL, and this can usually be avoided by lowering the bag of Ringer's solution before the entire liter has been instilled (thus preserving the "priming"

Table 13-3

Criteria for Positive Diagnostic Peritoneal Lavage

> $>100,000$ RBC/mm^3
>
> >500 WBC/mm^3, with a ratio of WBC to RBC $\times$ 100 > 1.0
>
> Amylase — lavage concentration $>$ serum concentration
>
> Bilirubin — lavage concentration $>$ serum concentration
>
> Presence of vegetable fibers or bacteria on microscopic exam

siphon function of the tubing). When poor fluid return is encountered despite this maneuver, instillation of an additional 500 mL of solution can often improve or restore flow. If the problem persists, conversion to open technique is required.

The most serious complication of DPL is injury to intra-abdominal organs or vascular structures, which often necessitates operative intervention. Late infectious complications are uncommon.

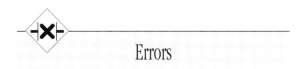

Errors

The initial resuscitation of the multiply injured patient, from a technical standpoint, is not difficult. The handful of procedures outlined above often represent definitive treatment or at least can temporize until definitive therapy is available. From a cognitive standpoint, the resuscitation also seems fairly simple on the surface — ensure an airway, provide adequate ventilation and oxygenation, and identify and control sources of shock.

However, there are pitfalls that frequently occur. Each can be avoided by having a thorough knowledge of injury patterns and their complications and by recognizing the times when a heightened sense of urgency is appropriate.

Inappropriate Focus on Single Injuries

It is often easy to focus on one injury that may seem the most serious, while failing to recognize the importance of an equally lethal injury in another body area or system. It is important to realize that injuries to multiple extremities or body areas tend to be a marker for high overall injury severity and high risk of occult injury. A diligent search for other injuries must be undertaken in this instance, especially if the response to resuscitation is not as good as expected. Two useful maxims in this situation are "when in doubt, start over and redo the ABCs of resuscitation," and "always assume the worst-case scenario until proven otherwise."

Inappropriate Emphasis on Obtaining Radiographic Studies

Although radiologic evaluation is important in all multiply injured patients, it is a mistake to send hemodynamically unstable patients outside of the resuscitation area to have radiographic studies. All of the important causes of shock can be assessed with a few portable plain x-rays and with bedside examinations such as DPL or ultrasound. Extensive radiologic evaluations only serve to take the patient away from the watchful eye of the clinical staff, and they delay definitive treatment or transfer.

The only exception to the rule of limiting radiologic evaluation comes in the angiography suite for treatment of major pelvic fractures. Exsanguination from a pelvic fracture can be rapid, and often the simple maneuvers such as wrapping the pelvis in a sheet to stabilize it are not sufficient to stop arterial bleeding. Therefore, early arteriographic embolization (or transfer to a facility that has that capability) is crucial to the successful treatment of the patient with a major pelvic fracture. This is especially true in the case of sacral fracture and sacroiliac joint disruption, as the risk of arterial injury is high in this area, and for pelvic fractures in elderly patients, in whom almost any pelvic fracture can injure fragile and inelastic pelvic arteries.

Inappropriate Reassurance from Normal Blood Pressures

It is important to realize that a normal blood pressure does not ensure that the patient is not hypovolemic. Compensatory mechanisms such as peripheral vasoconstriction and tachycardia can maintain relatively normal blood pressure after up to a 30% decrease in circulating blood volume, particularly in young individuals. Such mechanisms serve to maintain perfusion to the brain, heart, and kidneys at the expense of the splanchnic and musculoskeletal circulations. Because of this, even urine output may be maintained despite an ongoing hypovolemic state. Victims of multiple trauma must

be carefully monitored and continually assessed for the possibility of concealed hemorrhage.

Patients at the extremes of age can be especially difficult to assess because their physiologic compensation differs from the normal adult. Young children, in particular, have extraordinary circulatory compensatory reserve; they can maintain relatively normal vital signs right up until the moment they experience cardiopulmonary arrest from hypovolemia. The elderly, on the other hand, have almost no physiologic reserve. Injuries that in younger patients would seem minor can have devastating consequences in the older patient. It is crucial to have a greater sense of urgency when caring for the very old or the very young injured patient if there is any indication of significant injury or loss of blood volume.

Inappropriate Management of Intrathoracic Hemorrhage

Hemorrhage from injury to the lung parenchyma can rapidly become lethal. For bleeding from the pulmonary parenchyma to stop, the lung must expand fully, causing a tamponade and hemostatic effect against the chest wall. However, almost the entire circulating blood volume can rapidly be sequestered in the pleural cavity, with little opportunity for the lung to expand into apposition and achieve tamponade with the chest wall. Furthermore, such massive hemothorax leaves no room for gas exchange to take place, leading to hypoventilation and hypoxia.

Fortunately, such hemorrhage can be treated with a relatively simple procedure—tube thoracostomy. However, a common error is to assume that one chest tube is sufficient when, in reality, one tube is not always enough, especially with a large volume of intrathoracic blood that can occlude a tube with clot. Any retained blood or clot in the pleural space leaves a space into which hemorrhage can continue. Therefore, we recommend insertion of a second chest tube whenever initial output exceeds 500 mL. This increases the chances for complete evacuation of hemothorax, expansion of the lung, and cessation of bleeding.

Failure to Involve Appropriate Medical Personnel

Logistically, it is important to contact a surgeon as soon as it is apparent that a trauma patient will need to be admitted to the hospital. This determination can often be made in the prehospital phase, by listening to the paramedics' report of the patient's injuries. Having established criteria for activation of a "trauma response team," consisting of a surgeon, laboratory and radiology technicians, and nursing support staff, can simplify this decision and ensure that the essential personnel are available soon after the patient arrives in the emergency department. Similarly, once it becomes likely that the patient will require transfer to another hospital, that facility should be contacted and transport arranged immediately — time is of the essence in the care of the multiply injured patient. Further diagnostic studies serve only to delay transport and rarely contribute positively to the patient's ultimate outcome.

Controversies

Two important controversies in the management of trauma victims are worthy of discussion. One surrounds the type of fluid that should be used for resuscitation of trauma victims. The second is related to optimal management of traumatic rupture of the aorta.

Fluid Management

There has long been a debate over which type of fluids — colloid or crystalloid — are most appropriate for resuscitation of trauma patients who are in shock. As discussed earlier, a balanced crystalloid solution has been shown to adequately replace the extracellular, extravascular volume losses as cellular swelling occurs. Although many studies have been undertaken to explore the role of colloid, none have shown colloid to be superior to lactated Ringer's solution in terms of mortality, complications, or length of hospitalization in an intensive-care unit. Since crystalloid is at least equivalent and certainly much less expensive than colloid, it is the fluid of choice for most acute-shock resuscitations.

In recent years, there has been some interest in the use of hypertonic saline (often in combination with dextran) for resuscitations, with the theoretic benefit being the reduced volume of fluid needed to replace losses. Most studies, however, show no difference in the ultimate amount of fluid needed to completely resuscitate the injured patient. There may be some potential benefit to using hypertonic saline solutions in the early care of brain-injured patients, because of the fact that hypertonic intravenous fluids can decrease cerebral edema and reduce intracranial pressure. Furthermore, these is some evidence that hypertonic saline may partially inhibit neutrophil-induced organ injury during reperfusion insult. More study is necessary to determine if these theoretic benefits lead to improvements in clinical outcomes.

Aortic Rupture

Blunt thoracic aortic rupture has traditionally been evaluated using aortography as the definitive diagnostic test. Recently, however, the use of contrast-enhanced chest CT has been proposed as an alternative method of excluding such injuries. Proposed advantages of CT over aortography include its less invasive nature, as well as its rapidity and almost universal availability. However, proponents of aortography argue that CT has not been proven sensitive enough to support clinical decisions on its own. Several studies have suggested that newer-generation, helical CT scanners, as well as more radiologic experience, have begun to narrow the gap in sensitivity between CT and angiography.

Emerging Concepts

An important emerging concept in the management of victims of multiple traumatic injuries involves the ischemia-reperfusion syndrome discussed earlier in this chapter. It has been hypothesized that blocking the physiologic response to this syndrome at the cellular level might reduce morbidity and mortality from traumatic injuries. Following identification of the receptors responsible for the adherence-induced injury of the activated neutrophil in response to shock, researchers have developed antibodies that bind to these adherence molecules and competitively inhibit the neutrophil response. By preventing adherence of the activated neutrophil and release of its toxic reactive oxidative substances, the damage done to the microcirculation of the lungs and other organs is minimized. This so-called "trauma vaccine" has been shown in animal models to reduce the amount of volume resuscitation needed in the setting of severe shock, as well as to reduce the degree of pathologic change in the lungs. Clinical trials on human shock are currently under way, and such efforts may ultimately change the way in which trauma victims respond to their injuries.

References

Agolini SF, Shah K, Jaffe J, et al: Arterial embolization is a rapid and effective technique for controlling pelvic fracture hemorrhage. *J Trauma* 43:395, 1997.

Baker SP, O'Neill B, Ginsburg M, et al: *The Injury Fact Book*, 2nd ed. New York, Oxford University Press, 1992.

Bonnie RJ, Fulco CE, Liverman CT (eds): *Reducing the Burden of Injury: Advancing Prevention and Treatment.* Washington, DC, National Academy Press, 1999.

Bracken MB, Shepard MJ, Collins WF, et al: A randomized, controlled trial of methylprednisolone or naloxone in the treatment of acute spinal-cord injury. Results of the Second National Acute Spinal Cord Injury Study. *N Engl J Med* 322:1405, 1990.

Dalal SA, Burgess AR, Siegel JH, et al: Pelvic fracture in multiple trauma: classification by mechanism is key to pattern of organ injury, resuscitative requirements, and outcome. *J Trauma* 29:981, 1989.

Fry WR, Smith RS, Sayers DV, et al: The success of duplex ultrasonographic scanning in diagnosis of extremity vascular proximity trauma. *Arch Surg* 128:1368, 1993.

Healey MA, Simons RK, Winchell RJ, et al: A prospective evaluation of abdominal ultrasound in blunt trauma: is it useful? *J Trauma* 40:875, 1996.

Illig KA, Swierzewski MJ, Feliciano DV, et al: A rational screening and treatment strategy based on the electrocardiogram alone for suspected cardiac contusion. *Am J Surg* 162:537, 1991.

Jennett B, Teasdale G, Braakman R, et al: Prognosis of patients with severe head injury. *Neurosurgery* 4: 283, 1979.

Mackay M: Kinematics of vehicle crashes, in Maull KI (eds): *Advances in Trauma.* Chicago, Year Book, 1987, p 21.

Maier RV: Shock, in Greenfield LJ, Mulholland MW, Oldham KT, et al (eds): *Surgery: Scientific Principles and Practice.* Philadelphia, Lippincott-Raven, 1997, p 182.

Meyer DM, Jessen ME, Grayburn PA: Use of echocardiography to detect occult cardiac injury after penetrating thoracic trauma: a prospective study. *J Trauma* 39:902, 1995.

Mirvis SE, Shanmuganathan K, Miller BH, et al: Traumatic aortic injury: diagnosis with contrast-enhanced thoracic CT—five-year experience at a major trauma center. *Radiology* 200:413, 1996.

Root H, Houser C, McKinley C: Diagnostic peritoneal lavage. *Surgery* 57:633, 1965.

Shires GT, Coln D, Carrico J, et al: Fluid therapy in hemorrhagic shock. *Arch Surg* 88:688, 1964.

Shires GT, Cunningham JN, Backer CR, et al: Alterations in cellular membrane function during hemorrhagic shock in primates. *Ann Surg* 176:288, 1972.

Vassar MJ, Fischer RP, O'Brien PE, et al: A multicenter trial for resuscitation of injured patients with 7.5% sodium chloride. The effect of added dextran 70. The Multicenter Group for the Study of Hypertonic Saline in Trauma Patients. *Arch Surg* 128:1003, 1993.

Wiggers CJ: The failure of transfusions in irreversible hemorrhagic shock. *Am J Physiol* 144:91, 1945.

Wilberger JE: Diagnosis and management of spinal cord trauma. *J Neurotrauma* 8(suppl 1):S21,1991.

Winn RK, Mihelicic D, Vedder NB, et al: Monoclonal antibodies to leukocyte and endothelial adhesion molecules attenuate

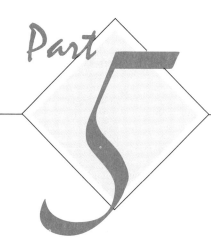

The Skin and Subcutaneous Tissues

Jimmy Y. Chung

Cutaneous and Subcutaneous Abscesses

Introduction

An abscess is a pathologic cavity filled with cellular and tissue debris, white blood cells, bacteria, and fluid, which forms as a result of an infectious process. An abscess can form within a body cavity (e.g., intra-abdominal, intracranial, or intrathoracic), an organ (e.g., liver, spleen, or lung), a joint space (e.g., septic joint), or a soft-tissue space (e.g., subcutaneous, intramuscular, or subfascial). This chapter will address the latter category only—soft-tissue abscess—as the other types of abscesses typically require specialized treatments. This chapter will focus particularly on common, soft-tissue abscesses and related problems that can be managed on-site by primary-care clinicians, as well as identify situations and complications that usually require referral to or consultation with a surgeon.

Pathophysiology

The content of an abscess forms a semiliquid substance, called pus, when the by-products of the host reaction against an infection accumulate, or when a previously existing sterile fluid collection (e.g., sebum in a sebaceous cyst, blood in a hematoma, etc.) becomes infected by a microorganism.

The body's defense mechanism isolates the infectious process by forming a fibrous wall around the pus—thus creating the abscess cavity. There is no blood flow into the cavity, and for this reason it is impossible to attain adequate levels of antibiotics in the abscess. Therefore, except for small cutaneous abscesses that sometimes rupture spontaneously, treatment always involves opening and draining the abscess cavity, rather than antibiotic therapy alone.

An abscess left unchecked can spread along tissue planes to cause necrotizing fasciitis or myonecrosis or can serve as the source of systemic infection and sepsis. Such progression in arms or legs can result in loss of a limb. Hematologic spread can seed distant organs to form intraparenchymal abscesses or can seed heart valves (usually the tricuspid valve) to cause endocarditis.

Microbiology

By far the most common pathogen responsible for cutaneous abscesses is *Staphylococcus aureus. S. aureus* binds to inflamed tissue and produces a catalase enzyme that protects the organism from hydrogen peroxide produced by neutrophils. It also produces a coagulase that can bind and activate fibrinogen, leading to formation of a fibrous wall that forms the boundary of the abscess cavity.

Various species of streptococcus are also found in cutaneous abscesses. Gram-negative rods such as *E. coli*, Klebsiella, Proteus, or Pseudomonas species cause incisional-wound abscesses after bowel surgery and cutaneous abscesses in hospitalized patients. Some abscesses contain multiple organisms, including anaerobic bacteria; mixed and anaerobic flora are especially common in abscesses that occur in immunocompromised individuals. Rare causes of abscesses include mycobacterium, fungal infections, parasites, and insects. Viruses do not cause abscesses.

Typical Presentation

Abscesses can present in any place in the body, and they are often given special names based on their anatomic location or pathophysiology. Various common types of cutaneous and subcutaneous abscesses are listed below, along with comments about their presentation, anatomy and etiology, and some brief remarks about treatment. Regardless of the anatomy or physiology involved in abscess formation, however, the end lesion—an abscess—is essentially the same, as is the basic approach to treatment—opening and draining the abscess.

Sometimes, patients present with significant induration and pain indicating cellulitis, but there is no evidence of an abscess and the patient is not febrile. For such patients, treatment with warm compresses and oral antibiotics can be administered until either the cellulitis improves or a true abscess develops that can be treated as described later in this chapter.

Furuncle

A furuncle is a cutaneous abscess of the skin glands and hair follicles that often begins as a folliculitis. Furuncles are frequently called "boils," and they most often occur in skin folds and areas afflicted by acne. When a local collection or group of enlarged furuncles appears on the back of the neck, it is called a carbuncle. Carbuncles are most common in men over the age of 40. Simple furuncles and carbuncles can be managed by incision and drainage under local anesthesia, but large or complex lesions may require extensive debridement and should be treated by a surgeon in the operating room under general anesthesia.

Sebaceous Cyst

Sebaceous cysts are subcutaneous collections of trapped skin debris and secretions that are surrounded by an epithelial sac. They can appear on any non–weight-bearing surface of the body—commonly on the back—and are usually filled with a white cheesy material. Patients may report a history of recurring sebaceous cysts that temporarily resolve after squeezing the cheesy contents out through a small opening in the surface of the cyst.

Definitive treatment involves complete excision of the epithelial sac, rather than expression of the cyst's contents, because sebaceous cysts usually recur unless the epithelial sac is removed. Sebaceous cysts may or may not be infected on presentation. If infected, they should be treated initially like any other abscess with incision and drainage; removal of the epithelial sac can be performed at a later date when the inflammation has subsided.

Pilonidal Cyst/Abscess

An abscess that appears in the gluteal cleft is called a pilonidal cyst; if there is a midline external opening with drainage, it is called a pilonidal sinus (Fig. 14-1). These lesions are not true cysts, however, but chronic granulomas.

The etiology of pilonidal cysts has been a subject of controversy, but they most likely are acquired lesions that arise from an infection of the hair follicles in the midline of the sacrococcygeal region. They occur most commonly in young hirsute patients, and the abscesses may contain an ingrown hair at their base, which serves as a nidus for chronic infection.

Figure 14-1

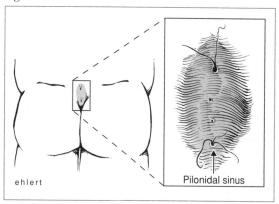

Pilonidal abscess. Pilonidal abscess occurs at the superior end of the gluteal cleft in the lower back. Hair may be protruding from the skin overlying the abscess.

Patients can present with an acutely inflamed abscess or a chronic draining sinus. Although the treatment for a chronic sinus can be complex and often requires surgical consultation, an acute abscess can be initially treated with incision and drainage like other abscesses, with subsequent surgical referral for definitive treatment. Postsurgical management includes meticulous hygiene and shaving of hair around the lesion.

Perirectal Abscess

Perirectal abscesses are thought to arise from obstruction of anal ducts. The predilection for obstruction of these ducts appears to be multifactorial, and various theories have been suggested to explain the genesis of perirectal abscesses, including congenital defects, androgen excess, and chronic constipation. There is a 3:1 ratio of men to women and a higher incidence in the fourth, fifth, and sixth decades of life. Certain individuals are at greater risk of developing a peri-

rectal abscess, including institutionalized elderly patients, patients with developmental delay, patients with spinal-cord injuries, and chronic opiate users. Patients with Crohn's disease are also at risk for perirectal abscesses; the abscesses typically result from fistulae between the ileum, colon, or rectum and the perirectal area.

There are four types of perirectal abscesses based on the specific anatomic location: perianal, ischiorectal, intersphincteric, and supralevator (Fig. 14-2). It is of note that the terms "perirectal" and "perianal" are sometimes used interchangeably, although erroneously, to describe any abscess in the rectal area; perianal abscess is simply one type of perirectal abscess.

In the majority of cases, an abscess in the anorectal region requires surgical consultation, because the pathophysiology of perirectal abscesses and the anatomy of the anal sphincter are complex, and mismanagement can lead to complications such as incontinence; chronic drainage; open, nonhealing wounds; strictures; and chronic pain. As a general rule, therefore, any abscess in

Figure 14-2

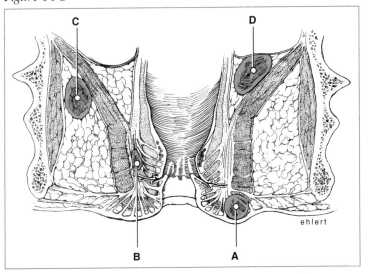

Perirectal abscesses. The figure shows the anatomic location of the four types of perirectal abscesses: perianal (**A**), interspincteric (**B**), ischiorectal (**C**), and supralevator (**D**).

proximity to the anus is an indication for surgical consultation. Of the four types of perirectal abscess, the only one that may be treated under local anesthesia in an office setting is the perianal abscess, which is a small lesion that forms superficial to the external sphincters. Other forms of perirectal abscess are almost always associated with a fistula-in-ano, and proper treatment includes a thorough examination under anesthesia, which is usually undertaken in the operating room.

Patients who have a perirectal abscess will typically present with an exquisitely painful mass around the anus. They often cannot tolerate a digital rectal examination without analgesia and sedation. The presence of a tender mass around the anus confirms the diagnosis, although deep abscesses may not be visible or even palpable, depending on their location. Dramatic relief of pain is often seen after removal of the pus under tension. Immediate incision of the abscess for temporary symptomatic relief is appropriate, followed by a surgical consultation on the same day. If the patient is febrile or ill, admission to the hospital for antibiotic therapy and immediate surgical consultation are indicated.

All perirectal abscesses should be drained at the time of diagnosis and never treated with antibiotics alone, because undrained perirectal abscesses can quickly extend into the deep tissues and cause necrotizing fasciitis or Fournier's gangrene. When draining perianal abscesses, the incision should be made on the anal side of the abscess to avoid a longer incision that might interfere with subsequent fistulotomy.

Finally, thrombosed external hemorrhoids are often mistaken for a perianal abscess. The management of hemorrhoids is discussed in Chapter 6.

Hidradenitis Suppurativa

Hidradenitis suppurativa is an extensive skin infection involving multiple apocrine sweat glands, often connected by complex sinus tracts. The condition always occurs after puberty and involves areas of the body in which apocrine glands are abundant—that is, the axilla, groin, and perineum.

Patients typically present with widespread, chronically draining lesions that have multiple openings. Small lesions can be treated with local wound care and occasional antibiotics and minimal debridement, and most will resolve in time, leaving scar tissue. Topical clindamycin, oral isotretinoin, and oral steroids may also be helpful in healing mild cases; CO_2 laser excision has recently been popularized as an alternative treatment. Surgical excision, however, is still considered definitive treatment and many experts advocate early surgical excision. Extensive disease may require wide debridement of the involved tissue. The resulting wound sometimes cannot be closed primarily and requires a skin graft or tissue flap.

Paronychia and Eponychia

An abscess that arises along the lateral edges of a fingernail or toenail is called a paronychia. Causes include hangnails and nail biting. An abscess that forms at the base of the nail is called an eponychia. Treatment involves incision and drainage and may require local elevation or excision of the nail from the nail bed (Fig. 14-3).

Figure 14-3

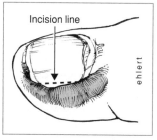

Drainage of a paronychia. Drainage of a paronychia usually involves elevation, and often removal, of a section of the nail adjacent to the abscess.

Figure 14-4

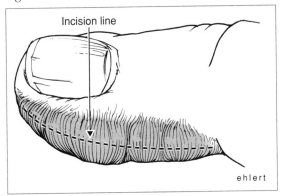

Incision and drainage of a felon. Note that the incision is made into the lateral aspect of the finger to avoid creating a scar on the highly sensitive fingertip pad.

Felon

An abscess that forms in the distal pulp of the finger is called a felon. The pulp area is divided into many small compartments by fibrous septae, so infection in this area usually does not form a single discreet abscess cavity. Incision and drainage of a felon is achieved with an incision along the lateral aspect of the fingertip to avoid scarring on the sensory pads (Fig. 14-4).

It is worth noting that hand infections can be deceptively more extensive than they appear, and complications can be disastrous. Thus, intravenous antibiotics and brief hospitalization is usually advised for anything more than a simple distal-pulp infection. Early surgical consultation should always be considered.

Surgical-Wound Abscess

Recent surgical incisions are at risk for developing infections, especially those resulting from contaminated or dirty procedures such as an operation for perforated appendicitis. Wound infections commonly occur 4 to 7 days after the procedure, but can also appear weeks to months later, occasionally resulting from retained suture material.

Devascularized fat in the subcutaneous space can become necrotic and infected, forming an abscess. Extension of the infection into the deeper fascia can cause dehiscence of the wound and further spread into deeper tissues. In the case of abdominal incisions, this process can result in wound dehiscence and evisceration, peritonitis, or incisional hernias. Therefore, wound infections should be treated like abscesses and drained by opening the incision over the inflamed area, and the integrity of the fascia should be examined.

Drug Injection Abscess

Abscesses in users of intravenous drugs are caused by injection of contaminated material into a vein, subcutaneous space ("skin popping"), or deep muscle tissue ("muscling"). The prevalence of these abscesses is higher in urban areas, but their prevalence is increasing in nonurban areas, parallel to the increased use of illicit drugs in nonurban communities.

The severity of abscesses in drug users is often exacerbated by the compromised immune system frequently found in these individuals and by injection of vasoconstrictive drugs that can cause tissue necrosis, which facilitates development of infection. The injected drugs are also frequently mixed with foreign materials that can elicit an intense inflammatory response. For example, abscesses are sometimes filled with a black necrotic material from injection of "black tar" heroin.

Abscesses in drug users are often multiple and deeper than they appear on the surface, and patients invariably have a low pain tolerance from chronic narcotic use. Therefore, local anesthesia may be inadequate for incision and drainage, and it may be necessary to treat these patients under monitored conscious sedation or general anesthesia. In addition, extreme care should be used in exploring these wounds because of the occasional presence of a broken needle within the abscess; one should always use instruments rather than fingers. A plain radiograph may be useful for detecting foreign objects in these abscesses.

When drug abuse–related abscesses are accompanied by fever, blood cultures should be drawn. If the cultures are positive, or if the patient has a heart murmur, the patient may have bacterial endocarditis. Appropriate screening for endocarditis (transthoracic or transesophageal echocardiography) should then be undertaken, and antibiotics should be administered as appropriate.

Necrotizing Fasciitis

Necrotizing fasciitis is a life-threatening bacterial infection that tracks along the fascia, causing extensive necrosis of the soft tissues and sometimes myonecrosis. Depending on the microbe involved, there may not be any pus produced. A variation of necrotizing fasciitis that develops in the perineum and scrotal area is called Fournier's gangrene.

Necrotizing fasciitis and Fournier's gangrene are difficult to diagnose because they usually do not exhibit cutaneous manifestations until the necrosis has progressed to the point of causing skin ischemia and or even death. Thus, a high level of suspicion must be maintained, especially when caring for patients at high risk for necrotizing fasciitis (diabetic, immunocompromised, or institutionalized individuals), or when a patient has severe pain, swelling, neurologic changes, unexpected systemic toxicity, or an unusually high leukocytosis, out of proportion to any visible infection.

Patients known or suspected to have necrotizing fasciitis should be seen immediately by a surgeon. Treatment includes antibiotics and wide debridement of affected tissue performed on an emergency basis, with scheduled reexploration of the infected area at a later date. Treatment failure and death are usually caused by inadequate debridement or delay in diagnosis.

Key History and Physical Examination

Patients with abscesses usually present with a warm, red, tender mass that demonstrates the hallmark signs of inflammation—heat (calor), red-ness (rubor), pain (dolor), and swelling (tumor). The mass may exhibit fluctuance on palpation, but lack of fluctuance does not rule out an abscess. A history of local trauma or insect bites may be present in a patient with a simple subcutaneous abscess, but most patients do not recall any precipitating events.

On the other hand, several risk factors should alert the clinician to the possibility that an abscess may be deeper, larger, or more serious than anticipated based on history and examination alone. As discussed earlier, patients with a history of intravenous drug use often have abscesses that are more extensive than they initially appear because of deep-tissue inflammation and necrosis. A history of diabetes mellitus should alert the clinician to potentially more extensive infections and a greater spectrum of causative microbes. Immunocompromising conditions such as infection with the human immunodeficiency virus (HIV) are also risk factors for serious skin abscesses.

A high level of suspicion for an abscess should also be present when examining febrile patients who have undergone recent surgery or invasive procedures. Any surgical skin incision that is red, fluctuant, or tender is likely to be infected and may already harbor an abscess. Tunneled access catheters (e.g., Hickman central lines, dialysis catheters, ventriculoperitoneal shunts) are common sites of abscesses that must be treated by incision and drainage and removal of the catheter. Epidural catheters and percutaneous endoscopic gastrostomy (PEG) tubes have also been reported to be sites of cutaneous abscesses. However, redness and yellow discharge around a PEG or feeding jejunostomy tube are common and, while frequently mistaken for signs of infection, are usually just chronic irritation.

For some patients, a cutaneous abscess can be a sign of a systemic disease. Systemic fungal infections such as aspergillosis, nocardia, or disseminated cryptococcosis in immunocompromised individuals (such as transplant or HIV-infected patients) may first present with cutaneous abscesses. An abscess on the chest wall may be a sign of empyema necessitatis, an encapsulated empyema discharging through the chest wall into the subcutaneous tissues; this is now rarely reported, but still occurs occasionally.

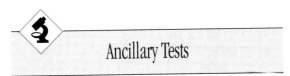

Ancillary Tests

Diagnosis and treatment of most cutaneous abscesses do not require any laboratory or imaging studies. In more serious infections, leukocytosis can be a good indicator of the extent of the infection, and, if present, antibiotics are usually indicated. Patients who are febrile should have blood cultures drawn and should be treated with antibiotics. Plain radiographs may help locate suspected foreign bodies or detect the presence of gas in the tissues if deep anaerobic infections are suspected.

If a fluctuant mass is not readily apparent on physical examination because of swelling or obesity, ultrasonography can be useful in locating deep fluid collections. If the presence of pus is not obvious, aspiration to determine if pus is present can be attempted using an 18-gauge needle on a syringe.

Gram stain and cultures of the abscess contents are unnecessary because the results will not change management plans—all abscesses require drainage regardless of the specific organism involved. Thus, routine cultures of abscess fluid incur additional costs to the patient without providing any useful clinical information.

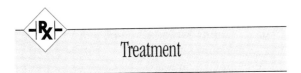

Treatment

Surgical Therapy

Incision and drainage (I & D) of the abscess cavity is the only treatment necessary in the majority of cases. The key concept is *adequate* drainage, and often a larger incision than initially expected

Figure 14-5

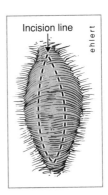

Elliptical incision for abscess drainage. It is essential to provide adequate drainage of the abscess cavity. This illustration demonstrates creation of an elliptical excision, rather than a simple incision, to ensure that the wound edges do not close until the abscess is adequately drained.

is necessary. Many clinicians make the mistake of simply aspirating or lancing the abscess, which is almost always an inadequate treatment. Adequate drainage can be obtained by creating a wide, elliptical incision such that the edges will not come together (Fig. 14-5), or by keeping the incision open with a wick of iodinated gauze or similar material.

EQUIPMENT

All the required equipment should be collected and arranged prior to beginning the procedure. Table 14-1 lists the suggested material necessary for a simple I & D.

Although the I & D procedure is inherently "dirty," it is good practice to observe sterile technique whenever possible to avoid introducing further contamination into the surgical field. If available, an assistant can be helpful in gathering the materials, administering systemic analgesics, and reassuring the patient. If sedation with a benzodiazepine is necessary for a very anxious patient, then, at minimum, pulse oxymetry and frequent blood pressure monitoring are recommended, with supplemental oxygen available to administer if oxygen desaturation is noted.

PREPARATION

Informed consent should be obtained, and documentation of informed consent should be part of the medical record. The patient should be warned that, although local anesthetic will be used, complete pain relief is generally not possible. The patient should be appropriately disrobed and gowned in a private procedure area and placed in a lying-down position in case of a syncopal event. Towels and absorbent pads should be placed under the patient. The skin should be cleansed widely with alcohol, iodine, or chlorhexadine and then draped.

ANESTHESIA

One-percent lidocaine has a fast onset, lasts 1 to 2 hours, and is suitable for I & D of most cutaneous and subcutaneous abscesses. The addition of epinephrine causes local vasoconstriction, which can help with hemostasis and lengthens the analgesic effect by slowing the removal of lidocaine by local-tissue blood flow. Epinephrine

Table 14-1

Material Necessary for Simple Incision and Drainage of a Cutaneous Abscess

Towels and absorbent pads
Alcohol/betadine swabs
Local anesthetic (e.g., Lidocaine 1%)
10-cc syringe, 18-gauge and 25-gauge needles
#11 or #15 scalpel
Sterile gloves
2 × 2 and 4 × 4 gauze pads
Packing material (gauze pads, or strips if the
   abscess is small)
Mosquito clamp
Scissors
Forceps
Irrigation fluid (e.g., bag of saline) with
   intravenous tubing
Basin

should not be used, however, in appendages (e.g., digits, nose, ears, penis) because of the risk of inducing ischemia.

Lidocaine is acidic in its injectable form, and the burning sensation associated with its injection may be partially alleviated with the addition of sodium bicarbonate into the mixture. In general, however, plain 1% lidocaine, without bicarbonate buffering, is adequate for all-purpose use.

If a longer anesthetic effect is desired, 0.25% bipuvicaine, which has a slower onset but a longer half-life, can be mixed 1:1 with the lidocaine. Caution should be used with bipuvicaine because, like lidocaine, if it is injected into the circulation in large doses, it can cause cardiac toxicity.

The anesthetic agent should be injected subdermally, directly over the most fluctuant point (or if fluctuance is unclear, the most tender point) of the abscess. Injection directly into the abscess cavity is ineffective and can exacerbate discomfort by increasing the intracavitary pressure. A nerve block may be appropriate in certain areas such as digits.

Despite all this, complete analgesia is usually not possible, and systemic narcotic administration may be helpful. "Freezing" the skin with ethyl chloride spray prior to incision is an option if additional anesthesia is required or if the patient is allergic to lidocaine.

PROCEDURE

A single, linear incision should be made along the longest axis of the abscess over the most fluctuant or tender area (see Fig. 14-5). The length of the incision depends on the size of the abscess and its location, but usually should be the length of the abscess cavity. Some clinicians prefer a cruciate incision, but this is unnecessary and can create disfiguring scars. In cosmetically sensitive areas (e.g., the face), a small slit into the abscess with a narrow gauze packing may be adequate.

When draining a large abscess, a basin can be used to collect the draining pus. If pus does not appear, it is usually because the incision is too shallow. Once the incision is made, a mosquito clamp can be used to explore into the abscess or "pop" through the abscess cavity wall if the incision is not deep enough.

Abscesses are usually loculated or contain multiple tracts that need to be opened up to create one large cavity that will drain adequately. This can be achieved by exploring the cavity with a clamp, a gauze sponge, or sweeping motion of a finger to ensure that all loculated areas have been opened. Exploration of the abscess cavity is usually the most painful part of the I & D procedure, but should not be omitted. As noted earlier, the examiner's finger should not be used to explore drug-injection abscesses because of the possible presence of a broken needle within the abscess cavity.

The resulting cavity should then be irrigated with sterile saline to remove all pus and dead tissue. While many clinicians perform this irrigation with a syringe and needle, an easier way to do this is to hang a liter bag of saline in a pressure device and irrigate the wound with intravenous tubing attached to the bag. If bleeding occurs, it will almost always stop with the application of gauze using manual pressure.

The cavity should be packed with gauze or a surgical drain, depending on the size of the wound. The wound should then be dressed with gauze and the dressing changed as often as needed. Frequent outer dressing changes should be anticipated since the wound will ooze for some time after the procedure. The packing should be changed the next day by the clinician and every day afterward by the patient until there is no further drainage from the abscess cavity.

The patient should be allowed to shower or bathe with the packing removed and let the water wash out the wound; the wound should then be repacked with gauze. Packing the wound with a moist, coarse gauze and allowing it to dry to the surface of the cavity before removing it will result in progressive debridement of bacterial overgrowth and cellular debris with each dressing change. Moistening the gauze prior to removal will defeat this purpose.

Nonsurgical Therapy

While I & D is adequate treatment for most simple abscesses, nonsurgical therapies are needed in some situations. If there is surrounding cellulitis or if the patient is febrile, or for facial and hand abscesses, antibiotics are indicated. Dicloxacillin (500 mg orally every 6 hours) or cephalexin (500 mg orally every 6 hours) are typically the first-choice antibiotics. If the patient has a penicillin allergy, erythromycin (500 mg orally every 6 hours) is an acceptable alternative.

If a patient is febrile or the cellulitis is extensive, the patient should be admitted to a hospital and treated with intravenous antibiotics. In most cases, immunocompromised patients or patients with prosthetic heart valves should also be treated empirically with intravenous antibiotics.

Finally, all patients with abscesses resulting from drug injection or a traumatic skin penetration should be given appropriate tetanus prophylaxis. Depending on the patient's immunization status, prophylaxis may require tetanus toxoid and tetanus immune globulin.

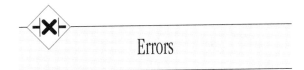

Errors

Inadequate Drainage

The most common error in the treatment of cutaneous abscesses is failure to achieve adequate drainage. Very often, the clinician will only lance or aspirate the abscess, which fails to drain the abscess cavity and frequently results in recurrence. Opening the entire abscess and removing all infected material will more likely result in complete resolution. An alternative for abscesses in areas where a large incision is undesirable (e.g., face and breast) is packing the cavity with narrow gauze through a small incision and leaving a wick of gauze protruding through the skin to prevent skin apposition.

Similarly, clinicians will sometimes treat an abscess with antibiotics alone, thereby failing to establish drainage of the abscess cavity. As noted, failure to drain an abscess increases the risk that the infection will spread from the abscess cavity to adjacent tissue planes and spaces. The increasing prevalence of antibiotic-resistant bacteria may make this scenario more likely, making antibiotic therapy without abscess drainage increasingly risky for patients.

Misjudging Severity

Misjudging the severity of the infection can lead to delayed or inadequate treatment and possibly death. Patients with a history of intravenous drug injection, diabetes, neutropenia, HIV infection, or an organ transplant should be monitored more carefully than usual. The potential for sepsis or necrotizing fasciitis should always be in mind when treating patients with any of these underlying conditions.

Rapidly progressing infections in otherwise normal patients should also raise concern about the possibility of a serious or complicated infection, and such patients should be considered for admission to a hospital. All patients presenting with an unusual history should be thoroughly examined for secondary abscesses.

Misdiagnosis

Another common but potentially disastrous mistake is misdiagnosis of another lesion as an abscess (Table 14-2). Many fluctuant masses are not abscesses, are not infected, and do not require drainage unless symptomatic. Examples are seromas, hematomas, lymphocoeles, and hydrocoeles. Contamination of masses through inappropriate incisions or aspiration can convert such masses into abscesses or other serious infection.

A tender mass in the groin or on the abdominal wall is likely to be a hernia, and needle aspiration should never be attempted on such a mass. A pulsatile mass anywhere, especially in the groin, popliteal fossa, axilla, antecubital fossa, or neck, should be considered a true or pseudoaneurysm until proven otherwise, as incision or aspiration of such lesions can cause life-threatening hemorrhage. An ultrasound duplex study and vascular surgery consultation should be obtained to help clarify the nature of such a mass. It is of note that nonpulsatile masses in these regions can also be aneurysms that may have thrombosed, and such masses should also undergo a duplex ultrasound examination.

Lymphadenopathy, benign or malignant tumors, bursitis, and cysts can also be mistaken for abscesses. Drainage and fluctuance in an abdominal incision from recent surgery may represent an infection, but these are also signs of fascial dehiscence. Such lesions should never be opened without surgical consultation because of the risk of evisceration and peritonitis.

Technical Complications

Certain areas of the body such as the face, neck, hands, joints, and anorectal region pose complex anatomic challenges to inexperienced clinicians. Incision and drainage of abscesses in these areas

Table 14-2

Common Lesions that Can be Mistaken for a Cutaneous Abscess

Abdominal wound dehiscence
Aneurysm
Benign or malignant tumor or cyst
Bursitis
Hematoma
Hydrocele
Inguinal or abdominal hernia
Lymph node
Lymphocele
Seroma

can result in poor cosmetic outcomes, failure to appropriately drain the abscess, and/or damage to nearby anatomic structures. Surgical consultation or referral should be obtained in such cases to increase the likelihood of a satisfactory outcome.

References

Callahan TE, Schecter WP, Horn JK: Necrotizing soft tissue infection masquerading as cutaneous abscess following illicit drug injection. *Arch Surg* 133:812, 7, 1998.

Connolly B, Johnstone F, Gerlinger T, et al: Methicillin-resistant *Staphylococcus aureus* in a finger felon. *J Hand Surg [Am]* 25:173, 2000.

Cook PA, Wilgis EF: Infections of the hand, in Cameron JL (ed): *Current Surgical Therapy*, 6th ed. New York, Mosby, 1998.

Dellinger EP: Surgical infection, in Sabiston D (ed): *Textbook of Surgery: The Biological Basis of Modern Surgical Practice*, 15th ed. New York, WB Saunders, 1998.

Frieden I: Infections and infestations, in Rudolph AM (ed): *Rudolphs's Pediatrics*, 20th ed. Stamford, CT, Appleton & Lange, 1996.

Friedland GH, Selwyn PA: Infections in injection drug users, in *Harrison's Principles of Internal Medicine*, 14th ed. New York, McGraw-Hill, 1998.

Hunt T, Mueller R: Inflammation, infection and antibiotics, in Way L (ed): *Current Surgical Diagnosis and Treatment*, 10th ed. Norwalk, CT, Appleton & Lange, 1994.

Keighley MRB: Anorectal disorders, in Nyhus L (ed): *Mastery of Surgery*, 3rd ed. New York, Little, Brown, 1997.

Knighton D, Locksley R, Mills J: Emergency procedures, in Saunders C (ed): *Current Emergency Diagnosis and Treatment*, 4th ed. Norwalk, CT, Appleton & Lange, 1992.

Spijkerman IJ, van Ameijden EJ, Mientjes GH, et al: Human immunodeficiency virus infection and other risk factors for skin abscesses and endocarditis among injection drug users. *J Clin Epid* 49:1149, 1996.

F. Frank Isik

Skin Lesions

Introduction

Accurate diagnosis of cutaneous and subcutaneous lesions can be challenging even for experienced dermatologists. Whereas most skin lesions are benign and can often be diagnosed by history and physical examination alone, diagnosing pigmented cutaneous lesions and subcutaneous masses can be difficult.

The purposes of this chapter are to present an approach to diagnosis and biopsy of the most common malignant skin lesions and to review several common benign skin lesions that can be confused with or precursors to those malignant lesions. This chapter cannot substitute for a dermatology text that describes the myriad of benign and malignant skin lesions, nor is this chapter a manual on reconstructive surgery following excision of large skin lesions. Rather, the intention is to provide a general approach to diagnosis and biopsy of common skin lesions and subcutaneous masses that a clinician in general practice might encounter.

Pathophysiology

The pathophysiology of most skin cancers is related to ultraviolet radiation–induced changes in the cellular biochemistry and ultrastructure of the skin. Skin malignancies generally arise in areas of heavy sun exposure, especially the head, neck, and extremities. Skin malignancy is more likely when individuals are fair skinned (poor tanning ability) and have significant vocational and recreational sun-exposure history. Additional predisposing conditions include radiation exposure, arsenic exposure, and immunosuppression.

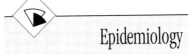

Epidemiology

Human worship of the sun is ancient. Solar mythology placed the sun at the center of religion and myth, and Sunday was designated as a day to worship the sun. The relationship between Apollo, the Greek god of the sun, and his son Aesculapius, god of medicine, provides evidence of the magnitude of the early belief that the sun had healing powers. The purported health benefits of the sun were further acknowledged in 1903, when Finsen was awarded the Nobel Prize in medicine for the treatment of infectious diseases with light radiation. This led to the Ecole au Soleil ("School of the Sun"), established in the Swiss Alps in 1910, to treat tuberculosis, anemia, chronic renal failure, syphilis, and septic wounds.

Worship of the sun was also embraced by the masses. Whereas 18th century Europeans coveted "porcelain paleness," by the early 20th century, tanning became associated with health and beauty. The resultant increase in sun exposure, coupled with the increased longevity of humans, has led to a rapid increase in the incidence of malignant skin lesions. Indeed, Coco Chanel's early 20th century dictum that the "1929 girl must be tanned" has done more to influence modern dermatologic epidemiology than she ever would have known.

Basal Cell Carcinoma

Between 1995 and 1997, there was an average of more than 500,000 new cases of skin cancer annually in the United States, with basal cell carcinoma representing 65% to 80% of these cases. Basal cell cancers arise from pluripotential cells residing in the basal layer of the epidermis. Whereas these tumors exhibit a wide variety of biologic behaviors, they are usually slow-growing lesions that have been present for many years with minimal risk (~0.05%) of metastases.

Squamous Cell Carcinoma

Squamous cell cancer is the second most common type of skin malignancy, with 100,000 new cases diagnosed each year. Squamous cell cancers arise from epidermal keratinocytes in areas of sun-damaged skin that are commonly referred to as actinic keratosis. Unlike basal cell carcinoma, squamous cell cancers grow more rapidly and can metastasize to local lymph nodes in up to 3% of cases.

Malignant Melanoma

The third most common skin malignancy is malignant melanoma, a potentially lethal neoplasm of neural crest–derived cells. The incidence of malignant melanoma has increased from 1:1500 persons in 1935 to 1:87 persons in 1996, and the mortality rate has increased by 2% annually in recent years. It was estimated in 1998 that there were over 40,000 new invasive cases and 50,000 new in situ melanomas in the United States.

Like squamous cell carcinoma, malignant melanoma tends to grow rapidly and metastasize to the lymphatic system. In contrast to squamous cell carcinoma, the rate of metastases, including distant metastases, is high in malignant melanoma. Early diagnosis can lead to a curative resection, but deep penetration with metastases is often incurable. Despite increased public awareness and a trend toward earlier detection, malignant melanoma is now the 5th leading cause of cancer deaths in the United States.

Benign Skin Lesions

There are a myriad of benign skin lesions, both pigmented and nonpigmented, some of which can be confused with skin cancers, and some of which can be easily distinguished from them. Several of the more common benign skin lesions are discussed in the following sections of this chapter.

Typical Presentation

Benign Nonpigmented Skin Lesions

The most common benign nonpigmented lesions arise from cells in the epidermis, including the epidermal appendages. A diagnostic characteristic of most benign nonpigmented lesions is that they have been present for many years and have changed little in nature.

Notable exceptions to the long-standing presence and slow growth of benign nonpigmented lesions are actinic keratoses and keratoacanthomas. Actinic keratoses are thought to represent premalignant changes induced by ultraviolet radiation. They are characterized by erythematous and often scaly appearing patches in sun-exposed areas.

Keratoacanthomas are rapidly growing lesions that mimic the growth rate and appearance of cutaneous squamous cell carcinoma. Though these lesions may spontaneously regress in a matter of weeks, the rapid growth warrants early removal to avoid missing a rapidly growing malignancy. Keratoacanthomas are generally regarded as nonpigmented lesions, but they can be pigmented at their center.

Benign Pigmented Lesions

Perhaps the major significance of benign pigmented lesions is that they can be confused with malignant melanoma. Indeed, as a general rule, any pigmented skin lesion, especially on an individual with significant sun exposure history, should raise suspicion that the lesion may be a melanoma rather than a benign pigmented lesion.

NEVI

A benign pigmented lesion with uniform color and smooth borders that appears on the skin between birth and 20 years of age is typically

Table 15-1

Benign Pigmented Lesions

TYPE OF LESION	CHARACTERISTICS
Junctional nevus	Flat, uniform color; pale to dark brown; sharply defined
Compound nevus	Darker surface may be smooth or rough; may have hair
Intradermal nevus	Raised, pale papule that distorts overlying normal skin; most without hair follicles
Blue nevus	Blue-black lump <5 mm in diameter; do not change in size with time
Spitz nevus	Usually in children: smooth dome-shaped red lesion <6 mm; rapid growth
Simple lentigo	Common brown-to-black mole; clinically indistinguishable from junctional nevi
Solar lentigo	Lighter tan lesion (a.k.a. "liver spot")
Seborrheic keratoses	Warty surface with "stuck-on" appearance
Pyogenic granuloma	Raised, painless, with surrounding inflammation

referred to as a nevus or mole. There are many types of nevi, more than the common kinds listed in Table 15-1.

DYSPLASTIC NEVI

Occasionally, a nevus that has been present for many years will acquire variegated colors, increase in size, and develop irregular borders, all of which suggest malignant change, but a biopsy does not show malignant melanoma. This clinical situation describes a type of degeneration called dysplastic nevi, which are considered potentially premalignant (Fig. 15-1). Some patients have large numbers of dysplastic nevi and may also have family members who are similarly affected—the so-called

Figure 15-1

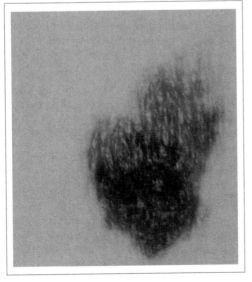

Dysplastic nevus. The lesion, which can be a precursor to malignant melanoma, has irregular borders and variegated color. (See also color plates.) *(Reproduced by permission from Fitzpatrick TB, et al:* Color Atlas and Synopsis of Clinical Dermatology: Common and Serious Diseases, *4th ed. New York, McGraw-Hill, 2001.)*

familial "dysplastic nevus syndrome," in which the lifetime probability of developing malignant melanoma is extraordinarily high.

Among individuals who do not have the familial dysplastic nevus syndrome, most dysplastic nevi never become malignant. Nonetheless, they warrant close observation and a biopsy if further change occurs in the lesion. It is always better to take a cautious approach and perform a biopsy than to provide a patient with blind reassurance, only to discover later that the lesion was indeed a malignant melanoma.

LENTIGO

In contrast to nevi, a lentigo is a pigmented macular skin lesion that develops in the later years of life after decades of sun exposure. Lentigo are the benign, flat, round brown "liver spots" commonly seen on the dorsum of the hands and on the head and neck. Occasionally, lentigo develop features of a suspicious pigmented lesion and can develop in to a lentigo maligna, also known as a Hutchinson's freckle. Lentigo maligna can arise on the cheeks of older individuals and represents a premalignant change and should be approached as such.

SEBORRHEIC KERATOSIS

Seborrheic keratosis is a benign and easily diagnosed condition seen in older individuals—especially those with a significant sun-exposure history. They appear as "stuck-on" scaly or greasy lesions. They are slow growing and need treatment or removal only for cosmetic reasons or if there is uncertainty about whether or not the lesion is, in fact, a seborrheic keratosis.

Malignant Nonpigmented Lesions

Most skin cancers fall in this category, with the vast majority being basal cell carcinomas of the superficial-spreading (Fig. 15-2A,B) or nodular type (Fig. 15-2C). These appear as slightly reddened, flat or raised lesions. The nodular variant has "pearly" borders and may have a "rodent ulcer" in the middle. The morpheaform, or sclerosing, variant has ill-defined borders and can be very aggressive, with a propensity for invasiveness and local recurrence after removal. Its key features include serpiginous margins with a flat, erythematous surface (Fig. 15-2D).

Squamous cell carcinoma of the skin often has features that distinguish it from basal cell carcinoma, but sometimes the two are confused. Squamous cell carcinomas have ill-defined borders and can appear scarlike with heaped-up edges or, more commonly, as a shallow ulcer with heaped-up edges (Fig. 15-3).

Malignant Pigmented Lesions

Table 15-2 presents a summary of some of the more common pigmented malignant skin lesions. Of these, malignant melanoma is the most important.

Diagnosis of melanoma can be facilitated by using the "ABCD" acronym, where the letters stand for Asymmetry, Border irregularity, Color variegation, and Diameter >6 mm (the diameter of a lead-pencil eraser) (Fig. 15-4). The surface of the lesion is unpredictable and may be flat, raised, or ulcerated.

When there is any possibility that a lesion is a melanoma, or if a pigmented lesion cannot be diagnosed with certainty as benign, it is essential that a biopsy be performed. Biopsy is a rapid and relatively simple procedure that can take less than 15 minutes and provides diagnostic and prognostic information. If the biopsy shows the lesion to be malignant, appropriate therapy can be instituted. If the biopsy shows it to be a dysplastic nevus, continued close observation of that patient is imperative.

Because the treatment and prognosis of melanoma depends on the depth of penetration (Breslow classification of <1 mm, 1–4 mm, or >4 mm), it is important that a biopsy of at least 4 mm depth be done every time, regardless of the level of suspicion that a lesion is malignant. Techniques for performing skin biopsies are discussed later.

Figure 15-2

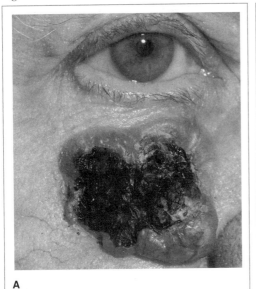

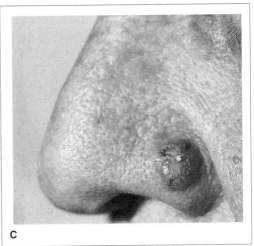

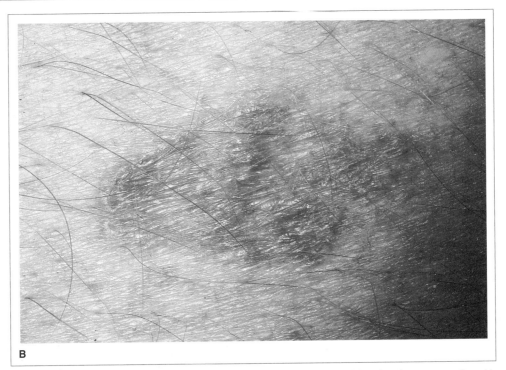

A,B. Basal cell carcinoma, superficial spreading type. The lesion is slightly reddened and may appear flat with a central ulcer **(A)** or pigmented **(B)**. **C.** Basal cell carcinoma, nodular type. The lesion appears as a firm nodule with telangiectasias. (See also color plates.) (*Reproduced by permission from Fitzpatrick TB, et al: Color Atlas and Synopsis of Clinical Dermatology: Common and Serious Diseases. 4th ed. New York: McGraw-Hill, 2001.*)

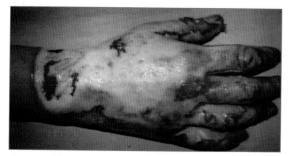

Plate 1 (Figure 9–1) Full-thickness burn Typical full-thickness burn with a white, dry appearance.

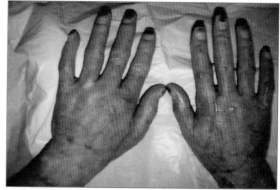

Plate 2 (Figure 9–2) Skin graft on full-thickness burn This figure shows the final outcome of a full-thickness burn treated with a skin graft. Both the cosmetic and functional results are good.

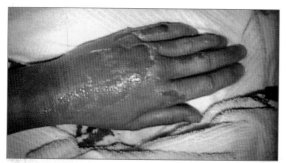

Plate 3 (Figure 9–3) Superficial partial-thickness burn The burned skin is moist and homogeneously pink and will blanch on application of pressure.

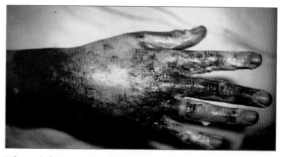

Plate 4 (Figure 9–4) Deep partial-thickness burn The burned area is a mixture of pale skin and a bright-red reticular pattern that does not blanch on pressure.

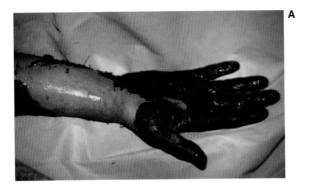

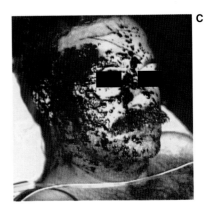

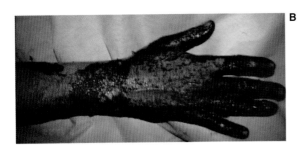

Plate 5 (Figure 9–5A,B,C) Asphalt burn Photo illustrates typical asphalt burn on **(A)** palmar surface of hand, **(B)** dorsum of hand, and **(C)** face. Note the sticky appearance of the asphalt, which is difficult to remove from the skin.

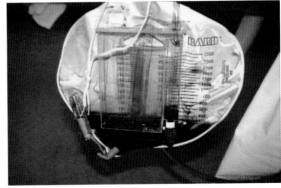

Plate 6 (Figure 9–6) Myoglobinuria Note the dark, reddish-brown color of the urine in the collection bag. This color is typical of myoglobinuria.

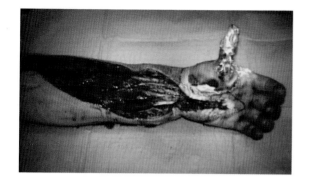

Plate 7 (Figure 9–7) Fasciotomy This patient has undergone fasciotomy and carpal tunnel release following swelling that occurred as a result of an electrical injury.

A

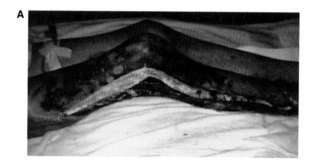

B

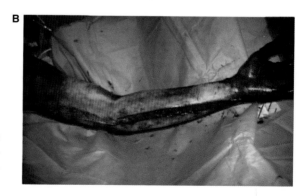

Plate 8 (Figure 9–8) Escharotomy Escharotomy is most often required in circumferential full-thickness burns of the extremities, shown here on the **(A)** leg and **(B)** arm.

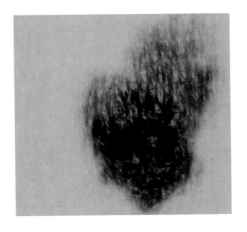

Plate 9 (Figure 15–1) Dysplastic nevus
The lesion, which can be a precursor to malignant melanoma, has irregular borders and variegated color. *(Reproduced by permission from Fitzpatrick TB, et al:* Color Atlas and Synopsis of Clinical Dermatology: Common and Serious Diseases, *4th ed. New York, McGraw-Hill, 2001.)*

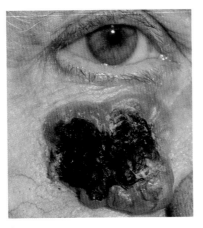

Plate 10 (Figure 15–2) Basal cell carcinoma, superficial spreading type. The lesion is slightly reddened and may appear flat with a central ulcer (**A**) or pigmented (**B**). *(Reproduced by permission from Fitzpatrick TB, et al:* Color Atlas and Synopsis of Clinical Dermatology: Common and Serious Diseases, *4th ed. New York, McGraw-Hill, 2001.)*

A

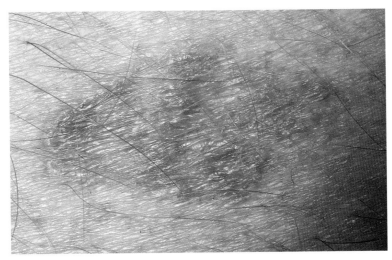

B

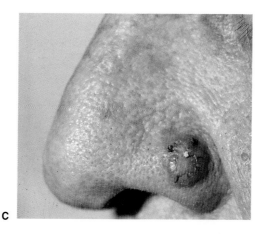

C

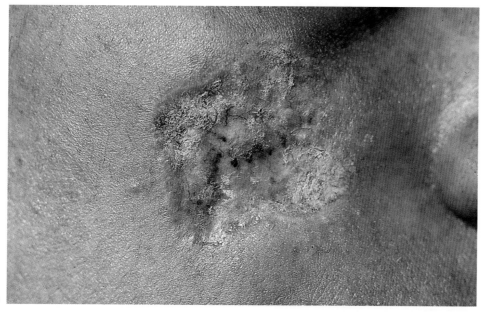

D

Plate 10 (Figure 15–2 Continued) **C.** Basal cell carcinoma, nodular type. The lesions appears
as a firm nodule with telangiectasias. **D.** Basal cell carcinoma, morpheaform variant. Key features
of this lesions are its ill-defined serpiginous margins and a flat, erythematous surface. *(Reproduced
by permission from Fitzpatrick TB, et al:* Color Atlas and Synopsis of Clinical Dermatology: Common and Serious Diseases, *4th ed. New York, McGraw-Hill, 2001.)*

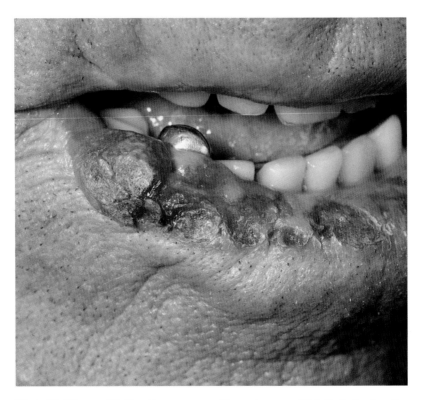

Plate 11 (Figure 15–3)   Squamous cell carcinoma   This lip lesion has the typical characteristic of a squamous cell carcinoma—an elevated ulcerating nodule. *(Reproduced by permission from Fitzpatrick TB, et al:* Color Atlas and Synopsis of Clinical Dermatology: Common and Serious Diseases, *4th ed. New York, McGraw-Hill, 2001.)*

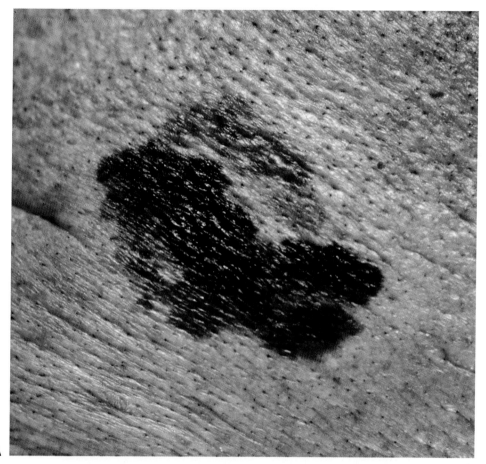

A

Plate 12 (Figure 15–4)   Malignant melanoma   The lesions are often asymmetric and have irregular borders and variegated color. **A.** Lentigo maligna melanoma growing inside a large lentigo maligna often seen in elderly patients. As in this case, these lesions often appear on the cheek. *(Reproduced by permission from Fitzpatrick TB, et al:* Color Atlas and Synopsis of Clinical Dermatology: Common and Serious Diseases, *3rd ed. New York, McGraw-Hill, 1997.)*

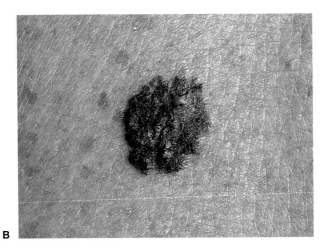

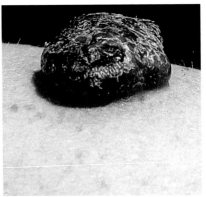

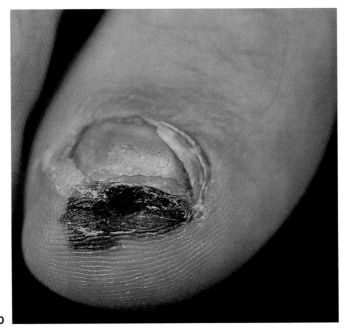

Plate 12 (Figure 15–4 Continued) **B.** Superficial spreading type, displaying the common findings of asymmetry, irregular borders, and variegated color. In this case, the melanoma (the darker, right portion of the lesion) developed in a dysplastic nevus (left portion of the lesion). **C.** Nodular melanoma, a red and black, round tumor with a markedly vertical growth potential. **D.** Acral lentiginous melanoma, showing the characteristic involvement of nail bed and skin, with variegated colors and asymmetry. The lesion often appears macular, with lateral growth. *(Reproduced by permission from Fitzpatrick TB, et al:* Color Atlas and Synopsis of Clinical Dermatology: Common and Serious Diseases, *3rd ed. New York, McGraw-Hill, 1997.)*

Figure 15-2 (continued)

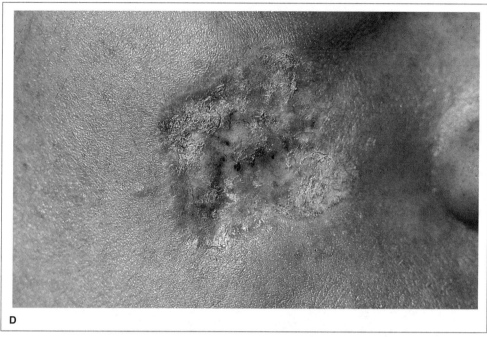

D. Basal cell carcinoma, morpheaform variant. Key features are ill-defined serpiginous margins and a flat, erythematous surface. (See also color plates.) *(Reproduced by permission from: Fitzpatrick TB, et al:* Color Atlas and Synopsis of Clinical Dermatology: Common and Serious Diseases, *4th ed. New York, McGraw-Hill, 2001.)*

Subcutaneous Lesions

The vast majority of subcutaneous lesions are benign. When removal of such lesions is performed, it is generally because of either cosmetic considerations or diagnostic uncertainty. The most common benign subcutaneous skin lesions are listed in Table 15-3.

Malignant subcutaneous masses, on the other hand, are rare and beyond the scope of this book. However, rapid growth, fixation, and pain in a dermatomal distribution are red flags suggesting

Table 15-2

Malignant and Premalignant Pigmented Skin Lesions

TYPE OF LESION	CHARACTERISTICS
Pigmented basal cell carcinoma	Common; may have a surrounding ring of smaller nodules
Pigmented squamous cell carcinoma	Rare
Dysplastic nevus	Intermediate between junctional nevus and melanoma in situ; wide variations in shape, color, and margins; usually >6 mm
Lentigo maligna	Hutchinson's freckle or senile freckle
Melanoma in situ	Continuum from dysplastic nevi to melanoma in situ

Figure 15-3

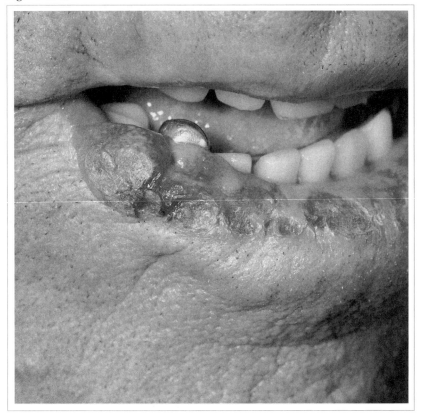

Squamous cell carcinoma. This lip lesion has the typical characteristic of a squamous cell carcinoma—an elevated ulcerating nodule. (See also color plates.) *(Reproduced by permission from: Fitzpatrick TB, et al: Color Atlas and Synopsis of Clinical Dermatology: Common and Serious Diseases, 4th ed. New York, McGraw-Hill, 2001.)*

Table 15-3
Subcutaneous Masses

TYPE OF LESION	CHARACTERISTICS
Lipomas	Soft, rubbery feel
Pilar cysts	Occur on the scalp
Epidermal inclusion cysts	Common in hands
Dermoid cysts	Common on the back
Ganglion cysts	Over joints or flexor tendon sheaths
Sebaceous cysts	Most common in head and neck; have a punctum
Neurolemmoma	Common along digital nerves

that a subcutaneous lesion may be malignant, and, in such cases, tissue diagnosis is essential.

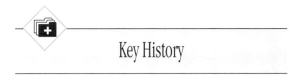

Key History

With cutaneous lesions, important points in the history are overall exposure to ultraviolet radiation, the onset of the lesion, and the rate of growth. Recent onset or rapid growth of a lesion in an individual with a significant history of sun expo-

Figure 15-4

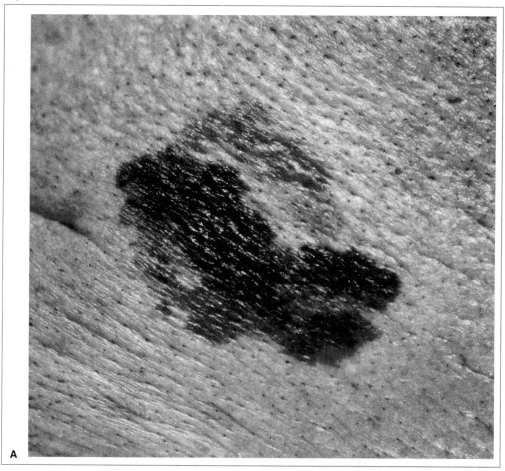

Malignant melanoma. The lesions are often asymmetric and have irregular borders and variegated color.
A. Lentigo maligna melanoma growing inside a large lentigo maligna often seen in elderly patients. As in this case, these lesions often appear on the cheek. (See also color plates.) (*Reproduced by permission from Fitzpatrick TB, et al: Color Atlas and Synopsis of Clinical Dermatology: Common and Serious Diseases. 3rd ed. New York: McGraw-Hill, 1997.*)

sure suggests the possibility of malignancy. Additional risk factors for cutaneous malignancy include chemical exposure (e.g., arsenic) or immunosuppressive medication (e.g., transplant patients). Finally, a family history of skin malignancy may indicate the presence of a familial syndrome, some of which are rare (e.g., basal cell nevus syndrome), and some of which are relatively common (e.g., dysplastic nevus syndrome).

When dealing with subcutaneous lesions, clinicians can be assured that the vast majority are benign. These lumps commonly have been present for many years, cause few symptoms, and patients usually seek care either for cosmetic reasons or because something has caused them anxiety about the possibility of skin cancer. Nonetheless, history can be useful in identifying subcutaneous lesions. Prior history of trauma in the region suggests an

Figure 15-4 (continued)

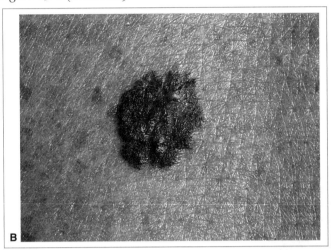

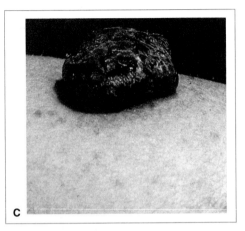

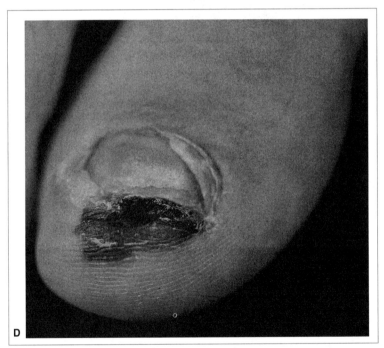

Malignant melanoma (*continued*). **B.** Superficial spreading type, displaying the common findings of asymmetry, irregular borders, and variegated color. In this case, the melanoma (the darker, right portion of the lesion) developed in a dysplastic nevus (left portion of the lesion). **C.** Nodular melanoma, a red and black, round tumor with a markedly vertical growth potential. **D.** Acral lentiginous melanoma, showing the characteristic involvement of nail bed and skin, with variegated colors and asymmetry. The lesion often appears macular, with lateral growth. (See also color plates.) *(Reproduced by permission from: Fitzpatrick TB, et al: Color Atlas and Synopsis of Clinical Dermatology: Common and Serious Diseases, 3rd ed. New York, McGraw-Hill, 1997.)*

epidermal inclusion cyst; secretion of sebaceous (cheeselike) material is typical of a sebaceous cyst; and a history of initial rapid growth followed by a long period of slow growth of a soft, mobile mass suggests a lipoma.

Key Physical Examination

Physical examination of patients with cutaneous and subcutaneous lesions should focus on the several characteristics of the lesions. The most important of these characteristics are location, color, texture, and mobility.

Location

Most skin lesions, both benign and malignant ones, occur in areas of heavy sun exposure; the face, shoulders, extremities, and back are the more common locations. Thus, location is not often a diagnostic characteristic of skin lesions.

For subcutaneous lesions, however, location is often very helpful in diagnosis because some subcutaneous lesions have characteristic locations. Common examples include ganglion cyst on the dorsum of the wrist, lipomas on the back, and epidermal inclusion cysts on the scalp.

Color

When a skin lesion is pigmented, consideration should always be given to malignant melanoma. Benign lesions, however, generally have uniform coloration with smooth borders, whereas multicolored lesions, especially those with irregular borders, signal the possibility of malignancy.

Clinicians should also keep in mind that, whereas pigmentation characterizes melanoma, basal cell and squamous cell carcinomas are occasion-

ally pigmented too. Conversely, lack of color does not rule out melanoma, since metastatic malignant melanoma may lose pigmentation, becoming an amelanotic melanoma.

Texture

A "stuck-on" appearance, characterized by grapelike or warty features, generally indicates a benign lesion. In contrast, a central ulcer in a raised nodular lesion suggests either a nodular basal cell carcinoma or a nodular melanoma.

Mobility

Mobility is not generally helpful for skin lesions, but it is an important characteristic to consider when evaluating subcutaneous lesions. Fixation of a subcutaneous mass to deeper structures and involvement of deeper structures such as vessels or nerves suggests malignancy, and such characteristics must be determined prior to biopsy by using imaging techniques such as computerized tomography or magnetic resonance imaging. This is essential to avoid injury to vital structures during excision of the lesion.

If malignancy is at all suspected, a full physical examination—including a complete skin survey— is mandatory. Meticulous palpation of the regional nodal basin near the lesion, assessing for presence, size, and mobility of lymph nodes, must be part of the examination.

Ancillary Tests

Other than biopsy, which is discussed in more detail below, ancillary studies rarely contribute to the diagnosis of cutaneous or subcutaneous masses. If a biopsy is positive for melanoma, screening for metastatic disease includes a chest x-ray and liver function tests. Routine use of computerized tomography (CT) scans, magnetic resonance imaging, and/or radionuclide scans is unjustified in the absence of history and physical examination evidence of metastatic disease. In fact, history and physical with the above-mentioned labs are more accurate than CT scanning for detecting metastatic malignant melanoma.

Treatment

This section of the chapter will review several techniques for biopsy and removal of skin lesions. However, removal is by no means the only treatment option for benign skin lesions or even for some malignant ones. Therefore, this section will begin with a brief overview of nonsurgical methods for treating several common skin lesions.

Nonsurgical Methods of Treatment

ABLATIVE THERAPIES

Ablative therapies, including cryotherapy and electrodessication and curettage are effective for many benign lesions. However, use of ablative therapy without obtaining any tissue for diagnosis demands extreme confidence in the diagnosis, and these modalities are virtually never appropriate for treatment of nevi.

Ablative modalities injure the lesion from outside to inside, without the ability to assess the depth of tissue involvement. Thus, if a malignant lesion is treated with an ablative modality, viable cancer cells deep in the skin may survive, proliferate, and metastasize, while the superficial surgical wound heals, masking the true growth of the deeper lesion. Although this happens rarely, it is an important consideration for any skin lesion being treated with ablation. A safe approach is to

restrict nonsurgical therapy such as cryotherapy to clearly benign lesions that can be easily diagnosed such as seborrheic keratoses, warts, and some actinic keratoses. Any suspicious skin lesion, or lesion that cannot be identified with certainty, should be biopsied using one of the simple surgical methods discussed later.

CHEMICAL AND RADIATION THERAPIES

Premalignant lesions such as widespread regions of actinic keratoses can often be treated with topical 5-fluorouracil creams. Results are good, and this therapy is better tolerated than cryotherapy for large numbers of skin lesions.

For patients with biopsy-proven basal cell carcinoma, radiotherapy offers a reasonable alternative to surgical excision, especially in technically challenging areas such as the tip of the nose. Fractionated radiotherapy is also being investigated as a treatment modality for malignant melanoma. Moh's chemosurgery is also a reasonable option for some nonmelanoma skin cancers that are not amenable to surgical excision. However, these treatment options first require an accurate diagnosis, which is usually made by a biopsy.

Surgical Methods for Biopsy and Excision

SHAVE BIOPSY

Most authorities feel that shave biopsy should be used only for seborrheic keratosis and then only if the diagnosis is 100% certain. The major reasons for not using shave biopsies in other situations are that shave biopsies (1) destroy tissue architecture, making histologic diagnosis difficult; (2) have inadequate depth to remove the entire lesion—an important consideration if the lesion proves to be malignant; and (3) with melanomas, any chance for accurate staging and treatment is eliminated. In addition, at least one recent study found that shave biopsies are only about 80% sensitive for diagnosis of basal cell carcinoma in comparison with excisional biopsy. For most cutaneous lesions, therefore, any of the other biopsy techniques is superior to shave biopsy.

PUNCH BIOPSY

Sterile, single-use punch biopsy instruments are inexpensive and are easy to use, even for the novice. For non–surgically inclined clinicians, this is the method of choice for skin biopsies.

Punch biopsies come in several sizes that reflect the diameter of the "punch," from 2 to 8 mm. A sharp blade defines the circumference of the instrument and allows a core of tissue to be easily removed. In general, a 4-mm or larger biopsy punch should be used, as smaller instruments do not usually provide adequate tissue for a diagnostic specimen. One can often remove the whole lesion with a 4 to 8-mm punch.

Informed consent precedes a punch biopsy, as it should any excisional or incisional procedure.

Then, after sterilization of the field with povidone-iodine solution, local anesthetic is infiltrated as a field block in four quadrants around the lesion. One-percent lidocaine with 1:100,000 epinephrine provides ideal hemostasis anywhere except the digits or tip of the penis, where lidocaine without epinephrine should be used instead. As a general rule, always wait 7 to 8 minutes prior to any incision to maximize epinephrine's vasoconstrictive effect.

The punch should be placed over the entire lesion or over the most concerning area of a larger lesion. With gentle downward pressure and repeating clockwise-counterclockwise rotation of the instrument, the blade will incise the skin and a tissue core will be created (Fig. 15-5). For all punch-biopsied lesions, it is vital to go at least 4 mm deep into the subcutaneous tissue. This ensures that if the lesion proves to be a melanoma, a biopsy of adequate depth will have been obtained. To gauge

Figure 15-5

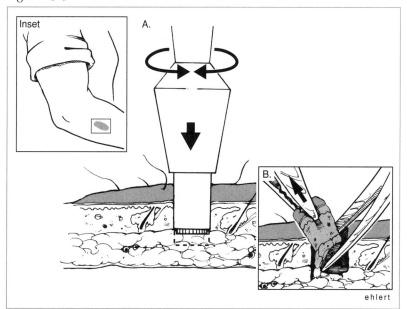

Punch biopsy. In **A**, the punch biopsy is obtained by applying gentle but firm pressure and repeating clockwise-counterclockwise rotations of the punch biopsy instrument. It is essential that the biopsy specimen be at least 4 mm deep. After the punch-biopsy instrument creates a core of tissue, the core is pulled upward with a forceps while the base is transected with a scalpel or scissor, as shown in **B**.

the depth of the biopsy, one simply removes the instrument and examines the depth of tissue that has been cored out. If deeper penetration is required, the instrument can be replaced over the core of tissue, and a deeper punch can be completed. Entering the subcutaneous fat for all lesions ensures a full-thickness biopsy of appropriate depth.

After removal of the instrument, a forceps is used for traction on the core of tissue while the base of the tissue is transected with a scalpel blade or scissors. Bleeding can be easily stopped with firm pressure using moistened gauze for 5 minutes. If bleeding does not respond to pressure, Monsel's (ferric subsulfate) solution, an electrocautery unit, or a handheld battery operated ophthalmic cautery will provide hemostasis. If necessary, the defect can be closed with one or two simple 4-0 or 5-0 nylon stitches across the defect.

Most tissue removed with a punch biopsy can be submitted to the pathology department in formalin. However, some pathologists prefer to receive suspicious pigmented lesions fresh, wrapped in saline moistened gauze.

The punch method is a good choice for most skin lesions, but is not generally useful for subcutaneous masses such as lipomas or cysts. In addition, anatomically sensitive areas such as eyelids should not be treated with deep punch biopsies; these are better suited to surgical excisions with a scalpel.

EXCISIONAL BIOPSY

An excisional biopsy provides the most complete diagnosis, and if the lesion is benign, the technique results in complete removal and treatment of the lesion. Excisional biopsy also provides definitive therapeutic resection for basal cell and squamous cell carcinomas, provided the margins of resection are negative for tumor (2-mm margins for basal cell, and 5-mm margins for squamous cell).

The technique of excisional biopsy requires that the resulting cutaneous defect can be closed primarily. A simple check to see if primary closure is feasible is to pinch the skin on either side of the lesion and determine how much tension is required to approximate two normal skin edges. If the tension required is minimal, an excisional biopsy is feasible. Informed consent is again essential.

MARKING THE LESION   With good lighting and a fine-tipped, nonerasable marker, a series of dots 2 to 3 mm around the perimeter of the lesion forms a useful boundary that can be connected to form a smooth line. The shape of the excision must be elliptical if suitable closure is to be achieved. If an irregularly shaped incision is created, it must be converted to a smooth ellipse that will close as a straight line. The ellipse should be oriented with the maximum width centered over the maximum width of the lesion. Generally speaking, the ellipse should be oriented perpendicular to the direction with the most cutaneous laxity, as this will result in the easiest closure (Fig. 15-6).

LOCAL ANESTHETIC   Only after skin markings are satisfactory should the field be prepped with povidone solution and should the local anesthetic (1% lidocaine with 1:100,000 epinephrine— except for digits) be administered, since the epinephrine will blur the margins between lesion and normal skin. It is important to wait for the epinephrine's hemostatic effect, because inadequate vasoconstriction can cause in a bloody incision and poor exposure, with the result being injury to underlying nerves or vessels.

THE INCISION   The scalpel (#15 blade) is held like a pencil between the thumb and index finger, as the opposite hand is used to apply firm, spreading pressure on opposing sides of the incision (Fig. 15-6). Spreading the wound makes it easier to determine how deep the incision is.

Once the circumferential incision is down to subcutaneous fat, the specimen is elevated with a forceps and the base severed using full-length strokes of the scalpel, at a uniform depth. Immediately after removal, place a stitch at an easily identifiable site on the lesion to be submitted (e.g., 12 o'clock) to mark the orientation of the lesion relative to the patient. The pathology request should clearly indicate how the marking

Figure 15-6

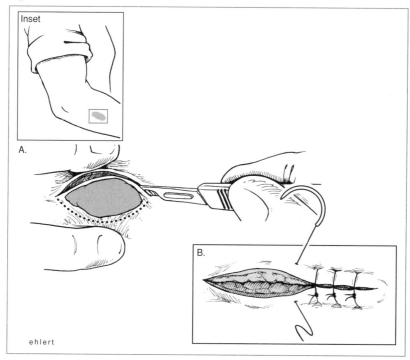

Excisional biopsy. The ellipse of the incision should be oriented with the maximum width centered around the maximum width of the lesion. Application of spreading pressure on opposite sides of the incision, as shown in **A**, will make it easier to monitor the depth of the incision. In **B**, the ellipse created during the excisional biopsy is closed with standard suturing techniques. Closure will be easiest if the ellipse of the incision is oriented perpendicular to the direction of the skin with the most cutaneous laxity *(inset)*.

stitch on the specimen is oriented. If a malignant lesion has positive margins, the pathologist can identify which margins are positive (e.g., 3 o'clock), which will facilitate identification of areas that require reexcision.

After the specimen is removed from the field, the base of the wound should be closely examined to verify that the lesion has been completely removed. Going down to the subcutaneous fat ensures that a full-thickness excision has been done.

The wound can be closed with 4-0 or 5-0 nylon simple stitches. Steri-Strips are then placed transversely across the wound to lessen the tension across the wound and stitches. Benzoin or Mastisol can be applied around the perimeter of the wound to facilitate adhesion of Steri-Strips to the skin.

INCISIONAL BIOPSY

Incisional biopsy is useful for larger lesions that, if completely excised, would require an incision that would be difficult to close. Whereas the setup and technical aspects are identical to those for excisional biopsy, an incisional biopsy is localized over part of the lesion and removes only a sample of the lesion—not the whole thing.

An ellipse is drawn around the area to be sampled. Under sterile conditions, a full-thickness skin and subcutaneous fat sample is removed as described above. It is important to include a margin of normal skin and subcutaneous tissue so that the pathologist can accurately orient the specimen and identify the pathology. If the lesion turns out to be malignant, referral to a surgeon is recommended for more complete resection and soft-tissue reconstruction.

A punch biopsy can often be a simpler and more acceptable alternative to incisional biopsy. Two or three punch biopsies over a single large lesion can provide the same information with less time, effort, and cosmetic defects than an incisional biopsy.

SUBCUTANEOUS BIOPSY/EXCISION

The following technique is for biopsy/excision of a subcutaneous mass that is suspected to be benign such as a lipoma or sebaceous cyst. If the history or physical examination suggests a malignant lesion such as liposarcoma or other sarcoma, this biopsy method should not be used. Instead, a deep punch biopsy in a thin individual, or a limited skin incision over the mass followed by a direct punch biopsy of the subcutaneous mass in more obese individuals, is appropriate. Shelling out a sarcoma, as described below for a cystic lesion, is inappropriate as it results in spread of tumor cells throughout the surgical field.

The biopsy technique for benign subcutaneous lesions involves an incision through the skin and removal of the lesion through the incision. Significant amounts of skin need not be removed, other than the need to remove the punctum present over a sebaceous cyst. Failure to remove the punctum of a sebaceous cyst can lead to recurrence of the lesion.

LOCAL ANESTHETIC   After prepping the site with povidone solution, local anesthetic (1% lidocaine with 1:100,000 epinephrine) should be infiltrated around the entire subcutaneous mass. This can be done effectively by infiltrating the area where the skin incision will be made and then all four quadrants, down to the depth of the lesion. As always, waiting for the lidocaine and epinephrine to take effect will facilitate the procedure.

THE INCISION   An incision slightly longer than the mass is made directly over it (Fig. 15-7). Using a skin hook on one side, the skin is lifted upward while curved scissors are used to spread the skin and cut around the mass, in essence "shelling" the mass out of its bed in the subcutaneous tissue. Once the benign mass has been freed laterally of normal skin and fat, the mass is picked upward with forceps, and the bottom is freed using combined blunt and sharp dissection. The specimen should be marked with a stitch to orient the specimen in the unlikely event that it is malignant.

After hemostasis is achieved with firm pressure or electrocautery, the skin can be closed in one or two layers. The two-layered closure using a deep, absorbable suture results in better scars since the stitches in the dermis reduce the tension on the epidermis. Benzoin and Steri-Strips should be applied after wound closure.

Postoperative Care

Patients who have undergone a skin biopsy should not shower or get the incision wet for 48 hours after the procedure. They should be instructed about signs of infection and how to apply pressure if the wound site continues to "ooze" blood. In 7 days (10 to 14 days on the back and extremities), sutures are removed, and benzoin and Steri-Strips are reapplied.

Complications

The usual complications following any surgical procedure are applicable to skin biopsy and excision. These include infection, bleeding, and wide or hypertrophic scars. Inadequate excision and/or recurrence of lesions may occur, which might necessitate repeat excision or biopsy. Therefore, it is important to inform patients about the possibility of recurrence. In particular, even adequately excised lipomas and cysts often recur. In the case of suspected malignant lesions, in which a biopsy is performed primarily for diagnosis, patients should understand preoperatively that they may need further surgery to remove the lesion entirely or to create wider margins around the lesion.

Figure 15-7

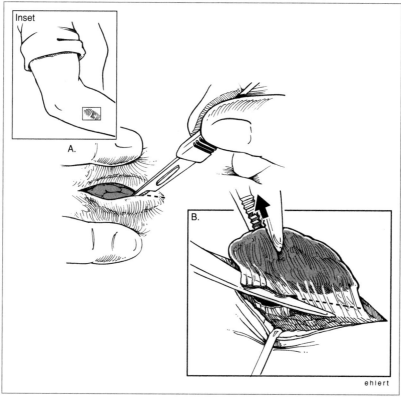

Exicison of a subcutaneous lesion. The subcutaneous mass is shelled out from its bed
(A), after which it is elevated with a forceps and freed from its bed **(B)**.

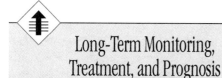

Long-Term Monitoring, Treatment, and Prognosis

By the time the patient returns for suture removal, the pathology report should be available, and discussion with the patient about the diagnosis, prognosis, and long-term plans should begin. The patient should be educated to monitor areas where malignancies were removed to detect recurrence early.

All patients with dysplastic nevi, previous skin malignancies, or extensive sun-exposure history should be followed every 6 months to 1 year. It is reasonable to photograph lesions or an entire region to monitor changes in the skin of patients with multiple dysplastic nevi. Polaroid or digital cameras are usually most useful for this purpose.

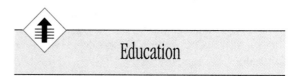

Education

In addition to the postoperative and follow-up instructions mentioned above, education of the patient should include discussion about sun protection. Patients should understand the potential risks of continued exposure to ultraviolet radiation.

Any sunblock with a rated sun protection factor (SPF) of 15 or above will provide reasonable protection, provided that a sufficient quantity of sunblock is used (1 ounce to cover the entire body). Patients using "safe" tanning salons should be warned that the actual safety of these salons is unknown.

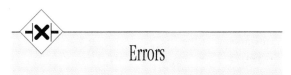

Errors

Clinicians make a variety of errors in the management of skin lesions. Three errors worthy of note are diagnostic errors in evaluating subcutaneous lesions in infants, performance of inadequate skin biopsies, and failure to biopsy pigmented lesions that are not clearly benign.

Subcutaneous Lesions in Infants

A benign-appearing subcutaneous mass in a newborn should not be attributed to a benign cyst or lipoma. Rather, subcutaneous masses in infants may represent a developmental anomaly or tumor.

A midline mass in the head or neck of an infant is especially concerning, because it may represent underlying neural tissue. Such lesions, which commonly present near the root of the nose or between the eyebrows, may represent the frontal lobe of the brain communicating through a defect in the skull (encephalocele). A mass could also be a branchial cleft cyst. A congenital, hairy, pigmented nevus over the thoracolumbar spine may be a clue to an unsuspected underlying myelomeningocele. None of these lesions should be biopsied with the techniques described in this chapter, as penetration of the skin may result in entry into the central nervous system.

Inadequate Biopsy

As discussed, the deep margin is especially important when performing a biopsy of a potentially malignant lesion. It is relatively straightforward to reexcise the lateral skin margins if these are inadequately excised or positive for residual tumor, but it is more difficult to reexcise positive deep margins. Therefore, the biopsy should always be full-thickness, and the deep margin of the excised lesion should always be examined to ensure that it looks grossly normal before closing a wound. Furthermore, if the diagnosis is melanoma, the depth of the original lesion will determine how wide the subsequent reexcision margins must be (1 to 3 cm, depending on melanoma thickness), as well as whether nodal dissection or adjuvant therapy will be necessary. These decisions will depend on the adequacy of the initial biopsy, and, therefore, inadequate biopsy specimens make treatment decisions more difficult.

Failure to Biopsy

It is impossible to overemphasize the importance of obtaining a definitive histologic diagnosis of pigmented skin lesions that are not unequivocally benign. For pigmented nevi, the distinction between benign and malignant lesions can be difficult. In fact, one study found that 3.8% of biopsied pigmented nevi diagnosed clinically by nondermatologists as benign were found to be malignant on histologic examination. The corresponding figure for dermatologists was 1.3%, indicating that clinicians of any specialty can mistake malignant melanoma for a benign pigmented nevus. Thus, the practice of some clinicians of "following" such lesions to see if they change over time exposes patients to the risk of undiagnosed melanoma.

Controversies

Initial reports had suggested that positive margins after excision of a basal cell carcinoma excision could be observed with little chance of recurrence. We now know that the recurrence rate is significantly higher (>60%) when the lateral margin is positive. Therefore, the current recommendation is to reexcise all positive margins of basal cell and squamous cell carcinomas, so those margins contain only normal skin.

Although the necessary margins of resection for basal and squamous cell carcinomas are well accepted, the margins of resection remain controversial for malignant melanoma. The most accepted recommendations are based on the depth of the initial lesion, emphasizing the importance of obtaining a good punch or incisional biopsy. Most melanomas under 1 mm in depth do not need further treatment, whereas deeper lesions may need between 2 and 3 cm of additional margins and, possibly, lymphatic mapping, nodal dissection, and adjuvant treatment. Further research will be needed to determine the ideal margins for excised malignant melanoma.

Emerging Concepts

Radiotherapy is emerging as a possible treatment for basal cell carcinoma and, perhaps, for malignant melanoma. As noted, for patients with biopsy-proven basal cell carcinoma, radiotherapy offers a reasonable alternative to surgical excision in technically challenging areas such as the tip of the nose. Fractionated radiotherapy is being investigated as a primary treatment modality for biopsy proven-malignant melanoma.

References

Ariyan S, Krizek TJ: Radiation effects: biologic and surgical considerations, in: McCarthy JG (eds): *Plastic Surgery,* 1st ed. Philadelphia, WB Saunders, 1990, pp 831–848.

Barksdale SK, O'Connor N, Barnhill R: Prognostic factors for cutaneous squamous cell and basal cell carcinoma. Determinants of risk of recurrence, metastasis, and development of subsequent skin cancers. *Surg Oncol Clin North Am* 6:625–638, 1997.

Cox NH, Aitchison TC, Sirel JM, et al: Scottish Melanoma Group. Comparison between lentigo maligna melanoma and other histogenetic types of malignant melanoma of the head and neck. *Br J Cancer* 73: 940–944, 1996.

Elwood M, Gallagher R: Skin cancer epidemiology in 1996: the Third Symposium on the Epidemiology of Melanoma and Non-melanocytic Skin Cancer. *Melanoma Res* 7:74–77, 1997.

Gloster HM Jr, Brodland DG: The epidemiology of skin cancer. *Dermatol Surg* 22:217–226, 1996.

Harris MN, Shapiro RL, Roses DF: Malignant melanoma. Primary surgical management (excision and node dissection) based on pathology and staging. *Cancer* 75:715–725, 1995.

Kittler H, Seltenheim M, Dawid M, et al: Morphologic changes of pigmented skin lesions: a useful extension of the ABCD rule for dermatoscopy. *Am Acad Dermatol* 40:558–562, 1999.

Pariser RJ: Benign neoplasms of the skin. *Med Clin North Am* 82:1285–1307, 1998.

Raasch BA: Suspicious skin lesions and their management. *Aust Fam Physician* 28:466–471, 1999.

Reeck MC, Chuang TY, Eads TJ, et al: The diagnostic yield in submitting nevi for histologic examination. *J Am Acad Dermatol* 40:567–571, 1999.

Rigel DS: Malignant melanoma: incidence issues and their effect on diagnosis and treatment in the 1990s. *Mayo Clin Proc* 72:367–371, 1997.

Rivers JK, Kopf AW, Vinokur AF, et al: Clinical characteristics of malignant melanomas developing in persons with dysplastic nevi. *Cancer* 65:1232–1236, 1990.

Russell EB, Carrington PR, Smoller BR: Basal cell carcinoma: a comparison of shave biopsy versus punch biopsy techniques in subtype diagnosis. *J Am Acad Dermatol* 41:69–71, 1999.

Mary Laya and
Benjamin O. Anderson

Palpable Breast Lumps

Introduction

There are many misconceptions in the clinical evaluation of breast lumps, the most common of which is the impression that breast cancers are difficult to diagnose. In reality, most cancers are simple to diagnose. An obvious palpable lump on clinical breast examination (CBE) or a spiculated mass on a mammogram generally tells the story. By contrast, it is difficult to demonstrate that an area of concern on physical examination or mammography actually represents normal breast tissue. Because the overarching purpose of evaluating a palpable breast mass or thickening is to identify or rule out breast cancer, when faced with such an abnormality one must decide how many tests to perform to "prove" the absence of cancer.

Unfortunately, there is no test or combination of tests that guarantees the absence of cancer cells somewhere in the breast, because all cancers have a "preclinical" phase before they can be appreciated by CBE, mammography, or other tests. In fact, the sensitivity of CBE is only 54%, and the sensitivity of mammography is about 85%. In addition, while mammography recognizes 85% of cancers, it misses 15% of cancers. Ultrasound also misses the diagnosis of breast cancer, because it generally does not distinguish the clinically significant microcalcifications of ductal carcinoma in situ (DCIS), nor does it image invasive cancers that fail to distort breast architecture. Even when a breast lump is known to be present, a diagnosis of cancer may be missed because diagnostic methods such as fine-needle aspiration (FNA) and core needle biopsy can have sampling error.

In many situations, the clinical uncertainties caused by less-than-perfect diagnostic tests are unavoidable. Partly for this reason, however, the most common reason that physicians in the United States are sued for malpractice is the alleged delay in diagnosis of, or the failure to diagnose, breast cancer. The purpose of this chapter is to provide a general outline on how clinicians can evaluate breast complaints such as breast masses in a minimally invasive fashion, while also minimizing the chances of missing a clinically subtle breast cancer.

Pathophysiology

Anatomy and Development

ANATOMY

The breast is a subcutaneous gland, lying between the fascial planes of the chest-wall muscles and the skin. It is comprised of hormonally responsive glandular/ductal tissue along with connective tissue (stroma) and fat. While masses can potentially arise from all three of these elements, it is the glandular/ductal elements that comprise the masses of greatest clinical significance.

The glandular/ductal network is organized like a tree (Fig. 16-1). This arborized structure consists of large, lactiferous sinuses at the nipple (the tree trunk) that branch into smaller and smaller ducts and ductules (the tree branches). The lobules are the microscopic termini (the leaves), where milk production occurs in the gravid breast. The "terminal ductal-lobular unit," which is a composite tissue of the terminal microscopic ducts and lobules and associated mesenchymal-stromal elements, is the site of most benign and malignant pathologic conditions of the breast.

FETAL DEVELOPMENT

Understanding breast development facilitates an understanding of the various conditions that present as breast lumps. In utero, the fetal mammary parenchyma derives from sweat gland-like tissue, and in the earliest stages of fetal life, mammary development is independent of sex-hormone stimulation. By the fifth week of gestation, the ectodermal "galactic band" or "milk line" has formed, extending from axilla to groin on the embryonic trunk. All but the thoracic portion regresses by

Figure 16-1

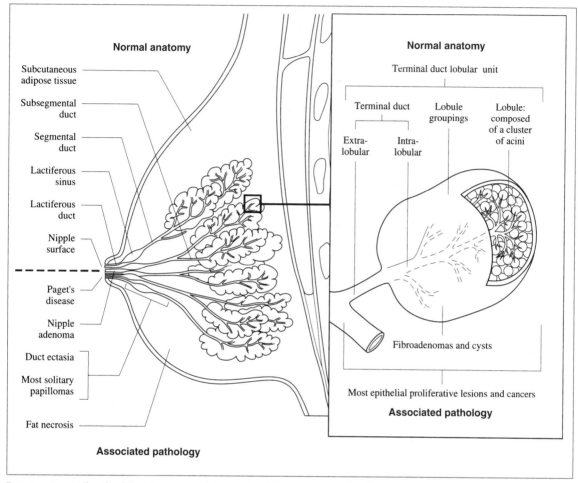

Breast anatomy. The glandular/ductal network is organized like a tree. Large lactiferous sinuses at the nipple (the tree trunk) branch into smaller and smaller ducts and ductules (the tree branches). The lobules are the microscopic terminus (the leaves), where milk production occurs in the gravid breast. The composite tissue of the terminal microscopic ducts and lobules is the site of most benign and malignant pathologic conditions. *(Reproduced from Hayes DF (ed). Atlas of Breast Cancer. St. Louis, Wolfe, 1993, with permission of Harcourt Publishers Limited.)*

apoptosis as development continues. Incomplete regression leads to accessory mammary tissue in 2% to 6% of adult women, most commonly in or near the axilla.

During the last trimester of fetal development, placental sex steroids enter the fetal circulation and stimulate breast-tissue differentiation. Under this hormonal influence, there is progressive development of branching ductules and the lobular alveolar structure in both males and females. At birth, alveoli are enlarged, and there is often detectable secretory activity stimulated by residual placental hormones. After withdrawal of sex hormones and prolactin at birth, involution occurs and the breast tissue enters a resting state until puberty. As might be predicted, therefore, breast cancers prior to puberty are all but impossible.

PUBERTAL DEVELOPMENT

At puberty, ovarian female estrogens initiate breast development by stimulating ductal sprouting and branching. The ductal system is a collection of approximately 20 discrete arborized structures called lobes. Estrogen potentiates an increase in the volume and elasticity of periductal connective tissue and also causes deposition of fat, which together form the substance of the developing adolescent breast. Progesterone promotes differentiation of the "terminal ductal lobular units," which are the microscopic grapelike secretory units with the functional lactational alveolar elements characterizing the mature human female breast.

DEVELOPMENTAL CORRELATES OF DISEASE

There are at least two features of breast development with pathophysiologic significance. First, in utero development is identical in males and females, and during this time rudimentary ducts, but not lobules, form. Because males develop ducts but not lobules, the 1% of breast cancers that occur in males are all ductal carcinomas. Male lobular carcinomas are rare if not impossible; such a diagnosis in a man should be suspected of being incorrect.

Second, the breast is a hormonally responsive tissue from the time of its inception. As a result, estrogens appear to play a permissive if not stimulatory role in breast oncogenesis. Breast tissues undergo dynamic cyclic changes during the course of the menstrual cycle analogous to those occurring in the endometrium. Patients who have uninterrupted estrogenic cycling (e.g., never interrupted for pregnancy) have a slightly increased risk for breast cancer development. Conversely, women who are oophorectomized at a young age and do not receive estrogen replacement will have a decreased chance of developing breast cancer.

Pathology

Palpable breast masses can arise in any of the tissues described above. The most important breast masses in clinical practice are carcinomas and sarcomas. However, a variety of benign breast lesions are also seen, including fibroadenomas, cysts, proliferative epithelial changes ("fibrocystic disease"), hamartomas, and disorders of fat tissue.

MALIGNANT BREAST LESIONS

CARCINOMAS   Invasive ductal carcinoma, ductal carcinoma in situ (DCIS), and invasive lobular carcinoma can all present as a palpable mass. Of these, DCIS is least likely to have a masslike presentation. DCIS is much more likely to present as a mammographic abnormality (cluster or field of microcalcifications), which is why the rate of DCIS diagnosis has increased since the early 1980s when screening mammography came into widespread use. Prior to mammography, DCIS was a rare diagnosis.

In general, breast carcinomas do not grow rapidly. Cancer growth models suggest that a palpable, 1-cm, invasive carcinoma has likely been present for 5 to 8 years. Invasive ductal carcinomas more commonly grow as enlarging, irregularly shaped spheres, with malignant fingers of fibrotic and malignant tissues that appear as starlike spiculations on mammography. Invasive lobular carcinomas can be more clinically subtle than invasive ductal carcinomas, because lobular carcinomas tend to grow in two-dimensional sheets rather than in three-dimensional masses. This can lead to clinically subtle thickenings rather than clinically obvious lumps. The microscopic margins of invasive lobular carcinomas commonly extend beyond the palpable extent of disease appreciated on CBE or during surgical excision.

SARCOMAS   Sarcomas of the breast occur, but are rare. These lesions usually have more in common with soft-tissue sarcomas elsewhere in the body than with breast cancers, per se. There is an increased chance of developing a breast sarcoma following radiation therapy for breast carcinoma, although the rate is still very low (approximately 0.1%). Sarcomas arising from the breast stroma (the supporting connective-tissue elements of the breast) are rare.

A stromal tumor unique to the breast is the "phyllodes tumor" (previously known as "cysto-sarcoma phyllodes"). Phyllodes tumors rarely metastasize, but they can be locally aggressive tumors with high recurrence potential. Thus, they require excision with wide surgical margins.

BENIGN BREAST LESIONS

FIBROADENOMAS Fibroadenomas are psuedoen-capsulated, sharply demarcated masses, which consist of disorganized but benign stromal and epithelial (glandular) elements. Their cause is unknown although they are considered abnor-malities of development.

Some data suggest that fibroadenomas will gradually reabsorb over a period of several years, which is why they are most common among women in their 20s and 30s but are relatively uncommon among women in their 50s and 60s. When diagnosing a fibroadenoma, which presents as a solid mass, it is most important to ensure that the mass is indeed a fibroadenoma and not a malignant breast tumor.

CYSTS Breast cysts arise from the terminal ductal-lobular unit, possibly as a result of ductal obstruction by cellular debris combined with active secretion from acinar cells in the lobule. The actual patho-physiologic origin of breast cysts is unknown, how-ever, with the possible exception that they appear to be potentiated by the presence of estrogen.

Breast cysts are thin-walled, fluid-filled struc-tures containing an opaque, proteinacious electro-lyte solution. Cysts are uncommon in postmeno-pausal women, unless they are on hormone replacement therapy (HRT). Like fibroadenomas, the only clinical concern about simple cysts is to confirm that the diagnosis is accurate.

PROLIFERATIVE EPITHELIAL CHANGES Proliferative breast disorders, often referred to incorrectly as "fibrocystic disease," may present as a thickened area or mass leading to the need for biopsy to identify the mass. More commonly, however, pro-liferative epithelial changes are biopsied after detection on mammography.

Proliferative epithelial changes are actually a spectrum of histologic designations ranging from adenosis and sclerosing adenosis, to mild or mod-erate hyperplasia without atypia, to atypical duc-tal or lobular hyperplasia. Once a mass is excised and the absence of invasive breast cancer is demonstrated, these lesions are only important inasmuch as they may be associated with an increased future risk of breast cancer. In addition, when a needle or core biopsy of the mass reveals atypical ductal hyperplasia, a complete excisional biopsy is recommended to confirm that the mass does not contain a region of DCIS or invasive can-cer that was not sampled with the initial biopsy.

HAMARTOMAS Breast "hamartomas," also known as fibroadenolipomas, are relatively uncommon. Histologically, hamartomas are an admixture of fibroglandular tissue and fat within a connective tissue capsule. Because they resemble normal breast tissue histologically, some breast clinicians question whether breast hamartomas are a real entity or whether they are merely normal breast tissue that feels like a lump on CBE or that stands out from surrounding fibroglandular tissue on breast imaging.

FAT TISSUE Fatty breast elements, though not the origin for malignant conditions, may be the source of a number of benign conditions that must be differentiated from cancers. While some textbooks describe "lipomas" of the breast, this has little meaning in clinical breast-mass manage-ment because lipomas are encapsulated nodules of mature adipose tissue, and the substance of the breast has nodules of fat interspersed throughout. Fatty tissue demarcated by stromal elements may also create a masslike effect, but if they are not truly encapsulated lesions in the breast, they are best referred to as fat lobules rather than lipomas.

A breast "lump" consisting of fat can be distinguished from fibroglandular tissue on mammogram by virtue of its low density. Because cancers are made of epithelial cells, which are more radiodense than fat, breast carcinomas cannot be confused with fat on a mammogram. Therefore, breast "lumps" with the density of fat on mammogram and/or ultrasound do not generally require additional evaluation. If needed, the presence of adipose cells on fine-needle aspiration will further confirm the benign nature of the lesion.

One exception to the easy distinction of fat from cancers occurs in the presence of fat necrosis following trauma. With significant trauma causing devascularization of a region of fat within the breast, the fat becomes dense and fibrotic and may remain so until the fat necrosis resorbs over a period of months. Fat necrosis can mimic a cancer clinically by becoming a palpable nodule, and radiographically it can appear as a density on a mammogram, though skilled mammographers can generally distinguish fat necrosis from carcinoma.

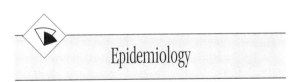

Epidemiology

Incidence and Prevalence

The four most common causes of breast masses are cancers, cysts, fibroadenomas, and focal proliferative epithelial (fibrocystic) changes. The proportion of breast masses that are caused by cancer increases with age, and breast cancer is uncommon in very young women. Nonetheless, breast cancer *does* occasionally occur in younger women—even in adolescents—and cancer must therefore be included in the differential diagnosis of a breast lump that occurs at any age beyond puberty.

Breast cancer incidence increases with age, and age is the strongest predictor of breast cancer

risk. The annual incidence of breast cancer increases from 127/100,000 for women 40 to 44 years of age to 450/100,000 for women 70 to 74 years of age. Nearly 80% of women diagnosed with breast cancer are 50 years of age or older.

Fibroadenomas present most frequently in patients between the ages of 20 to 50, presenting as multiple lesions in 10% to 15% of cases and undergoing involution after menopause. Cysts and focal fibrocystic/proliferative changes are hormonally driven phenomena of the reproductive years and become less common after menopause unless hormone replacement therapy is used.

Morbidity and Mortality

Breast cancer is the most common cancer diagnosed in women, accounting for 32% of all new cancers. Advances in detection and treatment have resulted in improved long-term survival or cure in most cases, but it remains the third most common cause of cancer deaths. Although 56% of breast cancer deaths occur in women 65 and older, breast cancer is also the leading cause of cancer mortality in women 15 to 54 years of age.

Risk Factors

TRADITIONAL RISK FACTORS

There are a number of well-established risk factors for breast cancer that include increased age, family history of breast cancer, early menarche, later age at menopause, later age at first term pregnancy, and a dense mammographic parenchymal pattern. Certain histologic changes are also associated with increased breast cancer risk; these include ductal hyperplasia, atypical ductal hyperplasia, atypical lobular hyperplasia, and lobular carcinoma in situ.

A number of mathematical prediction models can allow estimation of the absolute risk of breast cancer based on some of the aforementioned factors. The Gail model and Klaus model are the most widely used. Although these models may be useful in counseling patients regarding their future risk of breast cancer, they are not helpful in evaluating palpable breast lesions. The majority of women with breast cancer lack one or more of the traditional risk factors of breast cancer. The absence of risk factors should never dissuade the clinician from a full workup of a palpable mass or thickening.

GENETIC MUTATIONS

In the early 1990s, specific genetic mutations were identified in families with strong histories of premenopausal breast and/or ovarian cancers. These mutations, known as the BRCA-1 and BRCA-2 germ-line mutations, are responsible for only a small percentage of breast cancers, but women who carry mutations of these genes are at an especially high risk for breast cancer. In fact, women inheriting a mutation in one of these two genes have as much as an 85% chance of developing a breast cancer by the age of 70, and a 20% to 40% chance of developing an ovarian cancer. Breast cancer in these women often presents as a palpable mass, and it tends to occur in younger women in whom mammography is, in general, less sensitive for cancer detection because of the high glandular content of the breast in younger women.

Work is currently being done to elucidate how these mutation-associated breast cancers compare with sporadic breast cancers and with breast cancers in women with a family history of breast cancer but no abnormality of the BRCA-1 or BRCA-2 genes. It may be that a woman whose family does not have such a strong cancer history, but nonetheless is a mutation carrier, will prove to have lower cancer risks than originally thought. Also, some of the risk factors for cancer development may be different among women with BRCA mutations. For example, it recently was reported that BRCA mutation–positive women who have pregnancies earlier in life might have

increased risk for cancer development, unlike sporadic cancers for which early pregnancy tends to be protective.

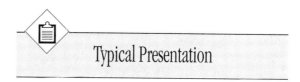

Typical Presentation

Common Signs and Symptoms

Breast masses or focal breast thickening may be discovered on routine physical examination or brought to the clinician's attention by the patient. At times, patients will identify a breast lump or thickening that is difficult for the clinician to palpate, but agreement on the location of any patient-discovered lesion is obviously important. Focal symptoms such as breast pain, localized itching, or a sense of fullness may also signify the presence of an underlying mass, and careful palpation and imaging of the symptomatic area is in order.

Uncommon Signs and Symptoms

Uncommon breast cancer symptoms include sensations of breast burning, pulling, tugging, and itching. Pulling or tugging in the breast can be the symptom of an invasive breast cancer that, by virtue of asymmetric contracture of the malignant mass, is causing distortion of the breast architecture that may or may not be apparent on physical examination or mammography. DCIS can cause significant, tenacious itching at the nipple.

All of these symptoms are nonspecific and relatively insensitive for breast cancer. That being said, a patient complaining of these symptoms, particularly if unilateral and localized, should undergo CBE and mammography, and possibly breast ultrasound. If these studies are negative for masslike or suspicious lesions, the patient still requires clinical follow-up with repeat CBE in 3 to 4 months to ensure stability of symptoms, rather than progression, over time.

Key History

As previously mentioned, the presence or absence of risk factors plays little role in driving the clinical workup of a palpable breast lump. There are also few historic items that distinguish benign from malignant masses with certainty.

Historic findings that are sometimes useful include the following. Increase in size of a palpable area is the most important historic fact suggesting that a lesion might be malignant, and a palpable mass that is stable in size over 2 years can be assumed to be benign. Although pain is more often associated with benign conditions, cancers can sometimes be painful. Focal breast pain warrants additional evaluation with CBE, mammography, and often breast ultrasound to ensure that the finding is not a subtle breast cancer presentation. Recent initiation of hormone replacement therapy or OCPs might suggest the need to evaluate the palpable mass after a trial cessation of hormone treatment. Disappearance of a mass following hormone withdrawal confirms a benign process.

It is also important to identify the possibility of pregnancy, as pregnancy may change the sequence of the diagnostic workup of a breast lump. As discussed later, however, pregnancy should not preclude or delay that workup.

Key Physical Examination

Physical examination of the breast and evaluation of breast lumps and thickenings are complicated by the marked variation in background tissue nodularity, consistency, and breast size among women. Careful examination is therefore required, and there is evidence that spending more time in the performance of a breast examination results in higher rates of detection of breast masses.

As paired structures, the two breasts can first be compared for symmetry on CBE. Palpation then follows. Palpable cancers may present as a thickening, as well as the more familiar mass or nodule.

Some physical examination characteristics are highly suspicious for malignancy. These include new or evolving nipple retraction, skin retraction, and obviously palpable axillary nodes. Other features suggestive of malignancy include a breast mass that has a hard consistency with irregular borders, is fixed to the chest wall or skin, and is painless.

It is critical to remember, however, that many cancers have none of the aforementioned characteristics, making it impossible to rule out cancer by physical-examination findings alone. Instead, multiple diagnostic studies are often needed, frequently in combination, to evaluate palpable breast masses. Once a mass is appreciated on the CBE, the question to ask is not "should I biopsy this mass?" but rather is "why should I not biopsy this mass?" That is, palpable masses should be biopsied unless convincing information from imaging and close clinical follow-up strongly suggest that the mass is a benign process like a breast cyst, fat lump, or small fibroadenoma.

Ancillary Tests

Modalities commonly used in evaluation of a palpable breast abnormality include mammography, breast ultrasound, and tissue sampling (fine-needle aspiration or core biopsy). None of these tests taken alone have performance characteristics (sensitivity, specificity, positive and negative predictive values) sufficiently accurate to distinguish benign from malignant lesions. When used in combination with physical-examination characteristics, however, sufficient accuracy can be achieved to determine the need for further evaluation or simply clinical follow-up.

Breast Imaging

MAMMOGRAPHY

Mammography should be ordered as the first diagnostic step in all women over the age of 30 and in selected patients aged 25 to 30. In a small percentage of cases, the diagnosis of a definitely benign lesion (e.g., a densely calcified fibroadenoma) can be made with a mammogram. In most cases, however, the mammographer will read the mammogram as normal, benign, indeterminate, suspicious, or malignant. The American College of Radiology now requires the use of this 1–5 scale, referred to as the Breast Imaging Reporting And Data System (BIRADS), which is described in the algorithms in Figures 16-2 and 16-3.

In the case of a suspicious or malignant finding, biopsy should be performed. Core needle biopsy is generally preferred to open surgical biopsy for cancer diagnosis. In all other cases (i.e., mammogram readings of normal, benign, or indeterminate), the next steps in the evaluation of palpable breast masses are fine-needle aspiration or core biopsy, and/or breast ultrasonography, depending on availability and local expertise.

Clinicians should be aware of the dangers of false-negative mammograms, which occur in 10% to 20% of palpable cancers. False-negative mammograms are probably related to the radiodensities of different breast tissues. Parenchymal and stromal elements of the breast are radiodense, while fat is relatively radiolucent. Women with less fat in the breast will therefore have radiographically dense breasts, and this generalized radiodensity can obscure the visualization of cancers. With the possible exception of cases in which a mammogram shows complete fatty replacement of the breasts, further studies are warranted in women with a palpable breast lump and a negative mammogram. Diagnostic options include breast ultrasound and fine-needle aspiration of the breast, with the choice of tests driven by the local availability of technology and personnel expertise.

ULTRASOUND

While breast ultrasound is not a substitute for tissue sampling, it can sometimes help the clinician select patients that can forego sampling as an initial diagnostic procedure. Simple cysts and small (< 2 cm) fibroadenomas with classic ultrasonographic features can generally be followed clinically by interval physical examination without tissue sampling. The downside of this approach is that ultrasonographic diagnosis of these conditions requires a skilled radiologist that is practiced in breast ultrasound. The clinician needs to be cognizant of the breast imager's experience in deciding whether to skip tissue sampling based on the results of an ultrasound study.

Ultrasonography of the breast is, however, the initial imaging study of choice in women under 30 years of age with a palpable mass, because the high frequency of mammographically dense breasts in this young age group makes mammography relatively less useful. The most important role of ultrasound in these women is to distinguish simple cysts from solid masses. Care must be taken to ensure that the ultrasonographically identified cyst corresponds to the palpable area of concern.

In expert hands and combined with mammography, ultrasound has been shown to have excellent performance characteristics for the identification of breast cancer with sensitivity of 78% to 97%, positive predictive value of 60%, and a negative predictive value of 99% in one series. When expertise in interpretation and close clinical correlation is lacking, confidence in the results should be adjusted accordingly. A clinically suspicious lesion should be removed regardless of imaging results.

Tissue Sampling

Aspiration of a palpable breast mass is most useful and accurate when used to evaluate a simple cyst. When nonbloody fluid is obtained and the palpable mass disappears completely, no further diagnostic studies are needed. If the aspirated fluid is

Figure 16-2

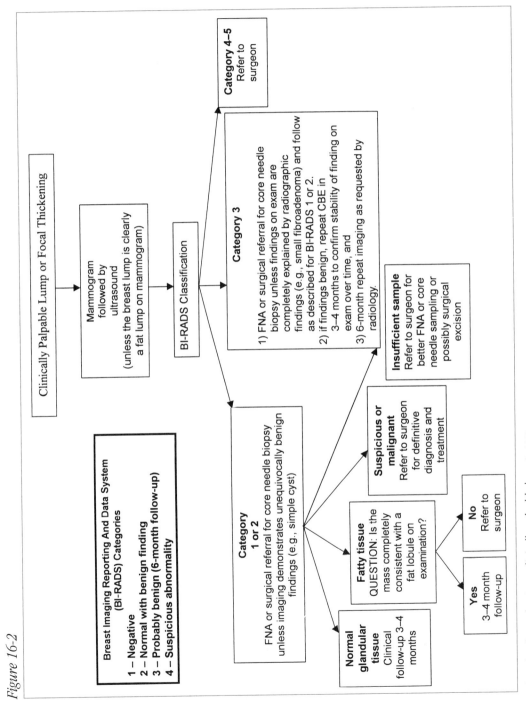

Algorithm for evaluating a clinically palpable breast mass.

Figure 16-3

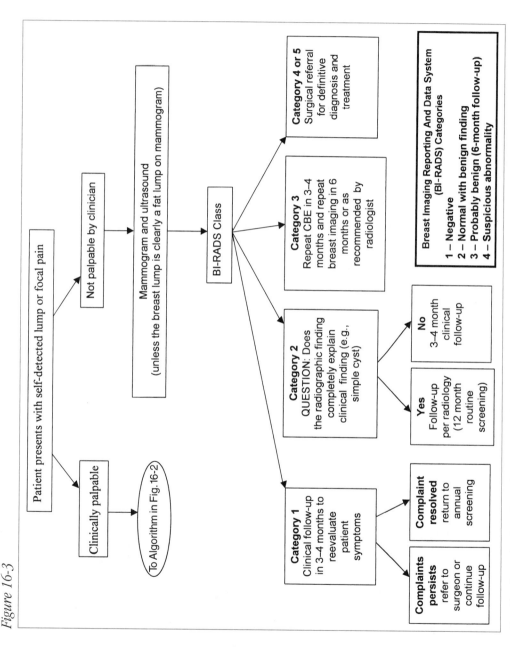

Algorithm for evaluating a breast lump or pain identified only by the patient.

typical of the normal content of breast cysts (serous, yellow, or greyish-green), it need not be sent for cytologic examination because such fluid almost never contains malignant cells. It can therefore be discarded. If bloody fluid (or fluid with the ruddy-brown appearance of old blood) is obtained, the fluid should be sent for cytologic examination and biopsy considered. If the palpable mass does not completely disappear, it should be evaluated further as if it were a solid mass.

With solid masses, the use of fine-needle-aspiration (FNA) cytology has become an important diagnostic adjunct (Figs. 16-4 and 16-5). Atypical or frankly malignant cells obtained by FNA demand further tissue diagnosis with an excisional biopsy. Adequacy of the FNA sample is operator dependent, and the experience of the breast cytologist is also critical. While a pathologist can be very experienced and comfortable with breast histology interpretation, the same individual may not be comfortable with breast cytology.

If no experienced breast cytologist is available, the clinician might be wise to preferentially perform a core needle biopsy, in which breast histology rather than cytology is obtained. In many centers core biopsy, rather than FNA, is the test of choice.

Other Tests

Stereotaxic localization and biopsy are appropriate for nonpalpable breast lumps that are discovered on mammographic screening. Such three-dimensional locating techniques are not generally needed for palpable breast lumps.

Magnetic resonance imaging (MRI) and nuclear medicine imaging (Sestamibi scans) of the breast are useful in the evaluation of known cancers and in the specialized evaluation of certain high-risk patients. In general, however, these studies do not play a role in breast cancer screening or evaluation of breast lumps.

Similarly, antigen blood tests like CEA and CA27-29 may be useful in following known cancers during and after breast cancer treatment, but

Figure 16-4

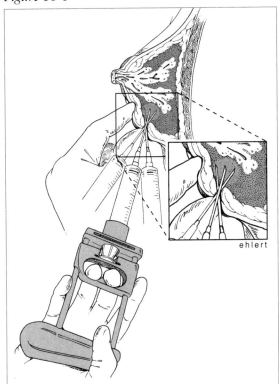

Fine-needle aspiration of a breast mass. The palpable lesion is held in position with the operator's nondominant hand. The breast skin and underlying fibroglandular tissue is anesthetized with lidocaine (*not shown*). The aspirating needle is then introduced into the lesion, with suction being applied to the needle to facilitate cell collection inside the needle shaft (not into the syringe). The needle is passed in and out of the mass in a few orientations (*inset*), with care to not pull the needle out of the skin, which can cause the cells to be pulled out of the needle shaft and into the syringe.

these tests are generally not useful for screening or diagnosing the nature of a specific breast lump. At this time, there is no clinically useful blood test for the detection of breast cancer.

Algorithms

In the past most breast masses were diagnosed by surgical excision. There are two problems with this

Figure 16-5

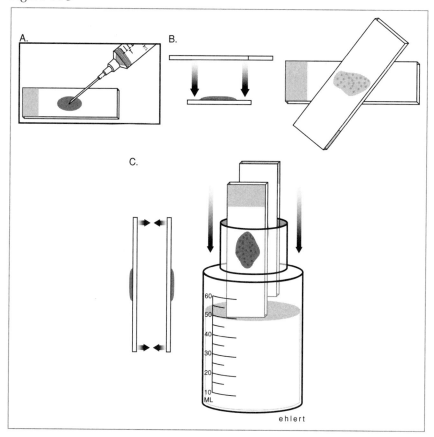

Cytology preparation of breast aspirate. The needle is unscrewed from the syringe *(not shown)*, and air is drawn into the syringe *(not shown)*. The needle is then reattached to the syringe, and, with the needle oriented bevel downward, the aspirate within the needle is forcefully expelled onto the glass slide **(A)**. The second slide is touched to the first to spread the material on the slide **(B)**. Quickly, to avoid air drying, the two glass slides are placed back-to-back and dropped in fixative **(C)**.

approach. First, surgical excision of benign breast tissue leaves a defect in the fibroglandular tissue that may complicate future CBE. Second, breast cancer diagnosed by needle sampling instead of surgical excision facilitates planning for subsequent surgical excision and the use of new techniques such as sentinel-node mapping. Thus, today most surgeons perform surgical excision of breast cancers after fine-needle aspiration or core biopsy has already provided a cytologic or histologic diagno-

sis. This "minimally invasive" approach to breast-mass diagnosis has become the primary way for establishing the diagnosis of cancer or for demonstrating the finding of benignity.

The algorithms in Figures 16-2 and 16-3 are offered as general approaches to the evaluation of a breast mass. Figure 16-2 describes an approach to a breast mass that the clinician can feel on CBE. Figure 16-3 describes an approach when the patient feels a mass or change in the breast, but the clinician cannot appreciate an abnormality on CBE.

To a certain degree, however, breast-lump evaluation defies an algorithmic approach. The problem is that cancers can present in a variety of ways, some of which are unusual and can mimic benign changes. How do we distinguish an atypical cancer from a mass thought to be benign by CBE and breast imaging? First, tissue sampling is critical to the evaluation of most breast masses, and the findings on that sampling must be consistent with the presumed breast diagnosis. Second, even if all of the findings on initial evaluation are consistent with a benign diagnosis, a palpable breast mass also needs to demonstrate a behavior over time that is consistent with that diagnosis.

When history, CBE, and breast imaging all suggest that a mass is a fibroadenoma, it still should be followed clinically to confirm that it is not growing appreciably. Because the end point of clinical follow-up is ill defined, many patients will choose to have palpable fibroadenomas excised (1) to definitively answer the question of diagnosis, and (2) to end the requirement for ongoing clinical follow-up. If a mass is thought to be benign, but is noted to grow on follow-up examination, it needs definitive histologic diagnosis. Low-grade phyllodes tumors can be indistinguishable from fibroadenomas on FNA and even core biopsy, but are distinguished clinically in that they tend to demonstrate fairly rapid growth over time.

Treatment

Appropriate treatment must be instituted when a breast lump is found to be malignant. A detailed summary of breast cancer treatment, however, is beyond the scope of this text. To summarize, the goal of breast cancer treatment is to minimize the chances of breast cancer recurrence in the breast (local); in the lymph nodes (regional); and at metastatic sites (distant), which are most commonly in the bone, liver, lung, and brain.

Treatment involves various combinations of chemotherapy, radiation therapy, and surgery. Medical oncologists usually direct the administration of chemotherapy. Radiation therapy is generally provided in specialized radiation centers, as the experience and technology for some techniques (e.g., electron-boost therapy) are available only at such facilities.

General surgeons perform most breast surgery in the United States. While breast surgery is a "bread-and-butter" aspect of general surgical practice, surgeons that specialize in breast surgery are more likely to be comfortable with breast conservation surgery and other new techniques such as sentinel-node mapping for breast cancer.

Primary-care clinicians working in conjunction with experienced medical oncologists may provided critical support to patients living in rural areas. Oncologists will often provide back-up for recognizing and treating chemotherapeutic complications.

Long-Term Monitoring and Prognosis

About 180,000 cases of breast cancer are diagnosed per year, and approximately 40,000 people die of the disease in the United States. This makes it evident that the majority of breast cancer patients are cured of their disease for the duration of their natural lifetime. At the same time, 10% of women will have an ipsilateral breast cancer recurrence, and 10% to 15% of breast cancer patients will develop a cancer in the contralateral breast. This means that ongoing surveillance is a cornerstone of breast disease evaluation.

After a breast cancer diagnosis and treatment, patients should have, at a minimum, annual CBE and mammography (of the remaining tissue in the diseased breast and also of the remaining breast) for the duration of their lifetime. Most breast specialists recommend 3- to 6-month follow-up clinical examinations for the first 5 years following diagnosis. Immediately following the diagnosis and treatment of a cancer, follow-up at more frequent intervals is generally recommended. After breast conservation therapy, a 6-month interval mammogram is recommended to obtain a new baseline image. The use of screening tests for metastatic disease (blood work, chest x-ray, bone scanning, CT scanning) is controversial but not widely recommended. Such testing is generally undertaken only when indicated by development of symptoms.

Special Situations

Breast Masses During Pregnancy or Lactation

The finding of breast lumps is common during pregnancy and lactation because of the physical and physiologic changes the breast undergoes during pregnancy. The evaluation of such breast lumps is complicated by the increased density of the breast associated with pregnancy, which interferes with interpretation of mammograms. In addition, some radiologists are reluctant to perform mammograms on pregnant women for fear of exposing a developing fetus to radiation.

Pregnancy-associated breast cancers have an increased likelihood to present at a more advanced stage (locally advanced disease) than breast cancers diagnosed in nonpregnant women. It may be that the hormonal milieu of pregnancy stimulates rapid cancer growth, or it may be that breast cancers are simply difficult to detect or are under-evaluated during pregnancy. The latter is a real possibility, because many clinicians make the error of delaying the evaluation of a breast lump until the completion of a pregnancy. A pregnant woman should be evaluated promptly if she has an asymmetric or dominant breast mass.

Breast ultrasound can be helpful in assessing whether there is mass effect in the breast, and tissue diagnosis by core needle sampling or FNA can be done with safety. Mammography can also be safely performed later in pregnancy with appropriate abdominal shielding. Because of the tendency for pregnancy-associated cancers to be aggressive and advanced, short-term follow-up is wise (3 to 4 weeks as opposed to 3 to 4 months) for a mass thought to represent a benign, pregnancy-associated breast change.

Mastitis

Infection or inflammation of the breast often occurs during lactation, but can also occur unrelated to pregnancy or lactation. The presumed etiology is obstruction of a lactiferous duct with subsequent bacterial infection of the proximal breast tissues. Mastitis generally resolves with antibiotic treatment, although it generally takes 3 to 4 weeks to do so because of the relatively poor blood supply in the breast. Mastitis can coalesce into an abscess, in which case surgical drainage is required.

Mastitis needs to be distinguished from inflammatory breast cancer. This latter process is an aggressive form of breast cancer that has the reddened appearance of inflammation, but which actually is not inflammation at a cellular level. Inflammatory breast cancers cause the breast to be reddened and swollen because the cancer metastasizes locally to the subdermal lymphatics. Lymphatic obstruction by cancer cells, not inflammatory cells, leads to redness and swelling of the breast with the "peau d'orange" skin from dermal edema.

Mastitis is common, while inflammatory breast cancer is rare, so the key to the diagnosis of inflammatory breast cancer is clinical suspicion. Clues to distinguishing the two conditions include the fact that mastitis tends to be excruciatingly painful, while inflammatory breast cancer tends to be painless or minimally painful. Furthermore, mastitis tends to be localized to one region of the breast, while inflammatory breast cancer tends to be diffuse and circumareolar. When a clinician suspects mastitis, it is appropriate to start antibiotic treatment, expecting significant improvement within the first week or two.

If there is no clinical response in the skin to antibiotic treatment, then a biopsy of the erythematous skin is indicated to look for subdermal lymphatic involvement by cancer. Full-thickness sampling is required. Unfortunately, a normal skin biopsy, while reassuring, does not definitively rule out inflammatory breast cancer. Up to 50% of skin biopsies can be normal with inflammatory breast cancer, which is why inflammatory breast cancer is generally considered a clinical diagnosis for which there may or may not be histologic confirmation.

Mammography should be performed if cancer is still suspected after a negative biopsy, or if all clinical findings of mastitis do not resolve completely after treatment. Mammography is also appropriate if the patient has other indications for mammography such as routine screening based on age.

Recurrent Breast Cysts

Ultrasonographic evaluation of breast cysts defines fluid-filled lesions either as (1) simple cysts having all of the homogenous, ultrasonographic characteristics of typical, benign breast cysts, or (2) complex cysts, which are fluid-filled lesions that fail to demonstrate all of the ultrasonographic findings of a simple cyst. Most complex cysts are not pathologic, but nonetheless have sonographic features (e.g., thick, cystic fluid with cellular debris) that cannot be reliably distinguished from features of cystic carcinoma, in which a cancer promotes fluid secretion and cyst formation. Thus, complex cysts require additional evaluation, usually by ultrasound-guided needle aspiration. The clues to a cystic carcinoma are that (1) some mass effect is generally seen on ultrasound in the cyst wall, (2) the cyst fluid on aspiration may appear bloody or have cancer cells on cytology, and (3) the cyst tends to recur after aspiration because the cancer is actively secreting fluid.

If the clinician appreciates a mass on CBE and is able to make the mass disappear completely by needle aspiration, then it probably was a benign breast cyst. However, clinical follow-up is warranted, because rapidly recurring breast cysts may be evidence of a subtle cystic carcinoma of the breast. For this reason, cysts that recur once or twice in 4 to 6 weeks should be evaluated by a surgeon for possible excision.

Breast Cancer in Men

One percent of breast cancers occur in males. For the reasons mentioned earlier, they are virtually always ductal in origin. Male breast cancer tends to be diagnosed at more advanced stages than female breast cancer. Part of the reason for this is that clinicians tend to fail to think of breast cancer when evaluating nipple abnormalities in men. Dominant breast masses and nipple erosions in men should be evaluated for cancer, just as they should in women.

Gynecomastia is common in comparison with male breast cancer, and the two can generally be distinguished on physical examination. If there is a question about the nature of the breast enlargement, mammography can be helpful because the mammographic appearance of gynecomastia and breast cancer differ. Tissue diagnosis can be used to resolve uncertain cases. It is of note that gynecomastia never causes erosions through the skin, and the presence of erosion mandates tissue biopsy for diagnosis of cancer.

Patient Education

Patients with breast lumps need to be aware that the majority of breast lumps are not cancers, but that breast cancer is always a possibility and that careful evaluation is important. They should also understand all tests have a certain percentage of "false-positive" results—meaning that some patients will have "abnormal" results but no cancer. Additional testing will need to be performed in such patients, strictly for the purpose of proving that the initial "abnormal" test was falsely positive. For example, some 10% of patients will require some studies (special mammographic views, breast ultrasound, or tissue sampling) after having an abnormal mammogram, even though only a fraction of these, less than 1%, will actually be found to have cancer after the evaluation is complete.

Patients diagnosed with breast cancer need to be educated to the fact that, while we cure the majority of beast cancers, a patient with a treated cancer is at increased risk for recurrence or development of a second breast cancer. Thus, ongoing surveillance is a lifelong, important aspect of their care. While they do not need to fear recurrence, they should be aware that it is a possibility. Cancer patients should receive care from knowledgeable health-care providers to minimize the chances of recurrence and to handle a recurrence in the event that it occurs.

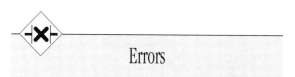

Errors

As noted earlier, delay in diagnosis of breast cancer is the most common reason physicians in the United States are named in malpractice suits. In fact, failure to diagnose breast cancer is the most frequent reason for malpractice actions against family physicians and is among the top three reasons for such suits against surgeons and obstetrician-gynecologists.

Certain errors are common among physicians sued for alleged delay in diagnosis of breast cancer, and in many cases these errors could have been avoided. While no algorithm or set of rules can guarantee freedom from litigation, it is instructive to review the common errors and misconceptions that lead to malpractice actions for delay in diagnosis of breast cancer.

Inappropriate Reliance on a "Normal" Mammogram

A normal mammogram does not exclude the possibility of breast cancer. In fact, mammography fails to identify 15% of cancers because of inter-ference from dense breast tissue that can obscure visualization of a cancer—a particular problem in younger women who tend to have dense breast tissue in comparison with older women.

While clinicians and patients with a palpable breast mass may feel some reassurance from a normal mammogram, the clinical evaluation should never stop simply because the mammogram is normal. Rather, the clinician should seek a triad or tetrad of clinical data to suggest that a breast lump is benign. Such data might include the combination of a negative mammogram, a negative ultrasound, a negative FNA or core biopsy, and short-term clinical follow-up indicating no change in the mass. Only then can the clinician and patient have a reasonable degree of certainty that a mass is benign.

Inappropriate Reliance on Physical Examination

It is far too common for clinicians to reassure patients that their lump is not a cancer because it "feels" like a cyst or a fibroadenoma. Clinicians may also be reassured by a patient's young age and, as a result, fail to obtain supportive data from breast imaging. While it is fine for a clinician to recognize that most breast lumps among young women are benign, the clinician must always obtain objective data supporting the clinical suspicion of benignity. A tissue diagnosis (cytology or histology) for a palpable mass should be obtained unless compelling evidence from history and breast-imaging suggests that this is not required. It may be appropriate to assure a patient that a lump is suspected to be benign, but it is also essential to inform the patient that the absence of cancer cannot be guaranteed and that appropriate diagnostics tests must be performed.

Failure to Document Appropriately

It is essential to maintain a complete and detailed medical record on patients being evaluated because of breast lumps. This point cannot be over-emphasized. Simply writing "normal breast exam" without further elaboration may be better than writing nothing at all, but not by much. The description of a breast examination does not need to be elaborate, but the clinician needs to be able to go back to the clinical note at the next visit and decide if the breast examination is stable, or if it has changed. If you feel a lump, measure it, and write the measurement down. Describe what the lump feels like, and state where it is located in the breast (e.g., 1.3-cm mass in left breast, 2 o'clock, 3 cm from the nipple-areolar complex). Describe the remaining breast tissue (e.g., smooth and homogeneous), state whether it is symmetric or asymmetric with respect to the opposite breast, and describe the axillary examination (e.g., no axillary masses appreciated).

As noted above, if a mass is detected and suspected to be a cyst, fibroadenoma, or benign breast tissue, it is appropriate to reassure the patient. However, it is also essential (1) to concomitantly explain that more diagnostic information is needed and that cancers cannot be excluded with 100% certainty, and (2) to document that cancer has been included in the differential diagnosis, along with recommendations made for further evaluation.

Failure to Listen to the Patient

While it seems self-evident that taking a good history is critical to any disease evaluation, a common complaint of patients who have elected to sue a physician for delay in breast cancer diagnosis is that "I told the doctor there was something wrong, but the doctor didn't listen." Patients feel both with their fingers and with their breasts, while clinicians feel only with their fingers. If the patient says, "it bothers me here" (a localized finding as opposed to a generalized breast symptom), it is the obligation of the clinician to evaluate the place the patient indicates. At a minimum, this evaluation consists of CBE and mammography, with consideration of breast ultrasound imaging of the area of concern. If CBE, mammography,

and breast ultrasound are all normal, then the patient should be reassured that cancer is unlikely (but not impossible). The clinician would be wise to see the patient in 3 to 4 months to confirm that the examination is stable.

Avoiding Errors

No clinician can guarantee the absence of cancer cells in the breast, because no test or combination of tests in medicine has 100% accuracy. The corollary to these statements is, of course, that all clinicians, no matter how experienced, will miss some breast cancers. The question is not, "how can I never miss a breast cancer?" but rather, "how can I keep the number of missed breast cancers to a minimum?" The reality is sobering.

Any patient with a breast mass (or without one for that matter) could come back 1 or 2 years later with a clinically obvious breast cancer at a site that previously was thought to represent normal breast tissue. How, at that time, can we best assure ourselves that we did what we needed to do to properly evaluate a mass, without doing too much or being too invasive?

A useful exercise for ensuring that the evaluation of a breast lump is appropriate is to apply the "prospective retrospectoscope" and see how you look. That is, imagine the patient returning in 1 or 2 year's time with a cancer in the area of the breast that you evaluated, and think about how your evaluation would look in retrospect. What did you do at the time of the first examination? Did you get a mammogram? Did you request a breast ultrasound? Did you or a surgeon or radiologist perform a FNA or a core needle biopsy? Did you tell the patient that you could not rule out cancer with 100% certainty and ask that she come back in a short (3- to 4-month) period to repeat her evaluation to confirm short-term stability? If the answer to all or most of the above questions is yes, then the evaluation was probably appropriate, and it would be difficult to argue that a breast cancer was missed through an error of omission. If, on the other hand, the patient was simply reassured on the basis of a physical examination and mammogram that everything was "fine" and sent on her way, then the evaluation was probably incomplete.

The purpose of this point is not to suggest that we should order extra tests for the purposes of defensive medicine. Unnecessary tests fail to be cost effective, do not provide reassurance to the patient, and fail to protect the clinician. Rather, the purpose of this point is to recognize that we have a limited number of tools for evaluating the breast (clinical history, physical examination, mammogram, ultrasound, tissue sampling, and short-term follow-up), and that it is appropriate and important to use as many of these tools as necessary to exclude the presence of breast cancer. Supportive evidence from multiple categories of tests is the most valuable evidence, and it avoids the need to perform an excisional biopsy of every palpable breast lump.

Emerging Concepts

Multidisciplinary Evaluation of Breast Lumps

Multidisciplinary approaches to breast health and disease management are the obvious wave of the future. Primary-care physicians perform the bulk of CBE in the United States, but they are often the least comfortable with difficult breast examinations or thorough evaluation of breast lumps, particularly in patients who have undergone prior breast surgery. Surgeons may be the most experienced in palpating breast lumps because they have the opportunity to see and feel the tumors at the time of operation, but they have little experience in radiologic evaluation. Mammographers are undoubtedly the most sophisticated in breast-imaging interpretation, but they are often uncomfortable with CBE. Pathologists know what is in the tissue or cytologic smear at which they are looking, but someone has to provide these specimens to the pathologist for a diagnosis to be rendered. Thus, no one field of breast disease evaluation holds all the cards.

To take advantage of the expertise of various disciplines, clinicians of all specialties are increasingly working together in teams to evaluate patients with breast lumps. Primary-care clinicians who consider the diagnosis of malignancy in all patients with breast complaints, who team up with skilled radiologists and surgeons, and who are backed up by a pathologist knowledgeable in breast-pathology diagnosis are least likely to err in the diagnosis of breast cancer. Such a team-oriented primary-care clinician will be providing the best care for patients and is most likely to avoid the personal and professional agony of an alleged "delay in diagnosis" breast-cancer lawsuit.

References

Albertini JJ, Lyman GH, Xoc C, et al: Lymphatic mapping and sentinel node biopsy in the patient with breast cancer. *JAMA* 276:1818, 1996.

Anderson BO, Petrek JA, Byrd DR, et al: Pregnancy influences breast cancer stage at diagnosis in women 30 years of age and younger. *Ann Surg Oncol* (2000 in press.)

Anderson BO, Senie RT, Vetto JT, et al: Improved survival in young women with breast cancer. *Ann Surg Oncol* 2:407, 1995.

Barton MB, Harris R, Fletcher SW: Does this patient have breast cancer? The screening clinical breast examination: should it be done? How? *JAMA* 282:1270, 1999.

Bodian C: Some limitations on studies about the relation between gross cystic disease and risk of subsequent breast cancer. *Ann N Y Acad Sci* 586:218, 1990.

Borgen PI, Wong GY, Vlamis V, et al: Current management of male breast cancer. A review of 104 cases. *Ann Surg* 215:451, 1992.

Burke W, Daly M, Garber J, et al: Cancer Genetics Studies Consortium. Recommendations for follow-up care of individuals with an inherited predisposition to cancer. II. BRCA1 and BRCA2. *JAMA* 277:997, 1997.

Carlson RW, Anderson BO, Benzinger W, et al: Update: NCCN practice guidelines for the treatment of breast cancer. *Oncology* 13:41, 1999.

Claus EB, Risch N, Thompson WD: Autosomal dominant inheritance of early-onset breast cancer. Implications for risk prediction. *Cancer* 73:643, 1994.

Colditz GA, Hankinson SE, Hunter DJ, et al: The use of estrogens and progestins and the risk of breast cancer in postmenopausal women. *N Engl J Med* 332:1589, 1995.

Daling JR, Malone KE, Voigt LF, et al: Risk of breast cancer among young women: relationship to induced abortion. *J Natl Cancer Inst* 86:1584, 1994.

Donegan WL: Evaluation of a palpable breast mass. *N Engl J Med* 327:937, 1992.

Duijm LE, Guit GL, Zaat JO, et al: Sensitivity, specificity and predictive values of breast imaging in the detection of cancer. *Br J Cancer* 76:377, 1997.

Dupont WD, Page DL, Parl FF, et al: Long-term risk of breast cancer in women with fibroadenoma. *N Engl J Med* 331:10, 1994.

Dupont WD, Page DL: Breast cancer risk associated with proliferative disease, age at first birth, and a family history of breast cancer. *Am J Epidemiol* 125:769, 1987.

Fisher B, Costantino JP, Wickerham DL, et al: Tamoxifen for prevention of breast cancer: report of the National Surgical Adjuvant Breast and Bowel Project P-1 Study. *J Natl Cancer Inst* 90:1371, 1998.

Fisher B, Dignam J, Wolmark N, et al: Tamoxifen in treatment of intraductal breast cancer: National Surgical Adjuvant Breast and Bowel Project B-24 randomised controlled trial. *Lancet* 353:1993, 1999.

Fisher B, Redmond C, Fisher ER, et al: Ten-year results of a randomized clinical trial comparing radical mastectomy and total mastectomy with or without radiation. *N Engl J Med* 312:674, 1985.

Fisher B, Redmond C, Poisson R, et al: Eight-year results of a randomized clinical trial comparing total mastectomy and lumpectomy with or without irradiation in the treatment of breast cancer. *N Engl J Med* 320:822, 1989.

Fitzgibbons PL, Henson DE, Hutter RV: Benign breast changes and the risk for subsequent breast cancer: an update of the 1985 consensus statement. Cancer Committee of the College of American Pathologists. *Arch Pathol Lab Med* 122:1053, 1998.

Greenlee RT, Murray T, Bolden S, et al: Cancer statistics, 2000. *CA Cancer J Clin* 50:7, 2000.

Habel LA, Moe RE, Daling JR, et al: Risk of contralateral breast cancer among women diagnosed with carcinoma in situ of the breast. *Proceedings of the Annual Meeting of the Society of Surgical Oncology*, Boston, 1995.

Hamed H, Coady A, Chaudary MA, et al: Follow-up of patients with aspirated breast cysts is necessary. *Arch Surg* 124:253, 1989.

Hartmann LC, Schaid DJ, Woods JE, et al: Efficacy of bilateral prophylactic mastectomy in women with a family history of breast cancer. *N Engl J Med* 340: 77, 1999.

Krag D, Weaver D, Ashikaga T, et al: The sentinel node in breast cancer—a multicenter validation study. *N Engl J Med* 339:941, 1998.

Layfield LJ, Chrischilles EA, Cohen MB, et al: The palpable breast nodule. A cost-effectiveness analysis of alternate diagnostic approaches. *Cancer* 72:1642, 1993.

Morrow M, Wong S, Venta L: The evaluation of breast masses in women younger than forty years of age. *Surgery* 124:634, 1998.

Newton P, Hannay DR, Laver R: The presentation and management of female breast symptoms in general practice in Sheffield. *Fam Pract* 16:360, 1999.

Osborne MP, Hoda SA: Current management of lobular carcinoma in situ of the breast. *Oncology* 8:45, 1994.

Osuch JR, Bonham VL, Morris LL: Primary care guide to managing a breast mass: step-by-step workup. *Medscape Womens Health* 3:4, 1998.

Petrek JA: Breast cancer and pregnancy. *J Natl Cancer Inst Monogr* 16:113, 1994.

Rosen PP: Proliferative breast "disease." An unresolved diagnostic dilemma. *Cancer* 71:3798, 1993.

Silverstein MJ, Lagios MD, Craig PH, et al: A prognostic index for ductal carcinoma in situ of the breast. *Cancer* 77:2267, 1996.

Skaane P, Sager EM, Olsen JB, et al: Diagnostic value of ultrasonography in patients with palpable mammographically noncalcified breast tumors. *Acta Radiol* 40:163, 1999.

Smart CR, Hartmann WH, Beahrs OH, et al: Insights into breast cancer screening of younger women. *Cancer* 72(suppl):1449, 1993.

Volpe CM, Raffetto JD, Collure DW, et al: Unilateral male breast masses: cancer risk and their evaluation and management. *Am Surg* 1999 65:250, 1999.

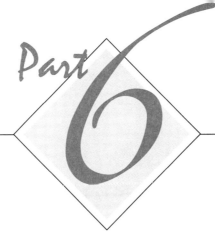

Genitourinary Problems

Bladder Outlet Obstruction

Introduction

bladder outlet obstruction is a disorder with varied presentations. Mild obstruction causes symptoms that are barely discernible. As the condition progresses, however, symptoms may include difficulty in initiating the urinary stream, interruption of the urinary stream, a decreased force or caliber of the urinary stream, and post-void dribbling. Urinary retention represents the "end stage" of bladder outlet obstruction, and the mild symptoms that initially were noted may progress to life-threatening infections and renal failure when acute retention persists without treatment.

The most common factor predisposing to urinary retention is bladder outlet obstruction caused by benign prostatic hypertrophy (BPH), and, therefore, urinary retention is most often seen in men. Other common etiologies include urethral strictures, bladder neck contractures, foreign bodies, prostate cancer, neurogenic bladder, and pharmacologically induced retention.

Determining the cause of bladder outlet obstruction and urinary retention is vital to successful long-term management. Acutely, however, the more pressing need is for intervention to decompress the bladder and relieve symptoms. This chapter will review techniques for intervening when acute urinary retention occurs, focusing on urinary obstruction in men.

Pathophysiology

Anatomy

The male urethra courses from the bladder outlet through the prostate gland, where it pierces the urogenital diaphragm before ending at the fossa navicularis in the glans penis (Fig. 17-1). The urethra is approximately 23 cm long and is divided into anterior and posterior segments. The posterior urethra is composed of the prostatic and the membranous (or sphincteric) urethra. The prostatic portion of the posterior urethra is 3 to 5 cm in length. The distal aspect of the prostatic urethra is defined by the verumontanum. This structure is located at the posterior aspect of the prostatic urethra and, together with the cristae plicarus, forms the prostatic fossa (Fig 17-2). The membranous portion of the posterior urethra contains the striated (or volitional) sphincter. The anterior urethra traverses the corpus spongiosum and terminates at the external meatus.

Etiology

BPH in humans is a nonmalignant hyperplastic process of the prostatic stroma. Hyperplasia begins in the transitional zone of the prostate with the formation of prostatic nodules (Fig. 17-3). As the nodules enlarge, the surrounding prostatic tissue is compressed. If the prostatic capsule is not pliable, the growing nodules eventually compress the prostatic urethra. A compliant capsule, on the other hand, permits prostatic hyperplasia to occur without a significant effect on urinary flow, so palpation of a large prostate during rectal examination is not necessarily predictive of obstruction. Similarly, a small prostate can cause complete obstruction if the capsule is tense.

Androgens (testosterone and dihydrotestosterone) are key to development of BPH, and men castrated before they reach puberty do not develop BPH. Testosterone, which is produced primarily by the testicles, diffuses into prostate cells where it is converted by the 5-alpha reductase enzyme to dihydrotestosterone. The action of dihydrotestosterone stimulates growth of prostate tissue leading to BPH.

Pathologic Consequences

Chronic urinary retention predisposes a patient to urinary tract infections, urosepsis, and death.

Figure 17-1

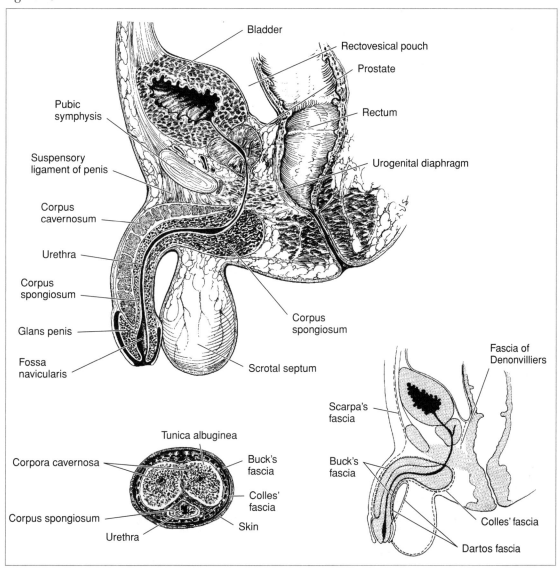

Anatomy of the male urethra. The urethra begins at the bladder outlet, travels through the prostate gland and urogenital diaphragm, and then courses through the penis before ending at the fossa navicularis in the glans penis. (*From Tanagho EA (ed):* Smith's General Urology. *Norwalk CT: Appleton & Lange, 2000, with permission.*)

Figure 17-2

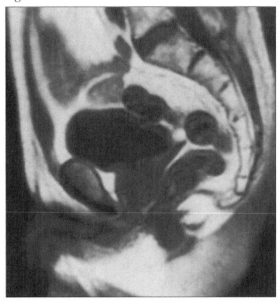

The posterior (prostatic) urethra. The prostatic urethra is proximal to the urogenital diaphragm. The verumontanum protrudes into the prostatic urethra, and the ejaculatory ducts enter the urethra through the verumontanum. (*From Walsh PC (ed):* Campbell's Urology. *Philadelphia, WB Saunders, 1992, with permission.*)

When outlet obstruction and urinary retention go untreated, increased intravesical pressures result in "back pressure" into the ureters with resultant hydronephrosis and subsequent renal dysfunction and renal failure.

Epidemiology

BPH is rare before age 40 and then becomes more common with increasing age. Some degree of bladder outlet obstruction affects about half of men by age 60, and 90% of men by age 85. A 50-year-old man who survives until age 80 has a 25% probability of requiring surgical intervention for bladder outlet obstruction at some point during his lifetime.

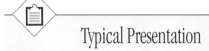

Typical Presentation

As discussed, bladder outlet obstruction is typically caused by compression of the urethra by BPH. It may also occur when a patient has urethral strictures, prostate cancer, paraphimosis, or other conditions outlined below. Patients typically present with symptoms that include hesitancy, decreased caliber of the urinary stream, a split or interrupted steam, and post-void dribbling. Some patients will complain of irritative bladder symptoms such as frequency, nocturia, urgency, and dysuria.

Figure 17-3

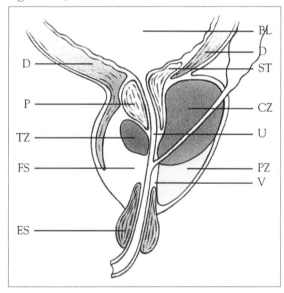

Benign prostatic hypertrophy. The diagram shows the various anatomic subdivisions of the prostate gland. Benign prostatic hyperplasia typically begins in the transitional zone of the prostate. *CZ*, central zone; *PZ*, peripheral zone; *TZ*, transitional zone; *V*, verumontanum; *FS*, fibromuscular stroma; *D*, detrusor muscle of the bladder; *P*, preprostatic urethra; *ES*, external urethral spincter; *ST*, superficial trigone of the bladder; *BL*, bladder lumen; *U*, urethral lumen. (*From Dixon JS, Gosling JA: Macro-anatomy of the prostate, in Kirby R (ed):* Textbook of Benign Prostatic Hyperplasia. *Oxford, Isis Medical Media, 1996, with permission.*)

A man experiencing urinary retention often presents with gradual worsening of previously identified obstructive symptoms. However, an acute inflammation of the prostate (e.g., prostatitis) or decompensation of the bladder's muscle function (e.g., from use of anticholinergic medications) can result in acute retention even in the absence of previous symptoms.

It is important to note that patients with urinary retention often do pass urine, despite the presence of obstruction. When the bladder is distended to capacity by urinary retention, urine may leak from the urethra in small frequent amounts without the patient feeling the urge to void or voiding normal amounts. This so-called overflow incontinence is a classic manifestation of urinary retention.

Finally, male patients with urinary retention, especially those who are frail or living in nursing homes, may present with atypical or nonspecific symptoms. Such symptoms can include confusion, weakness, agitation, delirium, and/or obtunded mental status.

Key History

In the initial evaluation of men with bladder outlet obstruction, a detailed medical history with particular attention to the urinary tract is essential. Previous urologic interventions, general health issues, and associated comorbidities should be reviewed. A voiding history is obtained, preferably by having the patient keep a voiding diary. Specifically, if the patient is producing frequent, small volumes of urine, or has not voided in 12 hours, the probability of urinary retention is high.

It is also important to determine whether obstructive symptoms were acute or gradual in onset. Progressive symptoms are consistent with BPH or urethral stricture disease. Acute symptoms, however, are more commonly noted with inflammatory disorders, paraphimosis, or drug side effects.

Another useful item in the history is to determine how the patient urinates. Frequently, a patient with chronic retention will have developed techniques to improve his urinary flow, and eliciting such a history facilitates the diagnosis of urinary obstruction. For example, a patient may state that he cannot urinate effectively while standing, but voids well when seated. This is consistent with BPH, in which sitting causes relaxation of the perineum and the sphincteric mechanism, thereby improving urinary flow. Other patients will report performing a credé maneuver (applying suprapubic pressure to expel urine from the bladder).

Finally, it is also important determine if the patient has had, or has risk factors for, sexually transmitted diseases. Even remote infections can lead to urethral scarring and strictures that result in acute urinary retention.

Key Physical Examination

Physical examination has a limited role in the evaluation of urinary retention. There are, however, four key areas to examine.

Anterior Abdominal Wall

One can often detect bladder distention by palpating the anterior abdominal wall. A markedly distended bladder is usually easily palpable. The bladder may also be tender, particularly to percussion, when urinary retention is of acute or recent onset. In obese patients, however, it may be difficult to palpate a distend bladder.

Rectum

Digital rectal examination is almost always performed in the evaluation of urinary retention.

However, it generally adds little to acute management because the correlation between prostate size, degree of obstruction, and symptoms is poor. Rather, the main purpose of performing a digital rectal examination is to palpate for prostate nodules that might indicate malignancy. Rectal examination should not be performed when there is a suspicion of acute prostatitis, as pressure on the prostate gland may result in bacteremia.

Foreskin

It is not uncommon for a phimosis or paraphimosis to cause urinary obstruction. Therefore, in uncircumcised men it is important to examine the foreskin to rule out these conditions.

Anterior Urethra

Palpation of the anterior urethra through the ventral surface of the penis may reveal nodularity or induration indicative of urethral strictures, particularly in men with a history of sexually transmitted diseases. Additionally, patients with a history of urolithiasis may have palpable stones in the urethra. Identification of either of these factors will alter treatment management.

Ancillary Tests

Several ancillary tests are useful in evaluating patients who have symptoms of bladder outlet obstruction. These include the International Prostate Symptom Score, urinalysis, blood testing, and measurement of post-void residual urine volume.

International Prostate Symptom Score (IPSS)

Patients with mild bladder outlet obstructive symptoms should complete the IPSS (Table 17-1). The score on the IPSS can be used as an objective indicator of treatment response or disease progression. It is important to note, however, that while the symptom index describes urinary symptoms and "bother" from BPH, it does not predict development of complications such as urinary obstruction.

Urinalysis

A urinalysis should be performed to detect hematuria, bacteruria, pyuria, and crystals. Presence of any of these elements in the urine may alter treatment decisions. For example, the presence of urinary tract infection in the face of urinary retention is an absolute indication for immediate intervention to relieve obstruction. However, such immediate intervention may not be necessary if the patient is not infected and has normal renal function with mild retention. In such situations, a patient may elect a trial of medical therapy prior to proceeding with interventions to relieve obstruction.

Blood Testing

Serum creatinine and blood urea nitrogen levels may be measured to assess for azotemia. These tests will permit detection of the 1% to 2% of male patients with bladder outlet obstruction who present with renal dysfunction.

In a patient with acute urinary retention, clinicians often measure the prostate specific antigen (PSA) level. Although baseline PSA levels are predictive of the risk for future development of urinary retention and can be used to screen for prostate cancer, PSA is not a useful test in the setting of acute retention. Furthermore, although prostate cancer in a patient with urinary retention may cause an elevated PSA, and since cancer is treated differently than obstruction from simple BPH, it is important to remember that urinary retention itself will elevate the PSA level. This invalidates the result of PSA tests for diagnosis of cancer during acute retention.

Table 17-1

International Prostate Symptom Score (IPSS)

	NOT AT ALL	LESS THAN 1 TIME IN 5	LESS THAN HALF THE TIME	ABOUT HALF THE TIME	MORE THAN HALF THE TIME	ALMOST ALWAYS
1. Over the past month, how often have you had a sensation of not emptying your bladder complete after you finished urinating?	0	1	2	3	4	5
2. Over the past month, how often have you had to urinate again less than 2 hours after you finished urinating?	0	1	2	3	4	5
3. Over the past month, how often have you found you stopped and started again several times when you urinated?	0	1	2	3	4	5
4. Over the past month, how often have you found it difficult to postpone urination?	0	1	2	3	4	5
5. Over the past month, how often have you had a weak urinary stream?	0	1	2	3	4	5
6. Over the past month, how often have you had to push or strain to begin urinating?	0	1	2	3	4	5
	NONE	1 TIME	2 TIMES	3 TIMES	4 TIMES	≥5 TIMES
7. Over the past month, how many times did you most typically get up to urinate from the time you went to bed at night until the time you got up in the morning?	0	1	2	3	4	5
Total IPSS Score						

The IPPS can be used to assess severity of symptoms caused by benign prostatic hypertrophy (BPH). The IPPS can be self-administered. Patients circle the most appropriate response for each question. The answers to each questions, which are scored from 0 to 5, are then summed to yield a total score. Scores can range from 0 (asymptomatic) to 35 (extremely symptomatic).

SOURCE: Barry MJ, Fowler FJ, O'Leary MP, et al: The American Urological Association symptom index for benign prostatic hyperplasia. The Measurement Committee of the American Urologicial Association. *J Urol* 148:1549–1557, 1992.

Post-Void Residual Urine Volume

The most useful test in evaluating patients with urinary retention is measurement of the post-void residual (PVR) urine volume. In fact, urinary retention is defined as an elevated PVR volume. Normal PVR volume is less than 50 cc, with the 25th and 75th percentile values for men being 2.5 cc and 35 cc, respectively. Volumes over 100 to 200 cc are diagnostic of urinary retention.

While the precise post-void residual volume is interesting to know, it is not essential to make an accurate determination of the PVR volume. Rather, simply establishing that the PVR volume is elevated provides sufficient information to diagnose urinary retention and justify initiation of treatment.

The easiest way to measure PVR in men with suspected bladder outlet obstruction is with ultrasound. This simple test is a noninvasive means to assess the degree of urinary retention and is easier than catheterization in men with an obstructed outflow tract. Alternatively, a urethral catheter may be placed to drain the bladder and determine the PVR. If ultrasound is unavailable and catheterization not feasible, yet another way to determine PVR is by injecting a small amount of intravenous contrast media, which will concentrate within the bladder and give an estimation of the PVR on an abdominal plain film.

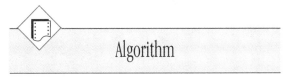

Algorithm

Figure 17-4 is an algorithm that outlines an approach to patients with urinary retention. If retention is mild and symptoms minimal, a trial of alpha blockade or 5-alpha-reductase inhibitors may be considered if no infection is present. If more severe retention, azotemia, or infection is present, acute intervention should be undertaken to relieve bladder outlet obstruction. The nature of the intervention will depend on whether retention is caused by BPH, urethral stricture, a foreskin problem, or a neurologically or pharmacologically induced hypocontractile bladder.

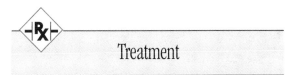

Treatment

Depending on the cause and severity of urinary retention, several options are available for treatment. These include both nonprocedural treatments and procedural treatments that include catheterization and surgical interventions.

Figure 17-4

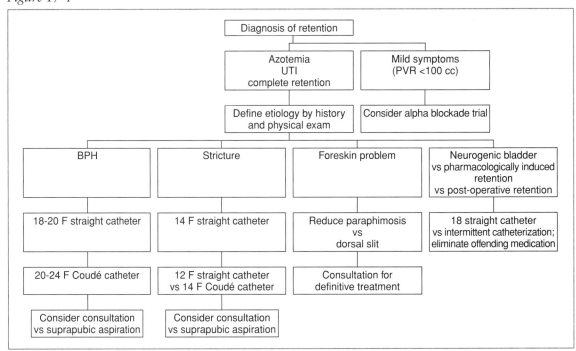

Algorithm for evaluation and treatment of urinary retention.

Nonprocedural Treatments

There are several nonsurgical treatment options for urinary retention, each aimed at a particular cause of retention. Therefore, it is essential to establish the cause of urinary retention before treatment is initiated. In particular, prior to treating BPH with pharmacologic therapy, one has to ensure that the etiology of the retention is not urethral stricture disease. This differential diagnosis can be made by inserting a catheter into the urethra. If the catheter (which should be larger than 14 F) slides easily into the bladder, it can then be removed with the assurance that a stricture is unlikely. In terms of specific approaches to management, there are several options depending on the cause of retention.

TREATMENTS FOR BENIGN PROSTATIC HYPERTROPHY

When a patient has mild symptoms of obstruction, no renal deterioration, and no urinary tract infection, one may consider medical management of the obstructive symptoms. Medical management involves drug therapy aimed at one of the two phases of BPH.

In the dynamic phase of prostatic obstruction, the muscular sheath surrounding the prostate compresses the hypertrophic gland into the urethral lumen, leading to obstruction of urethral flow. If contraction of this muscular capsule can be prevented, the urinary flow rate is often improved. The mechanism to achieve this muscle relaxation is alpha-adrenergic blockade. Medications that perform alpha blockade include generalized alpha-adrenergic blocking agents (e.g., prazosin), prostate-specific alpha-blocking agents (e.g., terazosin and doxazosin), and highly prostate-specific alpha-blocking agents (e.g., tamsulosin).

In the static phase, prostatic obstruction is caused by the growth of prostate tissue under the influence of androgens. By inhibiting 5-alpha reductase, androgenic activity is diminished, leading to a decrease in the size of the prostate gland. When using 5-alpha reductase inhibitors (e.g., finasteride), it is important to keep in mind that 5-alpha reductase inhibitors will artificially lower a patient's PSA level, thus eliminating the ability to use PSA as a screening tool for prostate cancer. In addition, the onset of action of 5-alpha reductase inhibitors is slow, so these medications have limited value if there is an urgent need to relieve obstruction and improve symptoms.

TREATMENTS FOR OTHER CAUSES OF URINARY RETENTION

Other causes of outflow obstruction also have specific medical treatments. For example, prostatic inflammation (i.e., prostatitis) can cause outflow obstruction and can be treated with antiinflammatory medications and antibiotics. Indeed, medical management of prostatitis is generally preferable to catheterization or other interventional treatments, as catheterization and urethral manipulation may exacerbate the problem.

Procedural Treatments

Procedural treatments for acute urinary obstruction include urethral catheterization, suprapubic catheterization, techniques for reduction of phimosis and paraphimosis, and urethral dilation for meatal stenosis.

URETHRAL CATHETERIZATION

Prior to making the decision to place a urethral catheter, it is essential to ensure that there is no obstruction in the anterior urethra. This determination is made by ensuring that meatal stenosis, phimosis, and paraphimosis are absent. Phimosis and paraphimosis are evident on physical examination, and meatal stenosis can be excluded by spreading the urethral meatus between the thumb and first finger; the typical adult male urethral meatus should appear wide enough to easily accept an 18 French catheter. Treatments for phimosis, paraphimosis, and meatal stenosis are reviewed below.

Once it has been determined that that the anterior urethra is patent, catheterization can proceed.

The procedure is conceptually divided into three phases.

PHASE 1—SELECTION OF AN APPROPRIATE CATHETER
Selection of a catheter, which should be based on the patient's history, often determines whether catheterization will be successful or unsuccessful. If a patient presents with a gradual increase in symptoms and the clinician determines that BPH is the likely cause of urinary retention, successful catheterization is most likely when the catheter is larger than 18 French in size. Conversely, if a patient presents with a history of previous urologic instrumentation or urethral disease, and, therefore, his retention is thought to be caused by a urethral stricture, a 12 or 14 French catheter is more likely to be successful. If a patient has a history of difficult catheterizations, a Coudé catheter is often ideal (see below).

PHASE 2—PRE-CATHETERIZATION PREPARATION   The keys to successful catheter placement are patient preparation and adequate lubrication.

PATIENT PREPARATION   In preparing the patient, the clinician should explain the procedure in detail, emphasizing that catheterization is not usually painful. The patient should be placed in a warm room in the supine position and should have his penis prepared with Betadine or other cleansing solution.

The clinician must recognize that strong abdominal-urethral muscular contractions can overcome the force of an attempted urethral catheterization. Therefore, relaxation is crucial for catheter placement. The patient should be encouraged to breathe in a regular pattern and to relax his abdominal musculature. Only necessary medical personnel should be present in the room before and during the procedure because when patients are exposed in front of multiple observers, they become tense and catheterization is more difficult.

LUBRICATION   Lubrication is essential to facilitate catheter placement and also to permit an assess-

ment of the ease with which catheterization will be accomplished. While some clinicians simply lubricate the catheter with a water-soluble lubricant (e.g., K-Y jelly) before insertion, a more effective method is to also inject viscous lidocaine directly into the urethra, assuming, of course, that the patient is not allergic to lidocaine.

Two-percent viscous lidocaine should be injected intraurethrally through an appropriate applicator such as the widely used jet applicator (Fig. 17-5). If a jet applicator is not available, then viscous lidocaine can be placed into a 10-cc syringe and injected into the urethra through a short, flexible angiocatheter. The patient should be reassured that the urethra will become anesthetized as the lubricant is placed, and the intraurethral injection should be made while the patient is breathing gently and deeply.

For successful catheterization, at least 20 mL of lidocaine should be used. A firm seal is important to prevent reflux of lidocaine out of the urethra. Such a seal can be obtained at the urethral meatus with the cone of the jet applicator or the base of the angiocatheter.

During injection of viscous lidocaine, the clinician can anticipate the ease with which catheter insertion will occur. If the lidocaine enters the urethra easily, a catheter should be easy to insert. If, however, lidocaine injection meets with a resistance, or is extruded when the meatal seal is

Figure 17-5

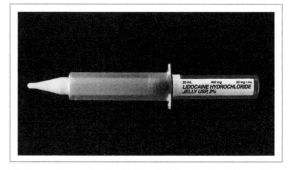

The jet applicator for instillation of lidocaine into the urethra.

removed, then the clinician should expect a more difficult catheterization.

PHASE 3—CATHETER INSERTION Catheterization with a straight Foley catheter is used to relieve acute urinary retention. Catheterization should begin by grasping the penis in the clinician's nondominant hand and holding it straight up toward the ceiling. The dominant hand is used to lubricate the catheter (with viscous lidocaine or water-soluble lubricant) and to place the catheter into the meatus.

The catheter should be advanced at a regular pace, but if resistance is encountered, the attempt should be aborted. If the catheter appears to "hang up" in the penile urethra, this is an indication that a stricture exists. The clinician should consider using a smaller catheter and attempt to navigate the stricture. If, however, the catheter appears to lodge in the prostatic urethra (i.e., beyond the penile urethra), this is an indication that a false passage exists and Coudé catheterization should be attempted.

A Coudé catheter is a device formed to navigate the anatomic curve of the urethra as it travels superiorly through the prostate gland (Fig. 17-6). The catheter is constructed so that the curl of the tip of the Coudé is aligned with the balloon port at the distal end of the tube. This alignment is important to remember as it allows the clinician to maintain orientation of the location of the curl (i.e., the catheter tip), even when it is within the penis. At all times during catheterization, the curl of the catheter should be pointing dorsally—that is, toward the patient's head. The Coudé catheter should be advanced in a similar fashion to the straight catheter. If resistance is encountered, the catheter is turned 45° to either side in an attempt to navigate the false passage. If this is unsuccessful, the patient should be asked to urinate while the catheter is placed. Urination may open the urethral channel and provide the catheter a route to the bladder. If this too is unsuccessful, the clinician needs to determine the relative risks and benefits of continued catheterization attempts.

If catheterization has failed after two attempts, further attempts at catheterization will often serve only to create deeper false passages. Therefore, after two failed catheterization attempts, a urologist generally should be consulted. If such consultation is not readily available, one may proceed with a third catheterization attempt, typically using a slightly larger Coudé catheter. If this catheterization attempt fails as well, a urologist will attempt catheterization using filiforms and followers or cystoscopic guidance. In a urethra that has had several previous catheterization attempts,

Figure 17-6

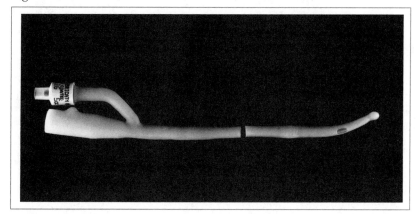

Coudé catheter.

suprapubic catheter placement or suprapubic aspiration may be necessary.

SUPRAPUBIC CATHETERIZATION

Suprapubic catheterization involves placement of one of several types of urinary drainage devices directly into the bladder through a percutaneous approach. Many types of suprapubic catheters are available, each of which requires a slightly different placement technique. In general, however, placement requires identifying the bladder using a spinal needle and then using an engaging system to place the catheter into the bladder.

While placement of a suprapubic catheter is a procedure usually performed by a urologist, suprapubic aspiration of the bladder to relieve acute retention may be performed by primary-care clinicians. The technique involves first identifying the appropriate landmarks (the midline, two finger-breadths above the pubic bone) for needle insertion. Then, with the patient in a supine position, a 3- or 5-inch, 18- or 20-gauge spinal needle is introduced, aiming slightly superiorly. A syringe is attached to the end of the spinal needle, and as the needle is introduced through the iodine-prepared skin, the plunger on the syringe is withdrawn. When urine is encountered, the syringe is advanced approximately 2 cm further. At that point, urine can be withdrawn from the bladder. Bladder aspiration is a temporizing measure until more definitive therapy can be instituted.

Caution should be taken in attempting this procedure in coagulopathic patients. The prostate and bladder have rich vascular systems, and a misguided needle, particularly in a patient with a bleeding diathesis, can result in significant bleeding. Patients who have undergone lower midline abdominal surgery should not have a suprapubic aspiration attempted without radiologic guidance. This is because such surgery often results in intestinal adhesions to the anterior bladder wall, and a needle inserted in such a patient may traverse the intestine.

Reduction of Paraphimosis

Paraphimosis is occasionally encountered as a cause of urinary retention. Typically, the patient is uncircumcised and has neglected to return his foreskin to its extended position after voiding or intercourse. When this occurs, the foreskin serves as a constricting band, impeding venous return from the glans penis. The glans then becomes engorged, edematous, and painful, and the foreskin can no longer be returned to its extended position.

Many techniques have been proposed for reducing paraphimosis, some of which are novel such as application of iced gloves, or using granulated sugar as an osmotic agent to reduce edema. These techniques are not recommended for general use, however, because they are not consistently effective and may delay institution of more effective treatments.

More commonly, one of two procedures is used, both of which rely on pressure to reduce edema in the engorged prepuce. In the first technique, the glans penis and prepuce are firmly grasped. Pressure is applied to the glans for 5 minutes. This is usually uncomfortable for the patient, and for this reason a penile block is commonly performed. To achieve the penile block, inject 1% lidocaine without epinephrine in a circumferential fashion at the base of the penis through a 25-gauge needle. While a circumferential block is usually adequate, a more effective penile block can be performed by infiltrating lidocaine into the dorsal penile nerves that run just below Buck's fascia at the base of the penis between at the 10 o'clock and 2 o'clock positions (Fig. 17-7).

A second technique can be used for paraphimosis that is particularly severe. After placing a 4 × 4 gauze dressing around the head of the penis, Coban is wrapped circumferentially, as tightly as possible around the glans penis, to remove edema from the head of the penis (Fig. 17-8). Over the course of the next 5 to 10 minutes, the Coban is wrapped around the glans penis tighter and tighter. After 10 minutes the Coban is removed,

Figure 17-7

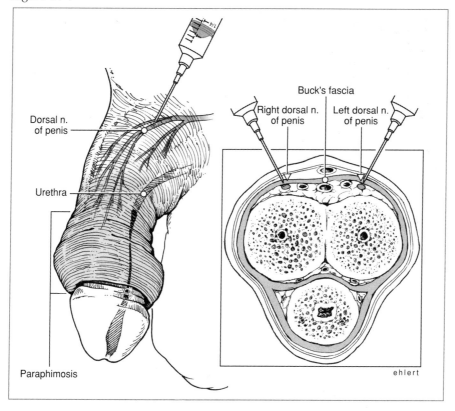

Dorsal penile nerve block. To anesthetize the penis prior to reducing a paraphimosis, a dorsal nerve block can be performed. Lidocaine without epinephrine is injected at the 10 o'clock and 2 o'clock positions of the penis, to a level just below Buck's fascia.

and most of the edema that had been present in the foreskin will have traveled proximally on the penis to allow reduction of the paraphimosis.

Reduction of Phimosis

Phimosis is most often encountered as a cause of urinary retention in a patient who is uncircumcised and has developed an episode of balanitis. The resulting inflammation results in the inability to adequately retract the foreskin, thus causing an obstruction to urinary flow.

The definitive treatment for phimosis is circumcision after resolution of the infection. As an acute treatment for severe phimosis, however, a dorsal slit of the foreskin can be performed. While this procedure is typically performed by urologists, other clinicians may need to perform the procedure in areas where a urologist is not available.

Following the placement of a penile block, the clinician makes an incision in the foreskin on the dorsum of the penis (Fig. 17-9). The incision is carried proximally on the foreskin until there is adequate visualization of the glans.

Figure 17-8

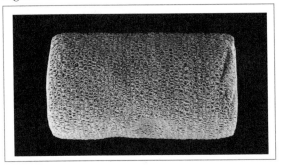

Coban bandage for wrapping the head of the penis to reduce paraphimosis.

Hemostasis is obtained by oversewing the cut edges of the prepuce using a 3.0 chromic suture. The patient is given a prescription for antibiotics (cephalexin is commonly prescribed). Several weeks later, when the inflammation and infec-

tion have receded, a formal circumcision is performed. Despite the dorsal slit, circumcision usually has a good cosmetic result.

Dilation of Meatal Stenosis

Meatal stenosis is encountered after urologic procedures that result in scarring of meatus. To treat this condition, a well-lubricated dilator (Fig. 17-10) is inserted into the urethra until an adequate lumen has been created. The patient may be given the dilator for self-dilations.

Follow-Up Care

Patients who have had an episode of acute urinary retention not caused by an obviously transient medical problem should be seen by a

Figure 17-9

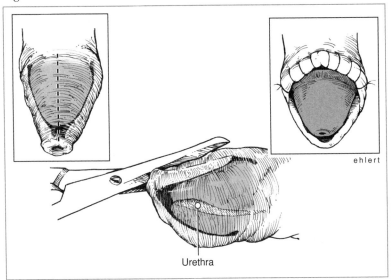

Dorsal foreskin slit and circumcision to reduce phimosis. Reduction of a phimosis is achieved by cutting a dorsal slit in the location shown by the dotted line, followed by suturing of the cut edges.

Figure 17-10

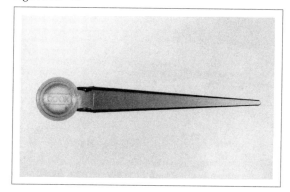

Dilator for dilation of meatal stenosis.

urologist to assess whether surgical intervention is necessary. A rough rule of thumb for determining the length of time the catheter can be left in place before urologic consultation is 1 week for every liter of urine that is retained in the bladder. The rationale for this rule is that, with larger volumes of urine retained in the bladder, the obstructive process is more chronic and acute intervention is less urgent; therefore, more time with a catheter in place is needed for the bladder to regain its muscular tone. Thus, if a patient had 1 liter of retained urine in the bladder, the catheter should remain in place and he should be seen by a urologist within a week; if 4 liters of urine were retained, the patient should be catheterized and should see a urologist within about 1 month.

However, patients whose urinary retention is thought to be the result of a reversible medical problem may be given a voiding trial prior to urologic consultation. For example, urinary retention may be caused by the use of an anticholinergic drug, or a patient who suffers from alcohol abuse may develop episodes of urinary retention caused by alcohol-induced neuropathy. In such situations, bladder function may improve after the causal problem is eliminated, and the patient may be treated with a voiding trial after an acceptable period of catheterization (using the same rule described above to determine the length of catheterization).

A patient who has not previously received alpha blockade can be started on an alpha-blocker to maximize the likelihood of a successful voiding trial. For patients that fail voiding trials after episodes of urinary retention, surgical treatment of their disease is often warranted.

Finally, the primary complication associated with short-term urethral catheterization is infection. Urinary tract infections are best avoided by placing an indwelling Foley catheter in a sterile fashion, by minimizing urethral manipulation, and by encouraging hygiene in the catheterized patient. Prophylactic antibiotics for simple indwelling Foley catheters are not routinely advised, as virtually all patients will have bacteriuria within a month of catheter insertion, and routine antibiotic treatment selects for resistant organisms. However, patients who develop systemic signs of infection while the catheter is in place should receive antibiotic therapy, with the selection of antibiotics guided by the results of urine cultures and sensitivity tests.

Long-Term Monitoring, Treatment, and Prognosis

Acute urinary retention represents the extreme in a range of symptoms associated with bladder outlet obstruction. In the past, urinary retention was an absolute indication for surgical intervention. Today, medical intervention may often be successful, thereby obviating the need for surgery.

For patients who are successfully treated with medical therapy, long-term monitoring remains key. Because urinary retention can be responsible for renal dysfunction, the patient's renal function should be assessed routinely. Additionally, a urinalysis should be periodically checked to ensure that a urinary tract infection has not developed.

Education

Educating patients with early obstructive symptoms may prevent the eventual need for urgent catheterization. Patients who should receive such education are those who are at risk of urinary retention such as those with BPH and a high IPSS score, known stricture disease, a history of multiple urethral instrumentations, or neurologic disorders (including diabetic neuropathy). Patients receiving anticholinergic medications should also be aware of the symptoms of urinary retention. Educating these patients about signs and symptoms of progressive urinary retention may allow early medical intervention and thus avoid the need for catheterization.

Errors

The most common error in catheterization is continuing to attempt urethral intubation despite multiple failures. Each unsuccessful attempt to catheterize the urethra makes eventual catheterization more difficult. Furthermore, uncontrolled or traumatic urethral manipulation can result in stricture disease. Therefore, it is important to minimize urethral trauma by limiting attempted catheterizations and obtaining urologic consultation when catheterization is unsuccessful.

References

Barry MJ, Fowler FJ, O'Leary MP, et al: The American Urological Association symptom index for benign prostatic hyperplasia. The Measurement Committee of the American Urological Association. *J Urol* 148:1549, 1992.

Bartsch G, Muller HR, Oberholzer M et al: Light microscopic stereological analysis of the normal human prostate and of benign prostatic hyperplasia. *J Urol* 122:487, 1979.

Berry SJ, Coffey DS, Walsh PC, et al: The development of human prostatic hyperplasia with age. *J Urol* 132:474, 1984.

Emberton M, Anson K: Acute urinary retention in men: an age old problem. *BMJ* 318:921, 1999.

Goldfischer ER, Cromie WJ, Karrison TG, et al: Randomized, prospective, double-blind study of the effects on pain perception of lidocaine jelly versus plain lubricant during outpatient rigid cystosocopy. *J Urol* 157:90, 1997.

Kerwat R, Shandall A, Stephenson B: Reduction of paraphimosis with granulated sugar. *Br J Urol* 82:755, 1998.

Kolman C, Girman CJ, Jacobsen SJ, et al: Distribution of post-void residual urine volume in randomly selected men. *J Urol* 161:122, 1999.

McConnell JD: Anti-androgen therapy for benign prostatic hyperplasia. In Stamey, Thomas A (ed): *Monographs in Urology*. West Point, PA, Merck, 1995.

Osterling JE: The origin and development of benign prostatic hyperplasia: an age-dependent process. *J Androl* 12:348, 1991.

Roehrborn CG, McConnell JD, Lieber M, et al: PLESS Study Group. Serum prostate-specific antigen concentration is a powerful predictor of acute urinary retention and need for surgery in men with clinical benign prostatic hyperplasia. *Urology* 53:473, 1999.

Susan Reed

Chapter 18

Spontaneous Abortion

Introduction

It is estimated that half of all pregnancies and 20% to 30% of recognized pregnancies end in spontaneous abortion. The number of identifiable spontaneous abortions is likely to increase as more pregnancies are diagnosed by inexpensive and simple tests, many of which detect pregnancy as early as 10 days after conception. Because of its frequency, spontaneous abortion is the most common reason why patients seek emergency gynecologic assessment. Therefore, the ability to evaluate and treat such patients is an important skill for primary-care clinicians.

This chapter will review the diagnosis and treatment of incomplete and inevitable abortion, including a description of the procedure for surgical dilation and suction curettage. It will also outline situations in which nonsurgical management may be the preferred treatment. The discussion will distinguish threatened abortions (50% of which will result in a live birth and which should be managed expectantly) from inevitable, incomplete, and complete abortions, and will also briefly consider conditions that may be confused with spontaneous abortion such as ectopic pregnancy. Lastly, the chapter will discuss indications for referral to a specialist and the necessary evaluation prior to transfer of care.

History

For decades, surgical evacuation of the uterus was universally accepted as the treatment of choice for spontaneous abortion. In the late 1800s when maternal death rates from sepsis exceeded 10%, the management of an incomplete spontaneous abortion focused on the use of uterine curettage to minimize blood loss and quickly remove the products of conception from the uterus to reduce the chance of infection.

In the early 1900s there was an increase in the prevalence of self-induced or illegally performed abortions. Indeed, a 5-year study of incomplete abortions managed at the San Francisco General Hospital in 1937 reported that 85% of the 730 cases of incomplete abortion resulted from self-induced abortion. The high risk of infection with incomplete self-induced abortions prompted practitioners to continue surgical management. While a 1953 follow-up study at the same institution found that the rate of illegally performed or self-induced abortions had fallen to only about 25% of incomplete abortions, the tendency to use surgical management strategies persisted.

In recent years, however, there has been a shift away from surgical evacuation of the uterus when patients undergoing spontaneous abortion are hemodynamically stable. The availability of effective antibiotics combined with the current low rate of self-induced abortion has markedly reduced the likelihood of infection. In addition, small, randomized, controlled trials have demonstrated the safety of expectant, rather than surgical management. Interestingly, a rarely cited descriptive study from the 1940s supports the practice of expectant management; Russell described 3739 cases of spontaneous abortion in Tennessee and did not find an increased complication rate among those patients treated medically or expectantly versus surgically.

Terminology

Proper understanding of the current management concepts for spontaneous abortion begins with a review of terminology. Regrettably, definitions and terminology are a mixture of lay language, antiquated obstetric terms, and legal jargon, including definitions from the 1973 US Supreme Court case of *Roe v Wade*. Table 18-1 contains the historic and current terms used by physicians, patients, and the legal system in describing states of pregnancy loss.

Because of religious and political connotations surrounding the term "abortion," it is recommended that care be taken when using this term in the presence of patients. Rather, the more acceptable lay terms, "miscarriage" or "pregnancy loss," can be substituted for "spontaneous abortion."

Table 18-1

Terms and Definitions Describing Pregnancy Loss

HISTORIC	
TERM	**DEFINITION**
Criminal abortions	All "nontherapeutic" induced abortions performed before 1973 (see therapeutic abortion)
Missed abortion	Prolonged retention of nonviable fetus *for longer than 8 weeks* and recognized before 20 weeks' gestation; this obsolete term should rarely be used
Therapeutic abortion	Pre–*Roe vs. Wade* (1973) terminology for an abortion performed to save the life of the mother

CURRENT	
TERM	**DEFINITION**
Abortion	Termination of pregnancy by any means before fetus is sufficiently developed to survive
Anembryonic demise, blighted ovum	Embryo degenerated or absent on ultrasound evaluation
Elective abortion	Induced abortion performed after 1973
Incomplete abortion	Expulsion of only a portion of pregnancy tissue at less than 20 weeks' gestation
Inevitable abortion	Less than 20 weeks' gestation with cramping, bleeding, rupture of membranes, and dilated cervix
Intrauterine fetal demise or IUFD	Fetal death in utero
Miscarriage	Spontaneous pregnancy loss, lay term
Septic abortion	Signs of intrauterine infection in conjunction with spontaneous or elective abortion
Spontaneous abortion	In utero fetal demise and expulsion at less than 20 weeks' gestation or less than 500 g fetal weight
Stillbirth	Greater than 20 weeks' gestation or greater than 500 g fetal weight, not living at time of birth
Threatened abortion	Bleeding or cramping in viable pregnancy before 20 weeks' gestation

Pathophysiology

Spontaneous Abortion Process

Expulsion of a pregnancy from the uterus occurs with cervical dilation and myometrial contractions. This process is mediated by alpha-adrenergic, hormonal, and prostaglandin stimulation. Oxytocin, released from the posterior pituitary gland, acts to mobilize calcium and initiate the myometrial contractile process. Inflammation, infection, or irritation, such as from blood within the uterus, will result in prostaglandin and cytokine release. The prostaglandins PGE_2 and $PGF_{2\alpha}$ are secreted by the endometrium and uterine cervix and result in activation or contraction of uterine myometrial fibers. These prostaglandins act to break down collagen fibrils in the cervix by increasing the water content, thereby breaking collagen cross-links, as well as mobilizing calcium stores. The mechanical force generated by uterine contractions and softening of the cervix ultimately leads to cervical dilation and pregnancy expulsion.

Hemorrhage occurs because of uterine atony (failure of the uterus to contract sufficiently, usually caused by either partial retained products of conception or infection). Atony can be exacerbated by lack of intrinsic prostaglandins or by an abnormality at the receptor level.

Anatomy

Management of the pregnant patient in the process of a spontaneous abortion requires an understanding of pelvic anatomy and the ability to assess uterine size and position. Prior to a surgical procedure, the practitioner should assess whether the uterus is anteverted, retroverted, or midposition as well as the angle of flexion between the cervix and the corpus (anteflexed, retroflexed, or nonflexed). Assessment of uterine size correlates with the number of gestational weeks or weeks from the last menstrual period. In general, an 8-week-sized uterus is approximately 8 cm in length (a small orange), a 10-week size is 10 cm in length, and a 12-week size is 12 cm in length (a medium-sized grapefruit).

The predominant uterine blood supply is through the uterine arteries that branch from the internal iliac or hypogastric arteries and the ovarian arteries that branch directly from the descending aorta. Control of these vascular structures, surgically or by arterial embolization, is imperative when patients have life-threatening hemorrhage associated with a spontaneous abortion that is unresponsive to other measures.

Pain occurring during a spontaneous abortion is mediated by activation of visceral sensory fibers from the uterus, cervix, and upper vagina, which travel through the hypogastric plexuses to the sacral, lumbar, and lower thoracic sympathetic chains to enter the spinal cord. Complete anesthesia for relief of pain during a spontaneous abortion at 20 weeks' gestation requires a T10–S5 block.

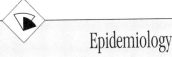

Epidemiology

Incidence

Approximately 50% of all pregnancies end in spontaneous abortion. Many of these spontaneous losses are subclinical with only 20% to 30% of recognized pregnancies resulting in spontaneous abortion. The incidence of spontaneous abortion increases with maternal age, partially corresponding to an age-related increase in the risk of nondisjunctional chromosomal abnormalities. The rate of spontaneous abortions is also increased in younger women with high gravidity.

Cause

Fifty percent of all spontaneous losses and 90% of losses occurring before 6 weeks have abnormal fetal chromosomes. The frequency of chromosomal abnormalities is related to the developmental stage, with very early losses more apt to be caused by chromosomal abnormalities or morphologic defects than losses that occur later in pregnancy. The most common chromosomal abnormality in spontaneous abortion specimens is trisomy 16.

Submucosal leiomyomas (fibroids) may interfere with implantation, especially when they are in a posterior fundal location, and have been implicated in very early pregnancy loss. Uterine anomalies such as bicornuate uterus, uterine septum, T-shaped uterus, and unicornuate uterus are more commonly associated with second-trimester and early third-trimester losses and are not generally associated with first-trimester spontaneous abortion.

Multiple infectious agents have been linked to early spontaneous abortion. Among the most common include mycoplasma, ureaplasma, listeria, herpes, brucella, rubella, cytomegalovirus, toxoplasmosis, and chlamydia. Maternal illnesses such as diabetes mellitus, hyperthyroidism, and hypothyroidism have also been implicated; however, thyroid disease is more apt to result in

Table 18-2

Maternal Morbidity and Mortality from Childbirth, Ectopic Pregnancy, and Spontaneous and Elective Abortions

	MORTALITY RATES	MORBIDITY RATES[a]
Childbirth	12/100,000	5/100
Ectopic pregnancy	100/100,000	Unknown
First-trimester abortion		
Elective termination	<0.5/100,000	0.5/100
Spontaneous loss	0.7/100,000	Unknown
Second-trimester abortion		
Elective termination	10/100,000	Dilation and evacuation 0.7/100
		Saline instillation 2/100
Spontaneous loss	2.3/100,000	Unknown

[a]Morbidities include fever, hemorrhage, infection, retained products of conception, and uterine perforation.
SOURCE: Data from Saraiya M, Green C, et al: Spontaneous abortion–related deaths among women in the United States—1981–1991. *Obstet Gynecol* 93:172, 1999.

anovulation with infertility than in early pregnancy loss. In addition, maternal chronic wasting diseases, including human immunodeficiency virus infection, carcinomatosis, tuberculosis, and severe malnutrition, can result in spontaneous pregnancy loss.

Lastly, trauma and teratogenic exposures are associated with pregnancy loss. Trauma data show that over 50% of pregnancies associated with major direct pelvic or abdominal trauma do not survive. Early pregnancy exposure to teratogenic substances typically results in first-trimester loss.

Morbidity and Mortality

Information on the natural history of spontaneous abortion and, concomitantly, morbidity and mortality figures related to spontaneous abortion are not well documented, as many women who have a spontaneous abortion do not seek medical attention, and no national reporting systems exist. However, using data on reported spontaneous abortion fatalities from the Centers for Disease Control (CDC) and Prevention's Pregnancy Mortality Surveillance System, and estimating the number of annual spontaneous abortions in the

United States, the overall mortality rate from spontaneous abortion is probably about 0.7/100,000. These data and other information about maternal morbidity and mortality of childbirth and ectopic and elective termination are available from the CDC and are summarized in Table 18-2.

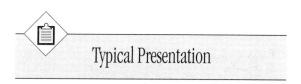

Typical Presentation

Patients presenting with cramping, bleeding, and a positive pregnancy test should be triaged based on severity of symptoms, physical examination, and ancillary diagnostic tests. Women with an inevitable or incomplete spontaneous abortion require specific management (expectant, medical, or surgical). Therefore, it is essential to distinguish patients with these conditions, especially those who are hemodynamically unstable, from those with threatened and completed abortions. It is also essential not to miss those who have an ectopic or molar pregnancy or fail to identify women with a viable pregnancy during a threatened abortion.

Inevitable Spontaneous Abortion

By definition, women having inevitable spontaneous abortions present with either a dilated cervix
or spontaneous rupture of membranes; severe
cramping and bleeding are also usually present.
Ultrasound most commonly demonstrates a nonviable intrauterine pregnancy, as shown in Figure 18-1. On occasion, despite significant vaginal
bleeding and full cervical dilation (the latter indicating inevitable abortion), fetal cardiac activity
may still be seen on ultrasound. Nonetheless,
even if fetal heart activity is identified, the presence of significant cervical dilation or ruptured
membranes before 20 weeks' gestation indicates
that pregnancy loss is inevitable.

Incomplete Spontaneous Abortion

Incomplete spontaneous abortions are those in
which the products of conception have been partially, but not completely, expelled. Women with
incomplete spontaneous abortions present with a
wide variety of symptoms, and not all patients

Figure 18-1

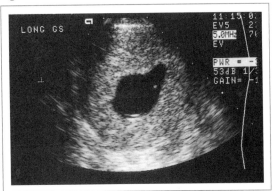

Inevitable abortion. Ultrasound showing nonviable, 8-week
intrauterine pregnancy in a patient who has an inevitable
abortion. Note that the gestational sac *(dark area)* is
irregularly shaped and contains only a speck of an involuting
embryo. (*Courtesy of Dr. Theodore Dubinsky, University of
Washington Medical Center.*)

Figure 18-2

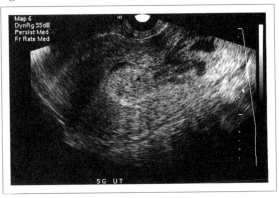

Incomplete spontaneous abortion. Ultrasound showing
products of conception in the uterus of a patient who has
had an incomplete spontaneous abortion. The uterus is filled
with material that has heterogencous echogenicity, and no
embryo can be identified. (*Courtesy of Dr. Theodore
Dubinsky, University of Washington Medical Center.*)

initially seek medical attention. Most commonly,
however, patients describe having passed tissue,
but they continue to have bothersome, intermittent cramping and bleeding.

The uterus is often tender and still enlarged,
even if tissue has been passed. The cervix may or
may not still be dilated, and the patient may have
a fever. However, patients can be afebrile with
a closed cervix and a nontender uterus and still
have retained products of conception demonstrated on transvaginal ultrasound (Fig. 18-2).

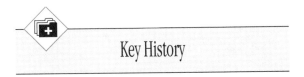

Key History

The presentation of inevitable and incomplete
abortions is discussed in the previous section. The
history is the key for distinguishing these two conditions (i.e., incomplete and inevitable spontaneous abortions) from threatened and complete
abortions and from ectopic and molar pregnancies (Table 18-3). The distinction must be made
because treatments for these conditions are quite

different from those for inevitable or incomplete spontaneous abortions. Treating a threatened abortion with interventions intended for incomplete or inevitable abortions can result in terminating a viable pregnancy. Intervening unnecessarily when patients have a completed abortion exposes the patient to unnecessary risks of treatment. Failure to identify an ectopic pregnancy or gestational trophoblastic disease (molar pregnancy) exposes the patient to the life-threatening effects of these conditions. Therefore, these four

important differential diagnoses are discussed in greater detail here.

Differential Diagnoses— Identification and Management

THREATENED SPONTANEOUS ABORTION

Threatened spontaneous abortion is defined as vaginal bleeding and/or uterine cramping in a woman who still has a potentially viable pregnancy with a closed cervix and intact membranes. Therefore, the typical history of patients with a threatened spontaneous abortion is light cramping and bleeding; these patients also have a closed cervical os and normal fetal cardiac activity on ultrasound. Patients with threatened abortions are generally clinically stable and should be followed expectantly, as 50% of these women will continue pregnancy without complication and will deliver at term.

COMPLETED SPONTANEOUS ABORTION

A completed spontaneous abortion is one in which the products of conception have been completely expelled from the uterus. Patients give a history of improving symptoms with decreased cramping and bleeding, following passage of tissue appropriate in quantity for the gestational age. Patients should always be requested to bring tissue passed at home for inspection in the office. If passage of tissue was recent, the cervix may still be open. If a patient reports passage of tissue, but presents with uterine tenderness and fever, an ultrasound can often distinguish between an incomplete abortion, in which tissue remains in the uterus, and a postabortal endometritis as a cause of the fever and tenderness. Completed abortions should be identified and followed expectantly.

ECTOPIC PREGNANCY

Ectopic pregnancies most commonly present with spotting rather than profuse vaginal bleeding, and the pain of ectopic pregnancy is more localized

Table 18-3

Key History and Symptoms for Diagnosis of Incomplete or Inevitable Spontaneous Abortion

HISTORY
Last normal menstrual period and interval from preceding menses
Length of menstrual cycles
Known conception
Date of positive pregnancy test and type of test
History of PID, IUD, prior ectopic pregnancy, tubal ligation
Previous history of pregnancy loss or history of birth defects
Desired or undesired pregnancy
Social support system

SYMPTOMS
Fever
Faint or dizzy
Shoulder pain
Pain or cramps: midline or lateral, bilateral or unilateral
Passage of tissue and description of tissue
Blood loss—duration, pattern, and volume[a]
Signs of pregnancy (nausea, bloating, breast tenderness)

[a]Estimated by the number of pads or tampons used/24 hours. A *soaked* pad ~20 cc blood and a *soaked* tampon ~10 cc blood. Soaked pads and tampons indicate heavy bleeding, as it is uncommon for women to soak their protection.

lateral pelvic pain than the generalized cramps of spontaneous abortion. Risk factors for ectopic pregnancy include a history of infertility or pelvic inflammatory disease, intrauterine device usage, prior ectopic pregnancies, tubal ligation, and multiple sexual partners.

Patients may present with dizziness, syncope, or shoulder pain, the latter resulting from irritation of the diaphragm caused by hemoperitoneum. Rarely will patients describe having passed significant tissue, and, if so, this is usually found on gross inspection to be clot or decidual cast, rather than placental or fetal tissue. Ectopic pregnancies require either surgical treatment or medical management with methotrexate; patients should be referred to a clinician with experience in these therapeutic modalities.

MOLAR PREGNANCY OR GESTATIONAL TROPHOBLASTIC DISEASE

Molar pregnancy may present with size greater than dates and several weeks or even months of persistent spotting or bleeding. On occasion, patients present with profuse vaginal bleeding and hemodynamic instability or with signs of hyperthyroidism. Recognition of a molar pregnancy is important because of the potential risk of choriocarcinoma with metastatic gestational trophoblastic disease.

Ultrasound findings are often diagnostic. If molar pregnancy is diagnosed, stable patients should be referred to a gynecologist for follow-up care and to monitor for ongoing, gestational trophoblastic disease.

Key Physical Examination

The triage of a patient for expectant or medical management, instead of surgical management, depends on establishment of a low-risk clinical profile on physical examination. Any patient with orthostasis, profuse blood loss, fever, purulent drainage from the cervical os, or uterine size larger than 11 weeks should not be considered for medical or expectant management. Table 18-4 lists the key components of the physical examination.

Ancillary Tests

Historically, no ancillary tests were available to help distinguish spontaneous abortion from other con-

Table 18-4
Key Components of Physical Examination

EXAMINATION COMPONENT	FINDING	SIGNIFICANCE
Vital signs	Fever	Infection
	Orthostatic hypotension	Excessive blood loss; sepsis
Abdomen	Distended, tender	Hemoperitoneum from ectopic pregnancy
Cervix	Amount of bleeding from os	Quantity of bleeding
	Cervical motion tenderness	Infection
	Os open	Inevitable abortion
	Purulent drainage from os	Infection
	Tissue in cervix or vagina	Incomplete abortion
Uterus	Uterine size and position	Establishes age of pregnancy
	Uterine tenderness	Infection or incomplete abortion

ditions for which it can be mistaken, and tissue obtained during dilation and curettage was the gold standard for diagnostic confirmation of spontaneous abortion. Today, diagnosis is aided by findings on transvaginal ultrasound, coupled with single or serial measurements of beta-human chorionic gonadotropin (β-hCG) levels. Additional tests that may be useful in differentiating spontaneous abortion from other conditions are auscultation with a Doppler stethoscope and performance of culdocentesis. Finally, baseline hematologic tests should be obtained to assist in the diagnosis and management of hemorrhage and to permit prevention of Rh fetal isoimmunization in future pregnancies.

Hematologic Tests

Baseline blood tests should always be performed for pregnant women presenting with cramping and bleeding. These tests include measurement of hematocrit plus typing and screening for assessment of blood type and Rh status. Blood typing and cross matching of blood for transfusion should be performed if extensive blood loss is suspected or

has occurred. If there is suspicion of infection, a white blood cell count is obtained.

Ultrasound and β-hCG

The diagnosis of spontaneous abortion, as well as its distinction from other conditions, has been revolutionized by the availability of ultrasound studies and β-hCG assays. The key ultrasound and β-hCG findings that distinguish threatened, inevitable, complete, and incomplete spontaneous abortion from one another and from ectopic, molar, and multiple gestation pregnancies are shown in Table 18-5.

At 6 weeks' gestation or later, and with a β-hCG level of greater than 1500 IU (Third International Reference Standard [IRS]), an intrauterine pregnancy should be visualized on transvaginal ultrasound. If a pregnancy is not visualized under these conditions, and the patient gives no history of passing tissue, she should be considered to have an ectopic pregnancy until proven otherwise. If she is stable and reliable without hemoperitoneum, serial β-hCGs can be followed to see if they double appropriately.

Table 18-5
Ultrasound and β-hCG Interpretations

DIAGNOSIS	ULTRASOUND FINDINGS	β-HCG (IU/L)
Inevitable abortion (nonviable intrauterine pregnancy)	Empty gestational sac >20 mm, fetal pole >5 mm without fetal heart tones	variable
Incomplete abortion	Endometrial thickness >5 mm and irregular	variable
Threatened abortion (viable intrauterine pregnancy)	Visible embryo with cardiac motion	>1500
Threatened abortion, unsure viability	<20 mm gestational sac, <5 mm fetal pole	<1500
Complete abortion	Endometrium thin and uniform	variable
Ectopic, possible or unsure viability	Empty uterus	<1500
Ectopic, definite	Empty uterus, ± adnexal pregnancy seen[a]	>1500
Molar pregnancy	"Snowy field"	variable
Multiple gestation	Multiple gestational sacs	>1500

[a]No tissue passed by history.

β-hCG, beta human chorionic gonadotropin, measured by Third International Reference Standard (IRS); IU/L, international units/liter.

In general, β-hCG should double every 48 to 72 hours in a viable pregnancy. Unchanged or falling β-hCGs suggest a nonviable pregnancy or an ectopic pregnancy. If spontaneous abortion was completed recently, β-hCG may still be quite high.

Most laboratories now use the 3rd IRS for computing β-hCG levels, but the 1st and 2nd IRS may still be used at some institutions. A general rule of thumb is that the 3rd IRS is roughly equivalent to the 1st IRS; and the 2nd IRS is equivalent to double the 1st or 3rd IRS. This rough correlation should be used in interpretation of the literature when reference standards from different institutions are used. Furthermore, because of variability in β-hCG assay techniques, it is important not to make clinical decisions using two levels analyzed at two different laboratories, even if both institutions use the same IRS.

If no intrauterine pregnancy is visualized on ultrasound, the patient does not describe having passed tissue, and the β-hCG level is less than 1500 IU (3rd IRS), she may have either a viable, early, threatened abortion (i.e., unsure viability of the pregnancy); a nonviable pregnancy; or an ectopic pregnancy. Unsure viability is further defined on ultrasound by the presence of a gestational sac of less than 20 mm or a fetal pole of less than 5 mm. A nonviable intrauterine pregnancy is defined by an empty gestational sac of larger than 20 mm on ultrasound or by a fetal pole of greater than 5 mm without fetal heart activity.

Completed spontaneous abortion can often be confirmed by transvaginal ultrasound when the endometrial lining is found to be uniform and thin and when serial β-hCG levels fall as demonstrated in Figure 18-3. Incomplete spontaneous abortion is suggested when endometrial thickness is irregular and heterogeneous (a very thickened irregular lining is highly suggestive of retained products of conception) and when serial β-hCGs do not fall appropriately.

Doppler Auscultation

If ultrasound is not available and the pregnancy is assessed to be greater than 10 weeks of gestation,

Figure 18-3

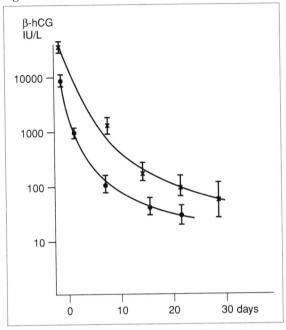

β-hCG levels in induced and spontaneous abortion. The top curve (x) shows levels seen with induced abortions. The lower curve (•) shows the levels seen with spontaneous abortions. Note that the scale is semilogarithmic and uses hCG units in the 2nd International Reference Standard (IRS). Most laboratories today use 3rd IRS units, which are approximately half of the 2nd IRS value. (*Adapted from Steier et al, 1984.*)

an attempt to confirm viability using Doppler for fetal heart tones is useful and important. Fetal heart tones are usually heard at 10 weeks, but are almost always heard by 12 weeks of gestation. In very large ectopic pregnancies, fetal heart tones may be heard by Doppler, but this finding is very rare.

Culdocentesis

Culdocentesis, the passage of a needle through the posterior vaginal fornix into the pelvic cavity to sample for blood, was once a key test in the evaluation of patients with possible ectopic pregnancy. It is now rarely needed because intraperitoneal fluid is easily quantified and assessed with ultrasound. If ultrasound is not available, however, or if fluid seen on ultrasound has an echogenicity not clearly consistent with blood, a culdocentesis may be appropriate to determine the presence and/or nature of intraperitoneal fluid.

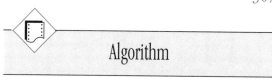

Algorithm

The algorithms shown in Figures 18-4 and 18-5 illustrate the general approach to diagnosis and management of first- and second-trimester spontaneous abortions. Table 18-6 lists information that

Figure 18-4

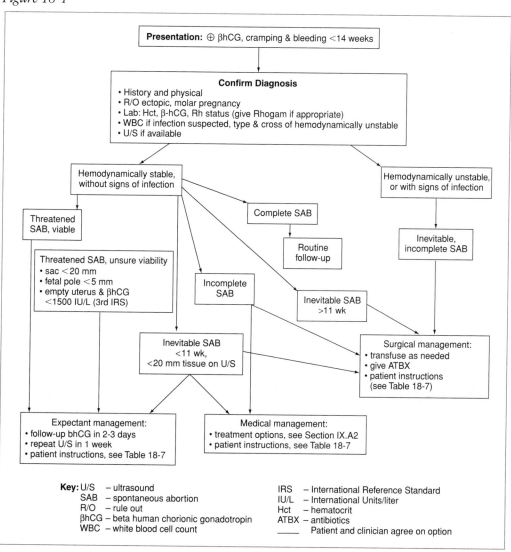

Algorithm for diagnosis and management of first-trimester spontaneous abortion.

Figure 18-5

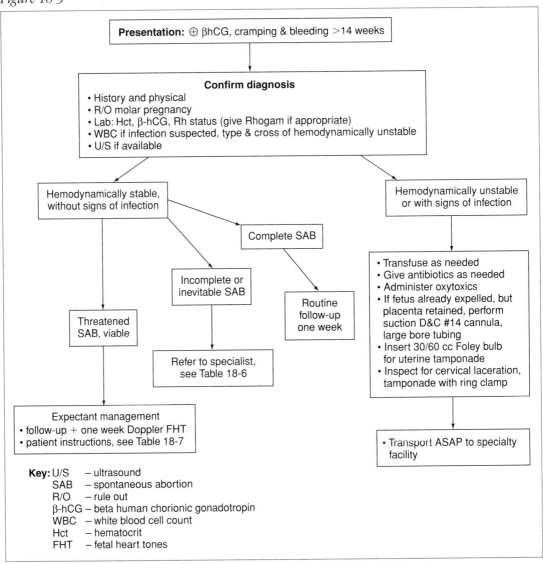

Algorithm for diagnosis and management of second-trimester spontaneous abortion.

Table 18-6

Information Needed When Referring Patients
to a Specialist Because of Spontaneous Abortion

1. Gestational age
2. Diagnosis
3. Hemodynamic stability (vital signs, including orthostatic blood pressure)
4. Infection present or absent
5. Ultrasound findings
6. Lab work (Hct, WBC, Rh status, βhCG)
7. Treatment attempted
8. Emotional state of patient and social support

will be needed when referring a patient with a spontaneous abortion to a specialist.

Treatment

First-Trimester Spontaneous Abortion, Nonsurgical Management

An inevitable or incomplete abortion in a patient who is stable, reliable, and without evidence of infection can often be safely treated with expectant or medical management. However, no large, randomized, controlled trials exist to compare the outcomes of expectant management with those of medical management.

EXPECTANT MANAGEMENT

Expectant management of inevitable or incomplete spontaneous abortion involves waiting for the patient to complete the abortion process by spontaneously expelling the products of conception. Recent studies suggest no increase in complications and a higher level of patient satisfaction when expectant management is undertaken. These studies also show no decrease in future fertility in comparison with women whose spontaneous abor-

tions are managed surgically. However, a woman is only a candidate for expectant management if she is hemodynamically stable, has no evidence of infection, and is deemed reliable to follow instructions. She should be fully informed of risks of expectant management, along with other options for management, including completion of the abortion using uterine curettage.

Sample instructions for patients undergoing expectant management of spontaneous abortion are given as in Table 18-7. In addition, Rh immune globulin (Rhogam) must be administered to all Rh-negative patients.

MEDICAL MANAGEMENT

Medical management refers to the use of medications to hasten expulsion of the uterine contents of patients with an inevitable or incomplete

Table 18-7

Sample Instructions for Patients Undergoing Expectant
or Medical Management of Spontaneous Abortion

Check back if you:
    Have a temperature exceeding 100.4°F
    Feel faint or dizzy
    Soak more than one pad per hour for 2 hours in a row
    Soak more than 8 pads/24 hours
    Have cramping and bleeding that continue beyond 5 days

We recommend that you:
    Take your temperature every 8 hours or if you feel hot
    Refrain from intercourse and strenuous exercise
    Increase fluid intake
    Rest in bed if contractions are severe
    Take ibuprofen 400 to 800 mg every 6 hours as needed for pain

Call your provider at _____ to get advice, to let us know how you are doing, or to schedule an appointment.

abortion. Medical management can be offered if the patient is stable, has no evidence of infection, and the pregnancy is less than 11 weeks' gestation. When medications are used, the same guidelines used in the expectant management scheme, as outlined in Table 18-7, should be followed to minimize the risk of hemorrhage or infection.

The prostaglandin, PGE_1 (misoprostol), has been used both in oral and suppository form for medical treatment of spontaneous abortion. Most commonly, the patient or provider places four 200 mcg tablets of misoprostol into the posterior vaginal fornix. Increased cramping is expected within the next 4 to 6 hours, with expulsion of tissue within 24 hours. If the tissue is not expelled, and the patient continues to be stable, the procedure can be repeated.

In many other countries, misoprostol therapy is combined with mifepristone (RU-486), an antiprogesterone agent. In the United States, however, mifepristone is only available in research settings and is not approved by the US Food and Drug Administration. Research suggests that mifepristone is most effective in anembryonic pregnancies. Preliminary research indicates that tamoxifen may also be effective for treating inevitable or incomplete spontaneous abortion.

Methergine can be used to evacuate the uterus after incomplete spontaneous abortion when only a small amount of tissue is retained and when there is no evidence of infection. It is given in 0.2-mg doses orally, intracervically, or intramuscularly every 6 hours for 24 hours.

First-Trimester Spontaneous Abortion, Surgical Management

Suction curettage is an alternative to expectant or medical management for treatment of incomplete or inevitable spontaneous abortions of less than 11 weeks' gestation. It is the treatment of choice for incomplete or inevitable spontaneous abortions from 11 to 14 weeks of gestation and is recommended at less than 11 weeks' gestation for patients who are hemodynamically unstable or show signs of infection.

Many primary-care clinicians perform suction curettage for spontaneous abortions at less than 12 weeks of gestation. After 12 weeks of gestation, however, complications such as uterine perforation are more common; for this reason, in more advanced pregnancies suction curettage is usually performed by a gynecologist. Preoperative measures and the suction curettage procedure are described below.

PREOPERATIVE MEDICATIONS

Preoperative medications to be considered for patients undergoing suction curettage are Rh immune globulin and antibiotics. As described later, sedation and analgesia are also frequently used.

RH IMMUNE GLOBULIN   Just as with patients undergoing expectant or medical management, patients undergoing suction curettage should be tested to determine their Rh status. Those who are Rh negative should receive Rh immune globulin.

ANTIBIOTICS   Antibiotics are administered if there are signs of infection. Antibiotic treatment can be given on an inpatient or outpatient basis, depending on the severity of infection and on whether the patient is a suitable candidate for outpatient treatment. A patient is considered a suitable candidate for outpatient antibiotic treatment if her childbearing is complete, if she is reliable and capable of complying with treatment, and if she is not systemically ill (defined as no or low-grade fever, no more than a slightly elevated white blood cell count, no tachycardia or hypotension, and only mild uterine tenderness). All other patients should be admitted for intravenous therapy. Antibiotic regimens are outlined in Table 18-8.

In the absence of infection, the need for antibiotics is less clear. No randomized controlled trials have examined antibiotic prophylaxis in the medical or surgical management of spontaneous abortion. It is well established that prophylaxis with doxycycline at the time of elective pregnancy terminations is effective in decreasing the risk of

Table 18-8

Antibiotic Regimens for Spontaneous Abortion Accompanied by Infection

	OUTPATIENT ORAL THERAPY[a]	INPATIENT INTRAVENOUS THERAPY[b]
Regimen A	Ofloxacin 400 mg po BID × 14 d *plus* Metronidazole 500 mg po BID × 14 d	Gentamicin 2 mg/kg IV load, then 1.5 mg/kg TID (single dosing may be substituted) *plus* Clindamycin 900 mg IV TID *followed by* Doxycycline 100 mg po BID × 10 d *or* clindamycin 450 mg po QID × 10 d
Regimen B	Cefoxitin[c] 2 g IV × 1 *plus* Probenecid 1 g po × 1 *plus* Doxycycline 100 mg po BID × 14 d	Cefoxitin 2 g IV QID *plus* doxycycline 100 mg po/IV × 14 d
Regimen C		Cefotetan 2 g IV BID *plus* doxycycline 100 mg IV/po × 14 d

[a]Outpatient treatment is only appropriate for stable, reliable patients who have only subtle signs of infection (see text).
[b]Inpatient therapy is indicated for patients who are systemically ill, septic, or not candidates for outpatient treatment.
[c]Can substitute any third-generation cephalosporin for cefoxitin.

postprocedure endometritis. Based on these data, and until studies are available on patients with spontaneous abortions who have no infection, most clinicians recommend antibiotic prophylaxis for patients undergoing suction curettage or other instrumented procedures. Data on outcomes of noninfected spontaneous vaginal deliveries performed without antibiotic prophylaxis would suggest that, similarly, prophylaxis is not warranted in the expectant or medical management of spontaneous abortion.

INFORMED CONSENT

Consent is obtained by explaining options for treatment (expectant, medical, and surgical) and by outlining known complications of the procedure (Table 18-9). The most important complications are infection, bleeding, uterine or cervical injury, and delayed complications such as Asherman's syndrome. In addition, some patients may

experience an adverse reaction to medications administered as part of the treatment regimen.

Table 18-9

Complications of First-Trimester Suction Curettage

	COMPLICATION	INCIDENCE
Immediate	Hemorrhage requiring transfusion	0.6/100
	Uterine perforation	0.1/100
	Anesthetic reaction	0.2/100
	Hematometra	0.1/100
	Laceration of cervix	0.2/100
Delayed	Retained products	<1/100
	Infection	1/100
Late	Asherman's syndrome	<<1/100
	Subsequent infertility	Unknown
	Rh sensitization (if no Rhogam is given)	2.6/100

An accurate description of the risks and benefits of the various treatment options is difficult to provide because there are no large randomized trials that compare expectant and medical management. However, a meta-analysis of observational and randomized trials involving 18 studies comparing expectant (545 pooled subjects), medical (198 pooled subjects), and surgical management (1408 pooled subjects) showed successful outcomes in 92.5%, 51.5%, and 93.6%, respectively. These data might lead one to conclude that surgical and expectant management outcomes are equivalent and that medical management is inferior. However, the studies included in the medical treatment arm varied greatly in gestational age and doses and types of agents used, and therefore it may be premature to draw conclusions from these data alone.

A further consideration in obtaining consent involves dealing with teenagers. In many states, pregnant teenagers are considered "emancipated minors" and can consent to dilation and curettage without the signature of a parent. Each state's Attorney General's Office can provide information regarding the statutes that govern consent and confidentiality in pregnant minors, as well as the state's definition of a minor.

CERVICAL DILATION

Before proceeding with suction curettage, the cervix should be dilated to at least the same mm diameter as the number of weeks of gestation and, ideally should be dilated by an additional 1 to 2 mm. In other words, a 10-week pregnancy should be dilated to 10 to 12 mm.

Dilation can be assessed with a digital examination of the cervix or by visual inspection of the cervix during a speculum examination. If the cervix is not dilated, one can proceed immediately with mechanical dilation or use chemical dilation. Chemical dilation is safer than mechanical techniques, but because it takes longer to achieve, it is not appropriate if immediate dilation is required (such as in a hemodynamically unstable patient).

CHEMICAL DILATION   Chemical dilation can be achieved by placing Laminaria (a natural product produced from seaweed) or a synthetic polymeric dilator such as Dilapan into the cervix. Use of these products for cervical dilation decreases the rate of uterine perforation and cervical lacerations by a factor of five. They can be used in the absence of hemorrhage or infection for patients who are not expected to expel the pregnancy within the subsequent 24 hours. A 2 mm laminaria results in 11 mm of cervical dilation over approximately 12 hours.

MECHANICAL DILATION   If immediate evacuation is required, one should proceed with mechanical dilation. Mechanical dilation is typically preceded by anesthesia, patient preparation, and a paracervical block described in the following section. Gentleness is the key to safe cervical dilation, along with the anatomic awareness that the cervix is 3 to 4 cm long and that mild resistance should be encountered at the cervicouterine junction or internal os. Thus, resistance felt at 3 to 4 cm is not caused by pressure against the uterine fundus.

Mechanical dilation is performed using sequentially larger cervical dilators until the cervix is dilated appropriately. Hegar or Sims dilators are most commonly used. Lubrication of the dilators with a water-soluble lubricant such as K-Y jelly will usually facilitate passage of the dilators through the cervix.

ANESTHESIA AND PATIENT PREPARATION

The patient is placed in dorsal lithotomy position and intravenous medications are administered. Fentanyl is recommended in doses described in Table 18-10, with or without midazolam or diazepam. If Laminaria or Dilapan have been placed, they are removed. Examination with attention to uterine size and position is performed. A sterile speculum is placed in the vagina, and the cervix is cleansed with an antiseptic solution. Local anesthetic is then injected into the base of the cervix at the 2 o'clock, 5 o'clock, 7 o'clock, and 10 o'clock positions. If the patient has significant hemorrhage, the paracervical block can be omitted.

Table 18-10

Instruments and Medications for Suction Curettage

INSTRUMENTS RECOMMENDED FOR FIRST-TRIMESTER SUCTION CURETTAGE
Graves medium vaginal speculum
Bierer atraumatic tenaculum
Foerster sponge forceps—curved and straight
Polyp forceps, De Lee
Hegar, Pratt, or Denniston cervical dilators, size 2–13 mm or 3–43 French
Uterine curette, Sims, size 2

EQUIPMENT THAT SHOULD BE IMMEDIATELY AVAILABLE
Vaginal retractors, Heaney
Needle holder, Heaney, long
Tissue forceps, long
Sopher forceps, large serrations (only used in second trimester)
Uterine sound
Uterine curette, Sims, sizes 3 and 4

DISPOSABLE EQUIPMENT AND SUPPLIES
Betadine
Chloroprocaine (2%) or lidocaine (1%) (15 mL—0.1 mg/kg)
Fentanyl, 50 mcg/mL in 2-mL ampule @ 1 mcg/kg dose
Atropine, 0.4 mg (1 mL)
Methylergonovine, 0.2 mg/mL
2 Syringes: 5 mL for intravenous administration of analgesic   20 mL for paracervical block
3 Needles: 20 g to draw up medications   25 g (1½″) for paracervical block   25 g (½″) for intravenous medications
Gauze sponges, 4″ × 4″ (5)
Cotton balls (5)
Clear plastic collection tubing with clear plastic handle, 11-mm inside diameter
Cannulas, uterine evacuation, rigid, clear plastic or flexible 6-mm through 14-mm outside diameter, straight and curved

SOURCE: Adapted with permission from Darney PD, Hurbach DS, Korn AP. *Protocols for Office Gynecologic Surgery*. Boston, Blackwell, 1996.

SUCTION CURETTAGE

INSTRUMENTS Two different equipment options are available for suction curettage. The handheld suction device, as illustrated in Figure 18-6, can be used for any pregnancy under 11 weeks of gestation with corresponding appropriate cannula. These handheld suction devices are portable and extremely useful in the office and in rural settings. They can generate suction pressures equal to and sometimes greater than traditional mechanical devices such as floor suction machines.

Instruments recommended for first-trimester suction curettage are listed in Table 18-10. A "no-touch" sterile technique is suggested, such that all instrument tips that enter the uterus are never touched and therefore remain completely sterile;

Figure 18-6

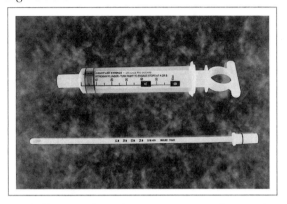

Handheld suction device for suction curettage. The cannula with syringe attached is directed into the uterine cavity after the tenaculum is placed. Suction is then applied by pulling back on the syringe plunger without changing the placement of the cannula. Suction curettage is then performed in multiple passes, reestablishing suction on each entry.

they are placed to the left side of the tray with handles to the right, or vice versa.

CURETTING THE UTERINE CAVITY   The anterior cervical lip is secured with a single-toothed tenaculum or ring clamp (Fig. 18-7, *A* and *B*). Slow, steady pressure during placement of the tenaculum or clamp results in less discomfort for the patient. If the cervix is not appropriately dilated, one should proceed with mechanical dilation, as described earlier.

It has been demonstrated that use of a traditional uterine sound instrument increases the risk of uterine perforation, and therefore sounding should not be performed. Instead, the suction cannula is inserted into the cervix and should pass smoothly into the lower uterine segment if the cervix has been properly dilated.

Once the cannula is within the lower uterine segment (Fig. 18-7*C*), suction is applied, and the cannula is not advanced further until amniotic fluid or products of conception are noted in the suction tubing. When amniotic fluid or products of conception are returned, the cannula is advanced to the fundus, and the uterine cavity is curetted with the suction cannula in a spiral fashion from fundus to internal os or with a gentle in-and-out

motion. The spiral technique is safer than an in-and-out motion for the inexperienced practitioner. Gentle traction on the cervix is important during suction curettage; it stabilizes the uterus and straightens the natural anatomic angle between the cervix and corpus allowing safe passage of instruments, thereby lowering the risk of perforation (Fig. 18-7*D*).

After suction curettage is complete, gentle, sharp curettage with a Sims curette will ensure complete removal of the products of conception. In pregnancies of less than 8 weeks of gestation, the tissue removed from the uterus should always be grossly inspected for confirmation that villi are present (Fig. 18-8). In more advanced pregnancies (9 weeks or greater), the products of conception should be inspected to ensure that all fetal parts have been removed from the uterus.

Second-Trimester Spontaneous Abortion

Spontaneous abortions at greater than 14 weeks of gestation are managed by dilation and evacuation (D&E). All such pregnancies should be referred to a specialist for treatment, unless the primary-care clinician has had specialized training and experience in surgical management of second-trimester spontaneous abortions.

In preparation for referral and transport, the clinician should ensure that the patient is hemodynamically stable and not bleeding excessively. Hypotension is managed with standard interventions, including intravenous fluids and, if necessary, blood transfusion and other modalities.

Excessive bleeding in a presumed empty uterus is initially managed with manual massage of the uterus, along with agents that induce uterine contractions such as oxytocin, Methergine, misoprostol, and prostaglandin 15-methyl $F_{2\alpha}$ (Prostin). Oxytocin 30 mIU, diluted in 1 liter of saline, can be administered through a wide-open intravenous infusion along with Methergine 0.2 mg intracervically or intramuscularly every 10 minutes for up to four doses or until bleeding is controlled. If hemorrhage is not controlled by these measures,

0.25 mg of prostaglandin 15-methyl $F_{2\alpha}$ is given intramuscularly every 10 minutes up to four doses.

If the uterus is felt to be evacuated of fetal parts with only a portion of placenta remaining in the uterus, gentle uterine curettage with a large Hunter's curette can be performed, followed by suction with a #14 cannula and large-bore tubing. An additional measure to control bleeding, when the above measures have failed, is insertion of a large-bore Foley catheter into the uterus with the balloon filled with 30 to 75 cc of saline for uterine tamponade.

Figure 18-7

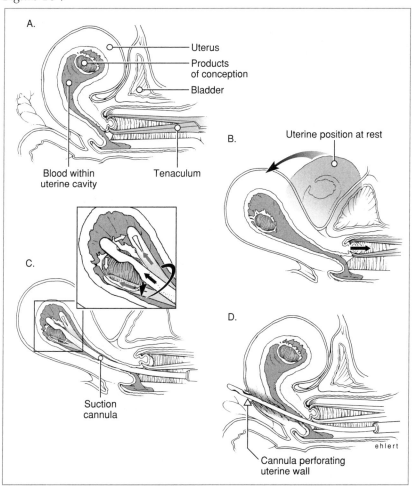

Passage of curette into uterine cavity. In most women, there is an angle of anteflexion or retroflexion at the cervicouterine junction; **A** illustrates anteflexion. In **B**, a tenaculum is applied to the lip of the cervix and traction is applied to straighten the cervicouterine flexure. This permits passage of instruments into the uterus with minimal difficulty, as shown in **C**. After insertion of the suction cannula, the instrument is rotated on its axis *(inset)* and moved inward and outward to retrieve tissue. Failure to apply traction can lead to perforation of the posterior uterine wall, as shown in **D**.

Figure 18-8

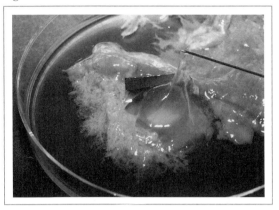

Chorionic villi. In pregnancies of 8 weeks or less, material removed from the uterus should be inspected to ensure that chorionic villi are present, thereby indicating that products of conception have been removed from the uterus. This photo shows the products of conception sitting in a glass dish. The pointer is lifting the wall of the 2.5-cm gestational sac. The fluffy tissue surrounding the gestational sac is chorionic villi. (*Courtesy of Dr. Alan Fantel, University of Washington Medical Center.*)

Finally, patients undergoing a second-trimester spontaneous abortion should be treated with antibiotics and Rh immune globulin, if appropriate. Indications for antibiotics and Rh immune globulin are the same as those for first-trimester spontaneous abortions.

Follow-Up Care

Normal follow-up involves emotional and supportive care from the clinician, with assistance from social workers, nurses, and other care providers. A check-back appointment should occur within 1 week after the abortion, with additional appointments as needed. Care should include attention to psychological and medical aspects of care.

PSYCHOLOGICAL CARE

A good understanding of the emotional meaning of pregnancy loss for each specific patient is imperative. It should not be assumed that all patients react with a sense of grief or loss. For example, if a pregnancy was unwanted, the patient may feel relieved, although she may feel guilty about the feeling of relief. Other patients react with a heavy sense of loss; most commonly, these are women with no prior pregnancy, with prior losses, or with a very wanted pregnancy. Some women may require psychiatric or counseling referral for severe grief, loss, mourning, or depression immediately following spontaneous abortion.

Care should be taken to involve the patient's partner, when appropriate, and to assess the partner's psychological needs. All patients/couples with these persistent symptoms at 8 weeks should be considered for antidepressant therapy or formal psychological counseling.

MEDICAL CARE

All patients with a completed abortion should receive instructions similar to those in Table 18-7. In addition, contraception should be discussed, as most patients will ovulate within 4 to 6 weeks from completion of spontaneous abortion, with an overall range of 2 weeks to 3 months. If the patient has not received prenatal or routine care prior to the spontaneous abortion, a Pap smear and screening for sexually transmitted disease is recommended.

Complications

Complications from surgical treatment of spontaneous abortion (Table 18-9) can be seen immediately after the procedure or be delayed for several weeks or months.

Immediate Complications

Immediate complications include hemorrhage, uterine perforation with potential for injury to pelvic and abdominal structures, and lacerations of the cervix. Anesthetic complications may also occur, but will not be discussed here. A review of anesthetic techniques is presented in Chapter 1.

HEMORRHAGE

Hemorrhage is most commonly caused by retention of products of conception, the presence of which can be confirmed with ultrasound. If ultrasound is not available, repeat curettage is performed as long as uterine perforation has not occurred.

Hemorrhage can also be caused from lacerations of uterine or cervical vessels, uterine perforation, or, most commonly, uterine atony. Uterine atony is usually treated with Methergine, 0.2 mg injected intracervically at the time of the procedure. Placement of a 30- to 75-cc Foley balloon into the uterine cavity, as described earlier, can be performed if other measures have failed. If a cervical laceration is visualized, it is tamponaded by grasping the bleeding laceration with a ring clamp and then performing a suture repair (see Chapter 20).

UTERINE PERFORATION

When uterine perforation occurs, the most common site is in the midline posteriorly. Perforations usually occur at the time of dilation as a result of forcing dilators through the cervix of patients with severe anteflexion or retroflexion of the uterus (see Fig. 18-7D). The risk of perforation can be reduced by applying traction to the cervix with the single-toothed tenaculum to straighten the cervicouterine axis. In addition, if difficulty is encountered in entering the uterus, ultrasound guidance and a flexible cannula can be used prior to insertion of rigid instruments.

Perforations can be managed expectantly if recognized prior to the use of suction or sharp instruments. Once suction or sharp instruments have been used, however, the possibility of damage to the gastrointestinal tract or other pelvic or abdominal viscera exists. If such injuries are suspected, or if the patient develops signs of hemorrhage or infection, laparoscopy or exploratory laparotomy should be performed immediately.

VASOVAGAL REACTION

A vasovagal reaction can occur because of cervical manipulation. Severe reactions should be treated immediately with intravenous atropine.

Delayed Complications

Delayed complications include infection and retained products of conception. Signs and symptoms of infection should always be treated promptly with antibiotic regimens similar to those described in Table 18-8. The complication of retained products of conception presents with delayed symptoms of fever and uterine tenderness. The diagnosis is usually made with uterine ultrasound, and the treatment is repeat suction curettage.

In exceedingly rare cases, patients with a uterine perforation and concomitant bowel or bladder laceration may develop uterine fistulae. Surgical repair is required.

Late Complications

Asherman's syndrome, Rh sensitization, and infertility are all rare, late complications of spontaneous abortion. Asherman's syndrome (formation of uterine synechiae that can obstruct or obliterate the uterine cavity) typically presents with amenorrhea or hypomenorrhea. Asherman's syndrome can be evaluated and treated with hysteroscopy.

Rh sensitization can occur when Rhogam either is not administered to an Rh-negative woman, or when an inadequate dose is administered in situations of severe hemorrhage. It is estimated that 2.6% of pregnancies in which Rhogam is not administered will have Rh sensitization in subsequent pregnancies.

Infertility from scarring of the fallopian tubes is an exceedingly rare complication of spontaneous abortion. It occurs from untreated pelvic infections that occur in association with the abortion or suction curettage.

Long-Term Monitoring and Prognosis

Most patients return to normal activities within 1 to 2 days following completion of spontaneous abortion whether it is managed expectantly, medically, or surgically. However, it can take 2 to 6 weeks before there is complete return to a nonpregnant state with normal hormone levels, resolution of emotional distress and fatigue, and normalization of anemia induced by bleeding. Mild cramping and bleeding can continue for several weeks following a spontaneous abortion. For most patients, complete physical recovery can be assumed by 4 weeks and emotional recovery is anticipated by 8 weeks.

As discussed earlier, ovulation should occur 2 to 12 weeks after spontaneous abortion. Appropriate counseling regarding contraception and the likelihood of subsequent pregnancy should be provided.

If the patient has had no prior miscarriage, the rate of recurrent miscarriage is approximately 15% to 20%, which is the same risk as in women with no history of spontaneous abortion. If she has had two prior spontaneous abortions, however, her risk of recurrence increases to approximately 30%, and with three miscarriages up to 40%. The risk of recurrence after more than six losses is approximately 50%.

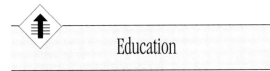

Education

Topics for education include self-management in the immediate period following treatment of spontaneous abortion (see Table 18-7). This information should be given in oral and written form, and should include instructions to call or return if fever, heavy bleeding, or uterine tenderness

develop. At some point after the spontaneous abortion is completed, patients should also receive information about the causes of spontaneous abortion (described earlier in this chapter) and about the risk of recurrence (described above).

Careful follow-up of teenagers is important, because their family and friends may not have been aware of the patient's pregnancy, and the patient may not tell family or friends about symptoms of postabortal complications she may be experiencing. Counseling about sexually transmitted diseases and birth control is essential in this age group.

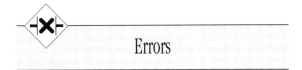

Errors

The most important errors in dealing with spontaneous abortions are misdiagnosis, overtreatment, miscalculation of the gestational age of the pregnancy, and failure to administer Rh immune globulin when indicated.

Misdiagnoses

The most important misdiagnosis is diagnosing spontaneous abortion when the patient actually has an ectopic or molar pregnancy. Such misdiagnosis can be life-threatening. This error can be avoided with appropriate use of ultrasound imaging, of which molar pregnancy has a classic appearance, and of which ectopic pregnancy can be suspected if products of conceptions cannot be visualized within the uterus.

Another diagnostic error is presuming that a spontaneous abortion is complete because the patient's bleeding has diminished and she reports passage of tissue, when, in reality, the abortion is incomplete and products of conception remain in the uterus. Missing an incomplete abortion can result in infection and hemorrhage. If the patient is not bleeding heavily and the cervix is closed, an ultrasound can be performed to document completion of the spontaneous abortion if the diagnosis is unclear.

Overtreatment

Overtreatment of completed spontaneous abortions involves use of suction curettage when expectant or medical management is a better alternative. Unnecessary use of curettage puts women at unnecessary risk from complications of dilation and curettage.

Overtreatment can also occur when a threatened spontaneous abortion with a viable pregnancy is treated with suction curettage or medical management, resulting in loss of the pregnancy. This error is avoidable with the use of ultrasound imaging to identify fetal heart activity or with monitoring β-hCG levels to assess the status of the pregnancy.

Miscalculation of Gestational Age

Miscalculation of the size of pregnancy can lead to misdiagnosis of a second-trimester abortion as a first-trimester abortion. This, in turn, can lead the clinician to inadvertently perform suction curettage on a second-trimester pregnancy, which, as discussed earlier, carries a substantially increased rate of complications when performed by an individual without experience in second-trimester procedures. Miscalculation of uterine size can also lead to perforation when instruments are passed into a uterus that is smaller that expected.

A related error is failure to correctly assess the position of the uterus. This can also lead to uterine perforation if instruments are passed through the cervicouterine junction or uterine fundus.

Failure to Administer Rh Immune Globulin

When faced with a patient who has had a completed abortion and no further complaints of bleeding, clinicians will sometimes assume that the patient is stable and fail to consider that fact that the patient might be Rh negative. As noted, all women with a spontaneous abortion should undergo a determination of their Rh status and receive immune globulin if they are Rh negative to lessen the risk of Rh sensitization during future pregnancies.

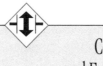

Controversies and Emerging Concepts

The most important trend in recent years has been the use of ultrasound as part of the evaluation of spontaneous abortions. It is no longer necessary to perform suction curettage to ensure that products of conception are not retained in the uterus, or to ensure that patients do not have a molar or ectopic pregnancy. These conditions can all be excluded with ultrasound, supplemented when necessary by measurements of β-hCG.

An important developing trend is the realization that evidence does not support the universal use of suction curettage or dilation and curettage for uncomplicated patients with inevitable or incomplete first-trimester loss. Patients who are hemodynamically stable with pregnancies less than 11 weeks' size, or who have uterine contents with an anterior-to-posterior diameter of less than 20 mm by ultrasound, can often be managed expectantly.

The most recent change in management of spontaneous abortions is medical treatment, which is now an option for patients with incomplete or inevitable spontaneous abortions who are hemodynamically stable without signs of infection and with uterine contents of less than 20 mm in the anterior-to-posterior uterine cavity diameter on ultrasound. As mentioned earlier, small studies suggest comparable complication rates in first-trimester incomplete abortions managed surgically and medically. Although patients have a subjective perception of increased bleeding with medical management, research has demonstrated a larger drop in hemoglobin levels following suction curettage.

Treatment should be tailored to the known risks and benefits at a given gestational age. Patient preference is respected in the absence of an obvious risk or benefit of one modality over another.

References

Alcazar JL, Baldonado C, Laparte C: The reliability of transvaginal ultrasonography to detect retained tissue after spontaneous first-trimester abortion, clinically thought to be complete. *Ultrasound Obstet Gynecol* 6:126, 1995.

Alloway T: The immediate use of the uterine scoop or curette in the treatment of abortions, versus waiting or the expectant plan. *Am J Obstet* 16:133, 1883.

Ambulatory Sentinel Practice Network: Spontaneous abortion in primary care. *J Am Board Fam Pract* 1:15, 1988.

Ben-Baruch G, Schiff E, Moran O, et al: Curettage versus nonsurgical management in women with early spontaneous abortions: the effect on fertility. *J Reprod Med* 36:644, 1991.

Blohm F, Hahlin M, Nielsen S, et al: Fertility after a randomized trial of spontaneous abortion managed by surgical evacuation or expectant treatment. *Lancet* 349:995, 1997.

Brier N: Clinical commentary: understanding and managing the emotional reactions to a miscarriage. *Obstet Gynecol* 93:151, 1999.

Cheney W: The treatment of incomplete abortion. *Occid Med Times* 6:684, 1892.

Chipchase J, James D: Randomized trial or expectant versus surgical management of spontaneous miscarriage. *Br J Obstet Gynaecol* 104:840, 1997.

Chung T, Leung P, Cheung LP, et al: A medical approach to management of spontaneous abortion using misoprostol. *Acta Obstet Gynecol Scand* 76:248, 1997.

Darney PD, Hurbach NS, Korn AP: *Protocols for Office Gynecologic Surgery.* Boston: Blackwell, 1966.

de Jonge E, Makin JD, Manefeldt E, et al: Randomised clinical trial of medical evacuation and surgical curettage for incomplete miscarriage. *Br Med J* 311: 662, 1995.

Dunn R: A five-year study of incomplete abortions at the San Francisco Hospital. *Am J Obstet Gynecol* 33:149, 1937.

Geyman JP, Oliver LM, Sullivan SD: Expectant, medical, or surgical treatment of spontaneous abortion in first trimester of pregnancy? A pooled quantitative literature evaluation. *J Am Board Fam Pract* 12:55, 1999.

Grimes DA, Schultz KF, Cates W: Prophylactic antibiotics for suction abortion. *Am J Obstet Gynecol* 150:689, 1984.

Haines C, Chung T, Leung D: Transvaginal sonography and the conservative management of spontaneous abortion. *Gynecol Obstet Invest* 37:14, 1994.

Hartman J: A comparative study of incomplete abortions at San Francisco Hospital. *Stanford Med Bull* 11:69, 1953.

Henshaw R, Cooper K, El-Refaey H, et al: Medical management of miscarriage: non-surgical uterine evacuation of incomplete and inevitable spontaneous abortion. *Br Med J* 306:894, 1993.

Herabutya Y, O-Prasertsawat P: Misoprostol in the management of missed abortion. *Int J Gynaecol Obstet* 56:263, 1997.

Hurd WW, Whitfield RR, Randolph JF, et al: Expectant management versus elective curettage for the treatment of spontaneous abortion. *Fertil Steril* 68:601, 1997.

Johnson N, Priestnall M, Marsay T, et al: A randomised trial evaluating pain and bleeding after a first trimester miscarriage treated surgically or medically. *Eur J Obstet Gynecol Reprod Biol* 72:213, 1997.

Jurkovic D: Modern management of miscarriage: is there a place for non-surgical treatment? *Ultrasound Obstet Gynecol* 11:161, 1998.

Kissinger DP, Rozycki GS, Morris JA Jr, et al: Trauma in pregnancy. Predicting pregnancy outcome. *Arch Surg* 126:1079, 1991.

Lelaidier C, Baton-Saint-Mleux C, Fernandez H, et al: Mifepristone (RU 486) induces embryo expulsion in first trimester non-developing pregnancies: a prospective randomized trial. *Hum Reprod* 8:492, 1993.

Li T: Recurrent miscarriage: principles of management. *Hum Reprod* 13:478, 1998.

Mansur MM: Ultrasound diagnosis of complete abortion can reduce need for curettage. *Eur J Obstet Gynecol Reprod Biol* 44:65, 1992.

Mishell DR Jr, Jain JK, Byrne JD, et al: A medical method of early pregnancy termination using tamoxifen and misoprostol. *Contraception* 58:1, 1998.

Nielsen S, Hahlin M: Expectant management of first-trimester spontaneous abortion. *Lancet* 345:84, 1995.

Nielson S, Hahlin M, Oden A: Using a logistic model to identify women with first-trimester spontaneous abortion suitable for expectant management. *Br J Obstet Gynaecol* 103:1230, 1996.

Osborn JF, Cattaruzza MS, Spinelli A: Risk of spontaneous abortion in Italy, 1978–1995, and the effect of maternal age, gravidity, marital status, and education. *Am J Epidemiol* 151:98, 2000.

Rulin M, Bornstein S, Cambell J: The reliability of ultrasonography in the management of spontaneous abortion clinically thought to be complete: a prospective study. *Am J Obstet Gynecol* 168:12, 1993.

Russell P: Abortions treated conservatively: a 12-year study covering 3,739 cases. *South Med J* 40:314, 1947.

Saraiya M, Green C, Berg C, et al: Spontaneous abortion–related deaths among women in the United States—1981–1991. *Obstet Gynecol* 93:172, 1999.

Steier JA, Bergsjo P, Myking OL: Human chorionic gonadotropin in maternal plasma after induced abortion, spontaneous abortion, and removed ectopic pregnancy. *Obstet Gynecol* 64:391, 1984.

Warburton D: Chromosomal causes of fetal death. *Clin Obstet Gynecol* 30:268, 1987.

WHO Task Force of Post-Ovulatory Methods of Fertility Regulation: Termination of pregnancy with reduced doses of mifepristone. *Br Med J* 307:532, 1993.

Wiebe E, Janssen P: Management of spontaneous abortion in family practices and hospitals. *Fam Med* 30:293, 1998.

Neil J. Murphy, Thomas J. Burke,
and Benjamin A. Garnett

Chapter 19

Cesarean Delivery

Introduction

Cesarean delivery is the most common surgical procedure performed in United States hospitals. The procedure has been part of Western and non-Western cultures since before the time of the Roman Empire. Cesarean delivery is mentioned in the Talmud, and, according to Greek mythology, Apollo removed Asclepius, founder of the Greek cult of religious medicine, from Coronis' abdomen.

The origin of the term "cesarean" is not entirely clear. It is often related to the birth of Julius Caesar. It is unlikely, however, that Caesar was born by abdominal delivery because abdominal delivery was almost universally fatal for the parturient during that era and Caesar's mother, Aurelia, is known to have survived his birth. Other possible origins of the term are the Latin verb *caedere,* which means "to cut," or *caesones,* the term used to describe the offspring of abdominal birth. Still others believe the term originated from the Roman law, *Lex Regis,* which mandated postmortem operative delivery when mothers died during childbirth, so that mother and child could be buried separately, a custom referred to as Lex *Cesare.*

The term cesarean "section" is also a matter of discussion, because both words refer to an incision. The proper name for the procedure is cesarean delivery.

Modern History

During the 19th century, cesarean delivery was transformed with the use of anesthesia, antisepsis, and silver wire for suture. Queen Victoria helped popularize the use of anesthesia for vaginal delivery when chloroform was administered for the births of two of her children in 1853 and 1857. The use of obstetric anesthesia then became popular among the wealthy and was subsequently applied to cesarean delivery. The increased use of carbolic acid and aseptic technique had a significant effect on reducing the incidence of postoperative puerperal infection. The introduction of silver wire sutures, popularized by North American frontier surgeons, made cesarean delivery even more acceptable by allaying the fears of surgeons who had abandoned suturing of blood vessels or the uterus because infection was almost inevitable with earlier suture materials.

The use of the transverse uterine incision and antibiotics in the 20th century led to further acceptance of cesarean delivery. Kerr developed the low-transverse uterine incision in 1926, which decreased the risk of subsequent uterine rupture. The discovery of penicillin by Fleming in 1928 and its subsequent purification in the 1940s eliminated the need for the extraperitoneal procedure described by Frank in 1907 to reduce peritonitis. Further advances led to the development of hospitals devoted to safer vaginal and operative deliveries. Further advances in research and technology influenced the regionalization of maternity care, which further decreased maternal and fetal morbidity and mortality.

Epidemiology

Frequency and Indications

The cesarean delivery rate increased from 4.5% in 1965 to 24.4% in 1987. As shown in Table 19-1,

many factors have contributed to the increasing rate of cesarean delivery. The increase occurred as the perceived need for cesarean delivery shifted from maternal to fetal indications. In North America the reason for most cesarean deliveries is previous cesarean delivery; other common indications include breech, dystocia, and nonreassuring fetal heart patterns. In Norway and Scotland the overall cesarean rate is approximately one-half that in North America, and the indications are reversed with previous cesarean delivery as a much less frequent indication.

Table 19-1

Causes of Increased Cesarean Rate

Medical advances diminishing maternal risks
Labor and delivery
  Repeat cesarean birth
  Continuous electronic fetal monitoring
  Dystocia diagnosis liberalized
  Epidural analgesia/anesthesia
  Macrosomia as indication for cesarean
    delivery (>4000 g vs >4500 g)
  Decreased use of forceps/vacuum
Maternal factors
  More older childbearing women/delay in
    childbirth
  More nulliparous women with attendant risks
  Increasing maternal risk
Fetal factors
  Fetus as a patient
  Less breech vaginal delivery
  Very-low-birth-weight fetus
  Active genital herpes
  Postterm pregnancy
  Multiple gestation (especially with nonvertex)
  Failed induction for fetal indication
Physician factors
  Fear of malpractice litigation
  Physician compensation (possible)
  Physician convenience (possible)

SOURCE: Reproduced with permission from Depp R: Cesarean delivery. In Gabbe SG, Niebyl JR, Simpson JL (eds): *Obstetrics—Normal & Problem Pregnancies.* New York, Churchill Livingstone, 1996, Table 19-3, p 564.

REPEAT CESAREAN DELIVERY

The single most-common indication for cesarean birth is repeat cesarean delivery. Studies have shown that most (60% to 92%) women who have had a cesarean delivery can successfully undergo vaginal-birth-after-cesarean (VBAC), yet less than 30% of these women will be delivered by VBAC. Older women and those of higher educational and socioeconomic status are less likely to undergo VBAC.

The best way to lower the cesarean rate in the long term is to reduce the rate of primary cesarean delivery. However, because so many cesarean deliveries are repeat cesareans, short-term efforts to decrease the rate of cesarean delivery should be aimed at increasing the VBAC rate.

ELECTRONIC FETAL MONITORING

Another factor responsible for the increased rate of cesarean deliveries is the widespread use of electronic fetal monitoring (EFM). EFM has been universally applied to women at low risk for complications during labor, despite a high false-positive rate in such women when fetal heart rate abnormalities are detected. In fact, the rate of primary cesarean delivery is at least 30% higher in low-risk women whose labors are monitored with EFM than for similar groups of women whose labors are not electronically monitored. The use of EFM and the increase in cesarean deliveries have not resulted in a significant decrease in fetal acidosis, long term neurologic complications for infants and children, or malpractice litigation.

EPIDURAL ANESTHESIA

The ready availability of epidural anesthesia is thought to contribute to the increased rate of cesarean deliveries. The rate of epidural anesthesia use has dramatically increased, with 90% of nulliparous parturients receiving epidural anesthesia in many communities. Women who receive epidural anesthesia during labor have higher rates of dysfunctional uterine contractions, especially when the epidural is begun prior to the active phase of labor. Inadequate uterine contractions may arrest the progress of labor, leading to the need for cesarean delivery. The fact that epidural anesthesia permits cesarean delivery with less anesthetic risk than with general anesthesia may make physicians more likely to respond to dysfunctional labor patterns by performing a cesarean delivery.

DELAYED CHILDBIRTH

Another factor contributing to the increased rate of cesarean delivery is the trend of delaying childbirth until later in life, leading to increasing rates of nulliparity and pregnancy at older ages. Age and nulliparity are strong independent predictors of cesarean delivery. Older mothers have higher rates of cesarean delivery because they have more medical risk factors and complications. Among nulliparous women, the primary cesarean rate is three times higher than of women having second or subsequent births.

OTHER FACTORS

Other factors contributing to the high cesarean rate include the increasing prevalence of obesity in the population (obesity is associated with an increased rate of cesarean delivery), concern about malpractice litigation, and the decreased use of forceps deliveries. Finally, progress in neonatal care has increased the survival rates of very-low-birth-weight infants, making clinicians more willing to deliver such infants by cesarean despite surgical risks to the mother.

Contraindications

There are few contraindications for cesarean delivery. A guiding principle is "what is best for the fetus is what is best for the mother." If the mother is medically unstable and the fetus is nonviable, then it is recommended that the maternal condition be stabilized regardless of fetal considerations, per se. If the fetus is of a gestational age consistent with viability, then the maternal condition should also be stabilized first and delivery considered only for obstetric indications. The exception to this dictum is a perimortem cesarean delivery, which is discussed later.

Regional Variation

There are regional variations in cesarean delivery rates in the United States. The southern region has the highest total and primary cesarean rates, followed by northeast, midwest, and western regions. Rates are higher for women with private insurance, those who deliver at for-profit hospitals, and those who deliver in hospitals with less than 100 beds. Some have suggested that these trends indicate that cesarean delivery rates may be influenced by financial/reimbursement considerations.

In addition to having the highest cesarean delivery rate, the southern region also has the lowest rate of VBAC, while the northeast has the highest VBAC rate.

Goals for Cesarean Delivery Rates

In 1990 the US Department of Health and Human Services published the *Healthy People 2000* objectives. This report targeted a goal of reducing the overall cesarean rate in the United States to 15% of all deliveries and the primary cesarean rate to 12% of all deliveries. Between 1991 and 1998 the overall cesarean rate declined from 22.6% to 21.2%. The primary cesarean rate also fell from 16.1% in 1989 to 14.9% in 1998. The only state to attain the *Healthy People 2000* objective of 15% was Alaska. In many other countries, cesarean rates are less than 15%, yet they have perinatal mortality rates lower than the United States, raising questions about the advantage of maintaining the high cesarean rate.

Table 19-2 offers benchmarks or "report cards" for cesarean delivery rates of women with dystocia and nonreassuring fetal heart tracing. Efforts to reduce cesarean delivery rates to meet these benchmarks have met with varying success. Several studies and a meta-analysis have confirmed that "active management" of labor can significantly shorten the length of labor, and in some studies it has been shown to decrease cesarean delivery rates. Other interventions shown to reduce cesarean delivery rates include the following:

1. Requirements for a second opinion before proceeding with cesarean delivery
2. Peer pressure from other clinicians
3. Public dissemination of physician-specific cesarean rates
4. Standardized guidelines for management of dystocia and nonreassuring fetal heart patterns
5. Changes in physicians' on-call schedules

Table 19-2

Benchmarking and "Report Card" Grade for Cesarean Birth in Nulliparas Using Epidural Analgesia

INSTITUTIONAL OR PRACTITIONER "REPORT CARD" GRADE	CESAREAN FOR DYSTOCIA IN NULLIPARAS WITH EPIDURAL BENCHMARK RATE (RANGE) IN PERCENTS	CESAREAN FOR NONREASSURING FETAL STATUS IN NULLIPARAS WITH EPIDURAL BENCHMARK RATE (RANGE) IN PERCENTS
A	5 (3–7)	2 (0–2.9)
B	10 (8–12)	4 (3–4.9)
C	15 (13–17)	6 (5–6.9)
D	20 (18–22)	8 (7–9.9)
F	25 (≥23)	10 (≥10)

SOURCE: Data from Thorp JA: Epidural analgesia during labor. *Clin Obstet Gynecol* 41:449–460, 1998.

6. Use of external cephalic version for breech presentation
7. Larger roles for midwives in the birthing process

In contrast, peer review programs and legislative mandates have not proved effective at reducing the rate of cesarean delivery.

Typical Presentation

The common indications for cesarean delivery can be divided into those primarily affecting the fetus, the mother, or both (Table 19-3). The most common indications for cesarean delivery are repeat cesarean, dystocia or failure to progress, breech presentation, and a nonreassuring fetal heart pattern.

The vertical transmission of human immunodeficiency virus (HIV) is significantly reduced by cesarean delivery in women who have not been treated with multidrug regimens. The need for cesarean delivery in HIV-positive women with such therapy is dependent on the viral load at the time of delivery. If the viral load is greater than 1,000 copies per milliliter, then cesarean delivery is indicated.

Key History

The key information needed prior to cesarean delivery is the same needed before any major surgery. Past medical, surgical, obstetric, gynecologic, family, drug-habit, transfusion, medication, allergy, and anesthetic histories are required. In addition, salient information about the current obstetric indication is essential such as length of labor and duration of ruptured membranes.

Vaginal trial of labor (VTOL) should be offered to all patients with a prior low-transverse cesar-

Table 19-3

Common Indications for Cesarean Delivery

INDICATION
Fetal
Nonreassuring fetal heart pattern
Other fetal indications
Malpresentation:
Transverse lie
Breech
Funic: cord prolapse
Brow
Face-mentum posterior
Human immunodeficiency virus
Active herpes virus
Immune thrombocytopenic purpura
Congenital anomalies
Macrosomia, relative
Low birth weight, relative
Maternal-fetal
Failure to progress in labor:
Arrest of descent
Arrest of dilation
Placental abruption
Placenta previa
Conjoined twins
Perimortem
Maternal
Repeat cesarean delivery
Contracted pelvis, e.g.,
congenital, fracture
Obstructive tumors
Abdominal cerclage
Reconstructive vaginal surgery,
e.g., fistula repair
Medical conditions, e.g., cardiac,
pulmonary, thrombocytopenia

ean delivery. The clinician should review all cesarean delivery operative reports to ensure that VTOL can be undertaken safely. The only contraindications for VBAC are those for any vaginal delivery (e.g., obstructed labor, previous classical incision or low-vertical incision that involved the active myometrium).

Informed consent for VTOL should be obtained and documented during pregnancy—ideally by 28 weeks of gestation. The discussion should include the risk of uterine rupture; hemorrhage; infection; and failure of VTOL with need for repeat cesarean delivery and its complications, including internal organ damage, hysterectomy, and death. The consent process should contrast these risks to those of a repeat cesarean delivery.

Key Physical Examination

The physical examination for cesarean delivery should address major medical, obstetric, and anesthetic concerns. The operating team must be cognizant that regional anesthesia may be converted to general anesthesia at any time during the procedure. A vaginal examination should be performed in all laboring patients just prior to surgical draping, to ensure that sufficient progress in labor has not occurred that would permit vaginal delivery and, therefore, preclude the need for cesarean delivery.

Ancillary Tests

Preoperative laboratory evaluation should include hemoglobin, blood type, and Rh factor. Because of the possibility that blood transfusion may be required, a blood clot tube should be present in the blood bank for blood typing and antibody screening on all patients undergoing cesarean delivery. HIV status should be known on all prenatal patients so that measures can be taken to decrease the risk of vertical transmission of infection.

If the cesarean delivery is being considered because of a nonreassuring fetal heart tracing, addi-tional testing is recommended to confirm that fetal distress is present because of the high rate of false-positive tests with EFM. Methods for confirmatory testing include measurement of fetal scalp pH or fetal response to scalp or acoustic stimulation.

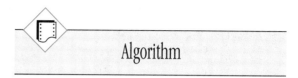

Algorithm

Figure 19-1 presents an algorithm for decision making in cesarean delivery and VBAC.

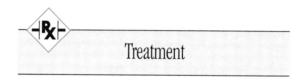

Treatment

This section will describe the cesarean delivery procedure, including preoperative considerations, surgical physiology and anatomy, options for the surgical approach, and the surgical procedure itself.

Preoperative and Nonsurgical Considerations

ANESTHESIA

For planned cesarean delivery, the patient should stop oral intake 8 hours before surgery. Preoperative administration of 30 mL of a non-particulate liquid antacid will minimize the risk of lung injury in the event that aspiration of gastric acid occurs during endotracheal intubation. Ant-acids should be routinely administered, even if surgery will be performed under conduction anes-thesia, because conduction anesthesia may be con-verted to inhalation anesthesia during the surgical procedure.

Positioning of the patient on the operating table is also important. Patients should be placed in a modified, left-lateral decubitus position to mini-mize aortocaval compression by the gravid uterus.

Figure 19-1

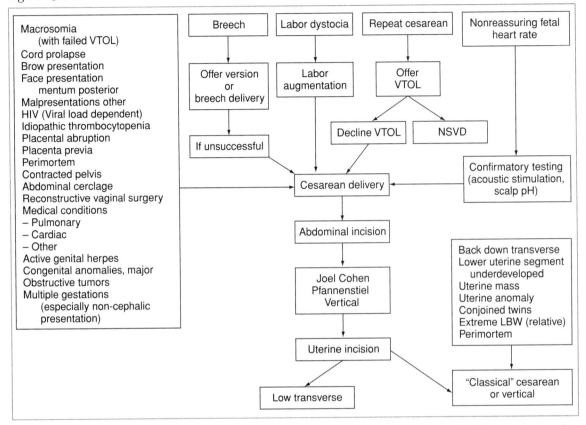

Algorithm for cesarean delivery and vaginal birth after previous cesarean delivery. VTOL: vaginal trial of labor; NSVD: normal spontaneous vaginal delivery.

INTRAVENOUS FLUIDS AND URINARY BLADDER

Pregnant women have a basal, physiologic fluid requirement of 2000 to 2500 mL per 24 hours. Fluids should be administered at a rate sufficient to cover this requirement, plus additional fluids for epidural anesthesia, increased insensible loss with labor, and insensible intraoperative loss of 1000 mL per hour caused by exposed viscera and blood loss.

Fluid administration prior to epidural or spinal anesthesia in normotensive patients usually involves a 1000 mL bolus of isotonic fluids such as lactated Ringer's solution or 0.9% saline. In the event of excessive bleeding, isotonic fluids are good first-line agents, but blood-product replacement is necessary for any ongoing blood loss greater than 1000 mL. A urinary catheter should be placed preoperatively to decompress the bladder and assist in fluid management.

ANTIBIOTICS

One to two grams of a first-generation or second-generation cephalosporin, or the equivalent dose of an extended-spectrum penicillin, should be available and given immediately after umbilical-cord clamping to decrease the risk of endometritis. Routine prophylaxis for prevention of bacterial endocarditis is no longer recommended in cesarean delivery.

SHAVING

Abdominal hair removal often is not necessary. If hair is removed, it should be removed in the operating room and not the evening before the procedure. The hair should be clipped and not shaved, because shaving with a razor causes breaks in the skin that increase the risk of wound infection.

INFORMED CONSENT

The operating surgeon should thoroughly discuss the risk and benefits of the procedure with the patient and a family member, if available. The counseling session is best documented in narrative form in the medical record, though a pre-printed form can be used. The discussion should be documented in both nonmedical and medical terminology. The consent should be signed and dated by the patient. Documentation should include diagnosis, procedure, common and important risk factors, alternatives to the proposed procedure, and other such procedures as found necessary in the best judgment of the medical staff during the procedure. The important risk factors can be simplified to bleeding, infection, internal organ damage, anesthesia risk, hysterectomy, and death.

Surgical Physiology and Anatomy

A woman's body undergoes numerous changes during pregnancy. Those most pertinent to performance of cesarean delivery are changes in maternal physiology and anatomy.

PHYSIOLOGY

The nonpregnant uterus is an almost solid muscular structure weighing 70 to 80 grams with a 10-cc cavity. By the end of pregnancy, the total volume of the uterine contents increases to an average of about 5 liters, but may be as much as 20 liters, so that the uterine capacity is increased by 500 to 1000 times. The uterine enlargement is a result of muscle hypertrophy, plus fetal and placental growth, and amniotic fluid accumulation.

In addition to changes in the uterus, many alterations in maternal cardiovascular physiology take place during pregnancy. These physiologic changes, which are shown in Table 19-4, increase maternal blood volume and flow in the pelvic organs, rendering the woman more susceptible to serious hemorrhage.

The cardiac output is higher when the parturient is in the lateral recumbent position because, in the supine position, the enlarged uterus compresses the inferior vena cava, thereby impeding venous return to the heart. Cardiac output can increase by over 25% when a pregnant woman moves from the supine position to her side and can decrease

Table 19-4

Maternal Cardiovascular Changes During Pregnancy

PHYSIOLOGIC PARAMETER	CHANGE DURING PREGNANCY
Cardiac output	Increases by 30% to 50%
Blood volume	Increases by 50%
Blood flow to uteroplacental circulation	Increased to 500 to 650 mL/min
Erythrocyte volume	Increases by 30%
Blood flow to uterus	Increased by 1000%
Systemic vascular resistance	Decreases (to variable degree)
Leukocyte count	Increased by 200%

correspondingly when she moves from a lateral to supine position.

ANATOMY

Anatomy pertinent to performing cesarean delivery involves the abdominal wall, the uterus, the adnexa, the urinary bladder, and the vascular supply of the pelvic organs.

ABDOMINAL WALL   The abdominal wall consists of five layers: skin, subcutaneous layer, musculoaponeurotic layer, transversalis fascia, and peritoneum. The subcutaneous layer contains Camper's and Scarpa's fascia, while the musculoaponeurotic layer contains the rectus sheath. The rectus sheath is formed by the conjoined aponeuroses of the external oblique, internal oblique, and transverse abdominis muscles.

The pyramidalis muscles arise from the pubic bones and insert into the linea alba several centimeters above the pubic symphysis. Their strong attachments to the midline can make separation of their attachments difficult by blunt dissection. There may also be tendinous attachments from the rectus abdominis to the rectus sheath that are difficult to separate during a Pfannenstiel incision.

UTERUS   The uterus has two portions—an upper muscular corpus and a lower fibrous cervix. In the first few weeks of pregnancy, the original pear shape of the uterus is maintained. The uterus then lengthens and assumes an ovoid shape. As the uterus enlarges, it reaches almost to the liver, displacing the intestines.

The uterine musculature is arranged in three layers. The muscle cells in the middle layer are interlaced such that when they contract after delivery, they constrict the perforating blood vessels.

The uterus is mobile during pregnancy. The abdominal wall supports the uterus when a pregnant woman is standing and maintains the relation between the long axis of the uterus and the pelvic inlet. When a pregnant woman is supine, however, her uterus falls back to rest on the vertebral column and the great vessels, especially the aorta and the inferior vena cava. With ascent from the pelvis as pregnancy progresses, the uterus usually undergoes dextrorotation, resulting in the left margin facing anteriorly. Levorotation can occur in the presence of a right-sided pelvic mass.

UTERINE LIGAMENTS   The broad, uterosacral, cardinal, and round ligaments surround the uterus. The broad ligaments have no supportive function, but are peritoneal folds that extend laterally from the uterus and cover the adnexal structures (Fig. 19-2).

Uterosacral Ligaments   The uterosacral ligaments hold the cervix posteriorly over the levator plate of the pelvic diaphragm. They lie on either side of the pouch of Douglas and are composed of smooth muscle, nerves, and connective tissue.

Cardinal Ligaments   The cardinal ligaments lie at the lower edge of the broad ligaments between the peritoneal leaves. They are composed of perivascular connective tissue and nerves that surround the uterine artery and veins.

Round Ligaments   The round ligaments are extensions of the uterine musculature, but offer little support to the uterus. Tension is exerted on the round ligaments as the uterus enlarges, which women sometimes experience as "round ligament pain."

ADNEXA   The lateral pole of the ovary is attached to the pelvis by the infundibulopelvic ligament, which also contains the ovarian artery and vein. Medially, the ovary is connected to the uterus through the utero-ovarian ligament. The fallopian tubes extend from the uterine cornua to the ovaries, and they provide ova with access to the uterine cavity. The ovaries vary in size, depending on the state of ovarian activity. The fallopian tubes are 8 to 14 cm long and are covered by peritoneum.

URINARY BLADDER   The urinary bladder can be divided into two portions, the dome and base. The base of the bladder, which rests on the upper vagina and cervix, contains the trigone and is contiguous with the muscle of the vesical neck and the urethra. The muscular dome of the bladder is relatively thin when distended. The bladder base is thicker and varies less with distention.

The surgeon encounters the bladder twice during a cesarean delivery—first, when opening the parietal peritoneum, which sweeps down onto the bladder, and, second, when taking the bladder flap down off the lower uterine segment, because the bladder spans the anterior cul de sac. The extent of the bladder may be confirmed by palpating for the Foley bulb or transilluminating the peritoneum.

BLOOD SUPPLY   An understanding of the blood supply of the uterus and vagina is essential for avoiding vascular injury during cesarean delivery. The vascular supply of the uterus originates primarily from the uterine and ovarian arteries (Fig. 19-2) while the vagina receives its circulation from a branch of the uterine artery.

Uterine Artery   The uterine artery, a main branch of the hypogastric or internal iliac artery descends for a short distance, enters the base of the broad ligament, and turns medially to the lateral aspect of the uterus. The uterine artery then crosses just anterior to the ureter (see Fig. 19-2). The inferior branch of the uterine artery supplies the upper vagina and the lower cervix, while the marginal branch traverses the lateral aspect of the uterus before dividing into three terminal branches: ovarian, tubal, and fundal. Throughout its length, the marginal branch is a convoluted vessel with numerous branches penetrating the body of the uterus, including one large branch that extends to the upper portion of the cervix.

Figure 19-2

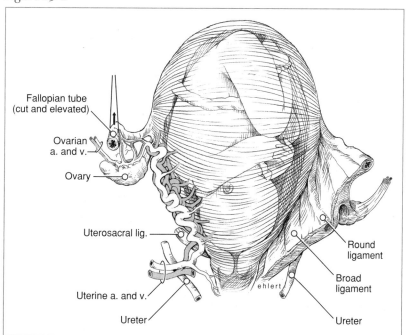

Uterine ligaments and blood supply. This illustration shows the uterine ligaments and blood supply to the ovary, fallopian tube, and side of the uterus. The ovarian and uterine vessels anastomose freely along the side of the uterus. Note the uterine artery and vein crossing over the ureter, which lies immediately adjacent to the cervix.

The relationship between the uterine artery and ureter is surgically significant. About 2 cm lateral to the cervix, the uterine artery crosses over the ureter. The ureter can be injured in the process of clamping and ligating the uterine vessels to control postpartum hemorrhage or during hysterectomy.

Ovarian Artery   The ovarian artery is a direct branch of the aorta and enters the broad ligament through the infundibulopelvic ligament. At the ovarian hilum, the ovarian artery divides into ovarian branches and a main branch that traverses the broad ligament. Near the upper lateral portion of the uterus, the ovarian artery anastomoses with the ovarian branch of the uterine artery.

Uterine and Ovarian Veins   The lateral uterus is composed largely of venous sinuses. These sinuses coalesce into arcuate veins that unite to form the uterine vein. Several large uterine veins accompany the uterine artery and empty into the hypogastric vein, which empties into the common iliac vein. The ovarian vein collects blood from the upper part of the uterus through a large pampiniform plexus in the broad ligament. The right ovarian vein empties into the vena cava, while the left ovarian vein empties into the left renal vein.

Vaginal Blood Supply   The vagina receives blood from the inferior extension of the uterine artery along the lateral sulci of the vagina and from a vaginal branch of the hypogastric artery. These form an anastomotic arcade along the lateral aspect of the vagina at the 3:00 o'clock and 9:00 o'clock positions. Branches of these vessels also merge along the anterior and posterior vaginal walls.

Surgical Procedure

The following section includes a step-by-step description of the operative procedures involved in cesarean delivery. The major steps in the procedure are listed in Table 19-5. Table 19-6 provides key considerations for clinicians who serve as surgical assistants for cesarean deliveries.

ABDOMINAL WALL INCISION

Options for the abdominal wall incision include the modified Pfannenstiel, the Joel-Cohen, and the midline vertical incisions, plus several variants of these incisions (Fig. 19-3). The midline vertical incision is said to be the quickest abdominal wall incision, but most experienced surgeons can perform either the modified Pfannenstiel or the Joel-Cohen within minutes.

MODIFIED PFANNENSTIEL   The modified Pfannenstiel incision is made 3 cm above the pubic symphysis. The incision is extended beyond the lateral borders of the rectus muscles in a curvilinear fashion to within 2 to 3 cm inferior and medial of the anterior superior iliac crests. In women with a large abdominal pannus, the incision may be placed under the pannus. However, the area is heavily colonized with bacteria. It may be difficult to prepare surgically, keep dry, and to inspect postoperatively.

The subcutaneous tissues are completely separated from the fascia of the abdominal wall muscles, and a transverse incision is made through the fascia. The fascial sheath is completely separated from the underlying rectus muscles by blunt and sharp dissection to the umbilicus and until the pubic symphysis is palpable. Any blood vessel perforating through the muscles can be ligated with electrocautery or can be cut and clamped. The transversalis fascia and peritoneum are elevated and sharply opened longitudinally in the midline.

JOEL-COHEN (MISGAV-LADACH MODIFICATION)   The Joel-Cohen abdominal wall incision, modified by surgeons at the Misgav Ladach Hospital, emphasizes stretching tissue within existing planes, rather than sharp dissection. This technique has particular advantages in remote or rural areas because it requires fewer instruments than other methods for opening the abdominal wall, and it is relatively easy to learn (Table 19-7).

The modified Joel-Cohen begins with a noncurvilinear (i.e., straight) transverse incision, 15 to 17 cm long, made 3 cm below the anterior superior iliac crests. The skin is opened superficially,

Table 19-5

Techniques of Cesarean Delivery

Prepare patient
　Informed consent
　NPO, nonparticulate antacid, anesthesia, bladder catheter
　Cleanse skin, clip hair, left lateral decubitus position
Abdominal wall incision
　Joel-Cohen (Misgav-Ladach modification)
　Modified Pfannenstiel
　Midline vertical
　Others: Maylard, Cherney
Fascial incision
　Misgav-Ladach: small midline fascial incision, stretch tissue
　Pfannenstiel: long transverse incision, separate rectus muscle/sheath, stretch
　　rectus muscles apart
Peritoneal incision
　Parietal
　　Longitudinal (Pfannenstiel)
　　Transverse (Joel-Cohen)
　Visceral
　　Transverse vesicouterine
　　Develop bladder flap
Uterine incision
　Low transverse
　Classical
　Low vertical
Delivery of fetal presenting part
　Elevate presenting part, maintain flexion if cephalic
　Assistant to dislodge presenting part, if deeply seated
Suction infant oropharynx
Apply fundal pressure
Clamp and cut cod, administer antibiotics and oxytocin, obtain cord blood
　Type and Rh,
　pH, stem cells (optional)
Delivery of placenta
　Assisted spontaneous
　Manual
Cleanse uterine cavity
　Place ring forceps at apices of uterine incision
Uterine closure
　Externalize uterus (optional)
　Inspect for possible extensions
　Single line of absorbable suture
　Imbricating suture (optional)
Inspect pelvic and abdominal contents
　Remove foreign material from peritoneal cavity
　Sponge and needle count

Continued

Table 19-5 (continued)

Techniques of Cesarean Delivery

Peritoneal closure (optional)
   Visceral (bladder flap)
   Parietal
Fascial closure
   Single, nonlocking
   Two lines of suture meeting in the midline, nonlocking (optional)
Subcutaneous (optional, if tissue >2 cm)
Irrigate subcutaneous tissue
Skin closure
   Subcuticular
   Staples
   Widely spaced mattress sutures
Apply sterile dressing

Table 19-6

Tips for Surgical Assistants at Cesarean Delivery

Exposure
   Focus on providing exposure of lateral aspects of the following
      Rectus fascia—on both opening and closing
      Vesicouterine peritoneum—opening only
      Uterus—on both opening and closing
Rectus fascia (with modified Pfannenstiel incision)
   Elevate fascia with Kocher clamps
   Blunt dissection of rectus muscle from fascia
   Provide countertraction on muscle while surgeon dissects fascia from muscle
   Recheck under fascia for bleeding before closure
Uterine incision
   Suction blood and fluid from incision as surgeon delicately scores uterus sharply
Delivery
   Apply fundal pressure when requested
   Assist with clamping and cutting umbilical cord
   Suction oropharynx, obtain cord-blood samples
If uterus is externalized after delivery
   Hold tension on fundus
   Keep the uterine incision dry for visualization of repair
   Maximize exposure with bladder blade
Uterine closure
   If surgeon is locking sutures, then loop suture over needle each pass
Knot tying
   Three throws for chromic
   Four throws for Vicryl, with first being a double throw or surgeon's knot

Figure 19-3

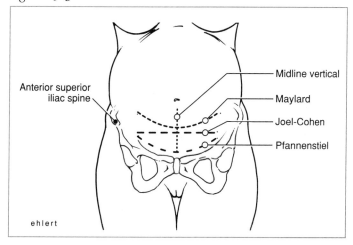

Abdominal wall incisions for cesarean delivery. There are several options for the abdominal wall incision.

followed by sharp dissection to open the fascia in the midline only (Fig. 19-4).

After opening the fascia, the remaining subcutaneous tissue, fascia, and rectus muscles are dissected bluntly. Because this technique simply stretches tissues transversely (Fig. 19-5), the incision is very rapid and results in less blood loss than other techniques. Because there is less bleeding and cutting, there is a decreased need for transfusion, less risk of HIV transmission, and easier modification or extension of the incision if complications arise. Decreased tissue damage also leads to less postoperative analgesia and early resumption of feeding and activity. Furthermore, there is shorter operative time, anesthetic time, and length of hospital stay, as well as, less febrile morbidity, wound infection, and adhesions.

MIDLINE VERTICAL The midline vertical skin incision extends from the pubic symphysis to within 2 cm of the umbilicus. The fascia is elevated and sharply dissected from the pubis to the umbilicus.

Table 19-7

The Misgav-Ladach Method of Cesarean Delivery

1. Modified Joel-Cohen opening of the abdomen
2. Parietal peritoneum opened transversely
3. No abdominal swab used
4. Lower uterine segment transverse incision
5. Uterus sutured continuously in one layer
6. Visceral and parietal peritoneum left open
7. Nonlocking, continuous closure of the fascia
8. Few widely spaced skin stitches

SOURCE: Reprinted from *Int J Gynecol Obstet* Vol. 57. Federici D, Lacelli B, Muggiasca A, et al. Cesarean section using the Misgav-Ladach method, p. 276, 1997, with permission from Elsevier Science.

Figure 19-4

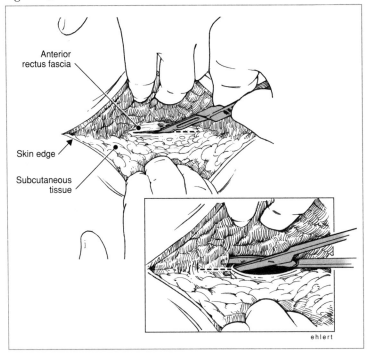

Joel-Cohen dissection of the fascia. The subcutaneous tissue is opened in the midline to the fascia. The fascia is opened transversely in the median aspect and extended under the intact subcutaneous tissue.

Figure 19-5

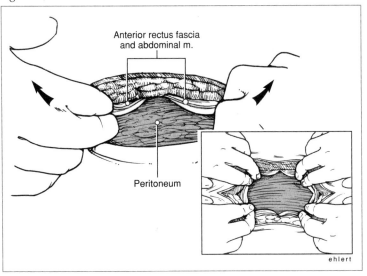

Stretching the incision. In the Joel-Cohen technique, after opening the fascia, the abdominal incision is stretched transversely.

This midline vertical abdominal wall incision can be performed rapidly and provides excellent exposure of the pelvis and sidewalls.

OTHER INCISIONS The transverse Maylard rectus-splitting incision begins with a curvilinear skin incision that extends 18 to 19 cm between the anterior superior iliac crests. The Maylard offers maximal exposure for abnormal lie, multiple gestation, or macrosomia. In the transverse Cherney incision, the rectus muscles are detached from their insertion at the pubic symphysis. The transversalis fascia and peritoneum are incised transversely in the Cherney, as opposed to the longitudinal Pfannenstiel approach.

PERITONEAL INCISION

In the Pfannenstiel and midline vertical incisions, the parietal peritoneum is sharply incised from the umbilicus to the bladder. In the Joel-Cohen, the peritoneum is stretched in a transverse direction (see Fig. 19-5). The visceral or vesico-uterine peritoneum is elevated and opened transversely 1 cm above the bladder reflection onto the lower uterine segment (Fig. 19-6). A bladder flap is bluntly and sharply developed transversely 10 to 12 cm, then inferiorly 5 cm, to the level of the bladder's apposition to the cervix.

UTERINE INCISION

Cesarean delivery is performed through one of several uterine incisions (Fig. 19-7). The most common is a low-transverse uterine incision through either a Pfannenstiel or a Misgav-Ladach (modified Joel-Cohen) abdominal incision. A less common surgical approach is the classical or vertical uterine incision. Each uterine incision can be performed through any of the abdominal wall incisions, although the midline skin incision may provide more exposure for the classic uterine incision.

Figure 19-6

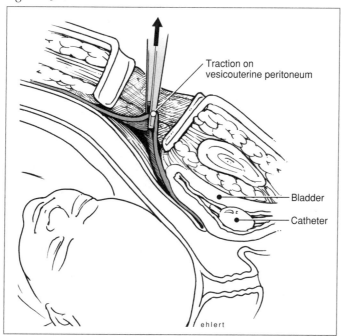

Traction on vesicouterine peritoneum

Bladder

Catheter

ehlert

Dissecting the vesicouterine peritoneum. To avoid injury to the bladder, the vesicouterine peritoneum is elevated off the bladder to expose the lower uterine segment.

Figure 19-7

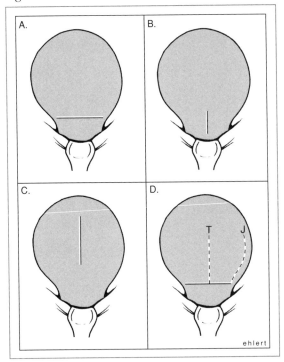

Uterine incisions for cesarean delivery. Uterine incisions include **(A)** low-transverse, **(B)** low-vertical, and **(C)** classical. In **(D)**, the low-transverse incision can be extended into a J-shaped or inverted T-shaped incision. The low-transverse incision is most common.

LOW-TRANSVERSE INCISION   The low-transverse (Kerr) incision, made in the inactive or noncontractile lower uterine segment, has a low rate of dehiscence. It also requires little bladder dissection and therefore is less likely to result in formation of adhesions to the bowel or omentum. In addition, the low-transverse uterine incision needs less surgical repair and results in less blood loss than a classical (vertical) incision.

The initial low-transverse uterine incision is made with a scalpel 1 to 2 cm from the upper margin of the bladder (Fig. 19-8). Score the median aspect of the uterus delicately with the scalpel. This and other sharp dissections should be performed with care to avoid injury to the fetus. If the lower uterine segment is very thin, fetal injury can be avoided by elevating the lower uterine

segment with Allis clamps or using blunt dissection with the tips of scissors.

The incision is extended 10 cm transversely, either bluntly with fingers (see Fig. 19-8) or sharply with bandage scissors if the uterus is thick. The incision should be large enough to avoid fetal injury and avoid unintentional extension into lateral vessels. If it is necessary to extend the uterine incision, then the first superior curvilinear incision should be to the right to avoid the lateral vessels because of the uterine dextrorotation.

Some operators place laparotomy sponges in the peritoneal cavity to minimize contamination from chorioamnionitis or thick meconium. The operator is ultimately responsible for retrieval of all foreign objects and must keep meticulous track of the sponge count and location.

VERTICAL INCISION   The classical uterine incision is made vertically and involves the active myometrium. The classical incision is indicated in a poorly developed, narrow, lower uterine segment; dense adhesions; or structural uterine abnormalities (e.g., myoma in the lower uterine segment or Bandl's contractile uterine ring). The classical inci-

Figure 19-8

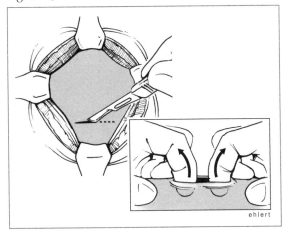

Low-transverse uterine incision. After incising the uterine wall with a scalpel and entering the uterine cavity, the incision should be extended by stretching laterally with the surgeon's fingers or with bandage scissors. In either case, care should be taken to avoid fetal injury.

sion is used in some cases of anterior placenta previa and malpresentation (e.g., back-down transverse lie and preterm breech).

The low-vertical incision begins as inferiorly as possible to avoid the active uterine segment. The incision is usually made about 2 cm above the bladder and is carried as far cephalad as necessary to allow facile delivery (Fig. 19-9). Superior extension is carried out either with bandage scissors or a scalpel.

MANAGEMENT OF AN ANTERIOR PLACENTA

If an anterior placenta is present, it should be dissected or separated from the uterine wall if necessary for rapid delivery. If the placenta is lacerated, then cut through it rapidly. Find the cord and clamp it immediately. A preoperative ultrasound may help anticipate placental location.

Figure 19-9

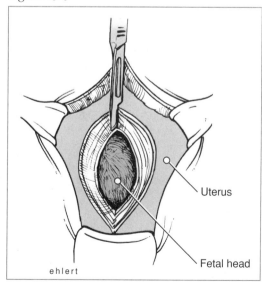

Vertical uterine incision. The classical uterine incision begins about 2 cm above the bladder, and is extended superiorly into the active uterine segment as necessary to facilitate delivery. The increased thickness of the uterine wall increases as the incision extends superiorly into the active uterine segment.

DELIVERY OF THE FETUS

CEPHALIC PRESENTATION   To deliver an infant from a cephalic presentation, it is necessary to remove the retractors and elevate the head with the surgeon's hand. The technique includes gently placing one hand into the lower uterine segment with small side-to-side movements to dislodge the head, but not injure the sometimes very thin uterus. After the head is elevated, the assistant should apply transabdominal pressure to the uterine fundus (Fig. 19-10). Flexion of the presenting part is desirable whether the fetus is occiput anterior or occiput posterior. If the head is deeply seated in the pelvis, an additional assistant may need to dislodge the head per vagina from under the operative drapes. If the head is high, then the surgeon may consider use of a vacuum extractor or forceps. The shoulders should be gently delivered one at a time while fundal pressure is continued. Before delivering the infant's torso, the oropharynx should be suctioned with either a bulb syringe or a De Lee suction device connected to continuous suction. The infant is transferred to an attendant after the umbilical cord is clamped and cut.

BREECH PRESENTATION   The presenting part should be confirmed preoperatively with ultrasound, as a breech presentation will require slightly larger abdominal wall and uterine incisions for adequate exposure. A vertical uterine incision may be necessary if the lower uterine segment is not well developed, such as in women delivering well before term.

The techniques for a breech cesarean delivery are similar to those used in a breech vaginal delivery. In a frank or complete breech, the infant's buttocks should be gently delivered in a manner similar to cephalic presentation noted above. In a nonfrank breech or transverse presentation, one foot should be grasped while the second foot is identified, and then both feet should be delivered at the same time while keeping the fetal back up. Compression of fetal organs during delivery should be avoided by grasping the pelvic girdle, rather than the abdomen.

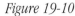

Figure 19-10

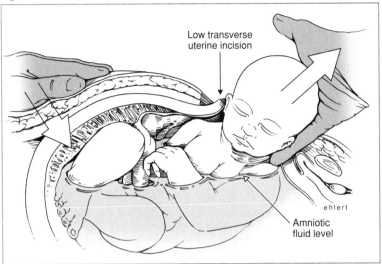

Delivery of the fetal head. Delivery of the fetal head is accomplished by lifting it anteriorly in the operator's hand while the assistant applies manual pressure to the uterine fundus.

It is essential to minimize hyperextension of the fetal neck. Hyperextension can be avoided by having an assistant suspend the infant's torso in a towel wrapped around the fetal body to maintain the proper alignment. The surgeon can maximize fetal head flexion with forceps or the modified Mauriceau-Smellie-Veit maneuver. The modified Mauriceau-Smellie-Veit maneuver uses one or two fingers anteriorly on the fetal maxilla and one finger posteriorly on the occiput to promote nuchal flexion. Any forceps will suffice (e.g., Simpson or Pipers) and should be readily available. The length and axis of Pipers may be a disadvantage in cesarean delivery.

The abdominal and uterine incisions can be extended if delivery of the fetal head is difficult. The uterine incision can be extended vertically into the active myometrium, perpendicular to the transverse uterine incision in an inverted "T" shape, or extended perpendicularly to the uterine vessels in a "J" shape. These extensions should be noted in the operative report and the patient informed about the risk of uterine rupture with future deliveries.

AFTER DELIVERY OF THE FETUS

After any delivery, the umbilical cord is clamped and cut. Cord blood should be obtained for infant blood type and Rh status. In addition, a 10- to 15-cm segment of umbilical cord may be saved for blood gas measurement. To ensure a good arterial specimen, the cord should be clamped close to the placenta. Cord blood pH values help document acid-base status in growth restriction, nonreassuring fetal status, breech presentation, preterm birth, amnionitis, thick meconium, or low Apgar scores.

DELIVERY OF THE PLACENTA

An infusion of 20 to 40 units of oxytocin in a liter of isotonic crystalloid is begun on delivery of the presenting part. Manual extraction of the placenta may be necessary on occasion; however, assisted spontaneous delivery of the placenta is preferred because it is associated with less blood loss and a lower risk of endometritis. It does not add significantly to operative time. Assisted spontaneous delivery of the placenta involves fundal massage and gentle traction on the umbilical cord (Fig. 19-11).

After delivering the placenta, the surgeon may externalize the uterus so the uterine cavity can be inspected and cleansed with a moist laparotomy sponge. When the cervix has not dilated from labor, the surgeon should consider dilating it to allow egress of lochia. This may be accomplished with a ring forceps dropped down through the uterine incision and passed through the cervix "from above." The instrument should then be discarded from the sterile field. Alternatively, after the abdomen is closed, the cervix may be dilated manually "from below" if adequate anesthesia is present.

REPAIR OF THE UTERUS

The uterus can be repaired within the peritoneal cavity or while externalized. Externalization offers increased exposure of the uterus and adnexa, plus ease of fundal massage. Neither febrile morbidity nor blood loss is increased by externalization, but externalization may cause discomfort and vomiting when the cesarean delivery is being performed with regional anesthesia.

Significant bleeding points should be clamped with ring forceps and the fundus of the uterus covered with a moist sponge. The margins of the uterine incision should be identified before repair, because the caudal margin of a thinned-out lower uterine segment can be confused with the posterior uterine wall ballooning into the operative field.

The uterine incision is closed with a single layer of 0 or #1 absorbable suture in a running-locked manner. The traditional closure begins just beyond one apex of the incision and proceeds just beyond the other apex. Some operators add a second line of sutures to imbricate the incision, but a double-layer closure does not improve postoperative

Figure 19-11

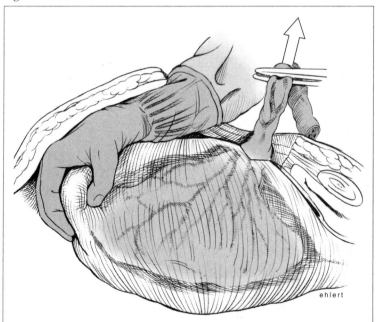

Delivery of the placenta. The placenta is delivered in assisted fashion by placing gentle traction on the umbilical cord, along with fundal massage. In the illustration, the placenta is bulging through the uterine incision.

outcome or reduce the risk of uterine rupture in subsequent VTOL.

Closure of a vertical incision requires a layered closure, using successive layers of 0 or #1 absorbable suture. Repair of a thick uterine wall may require three layers.

EXPLORATION OF THE PELVIS AND ABDOMEN

After repair of the uterine incision, the surgeon should explore the pelvis and abdomen—not just to inspect for surgical injuries but also to detect unsuspected pathology. The true pelvis should be inspected, and the adnexa should be palpated. If anesthesia and maternal condition permit, the vermiform appendix omentum, liver edge, spleen, kidneys, and para-aortic region can also be palpated and/or delivered for visual inspection. However, for patients receiving epidural anesthesia, palpation in the upper abdomen and traction on the viscera can be painful.

Following exploration of the pelvis and abdomen, remove all foreign material from the pelvis, and, if chorioamnionitis is present, the pelvis should

be copiously lavaged. Finally, it is essential to confirm that needle and sponge counts are correct.

CLOSURE OF PERITONEAL, FASCIAL, SUBCUTANEOUS, AND SKIN LAYERS

In the past, the vesicouterine and parietal peritoneum were closed with a 2-0 absorbable suture. Studies have shown, however, that closure of the peritoneum offers no advantage and increases operative time, febrile morbidity, cystitis, narcotic use, antibiotic use, and length of stay in the hospital.

The fascia is closed with a 0 or #1 nonlocking, continuous, long-lasting absorbable suture (e.g., polyglactin). Traditionally, the closure proceeded from the distal aspect of the incision to proximal, with sutures placed at 1.0-cm intervals that are 1.5 cm from the margin of the cut fascia. Some surgeons close the fascia with two lines of suture that meet in the midline. In the modified Joel-Cohen fascia closure, sutures are placed away from the surgeon. Many surgeons perform a Smead-Jones mass closure (Fig. 19-12) with a #1 nonabsorbable suture for wounds at high risk of dehiscence (e.g.,

Figure 19-12

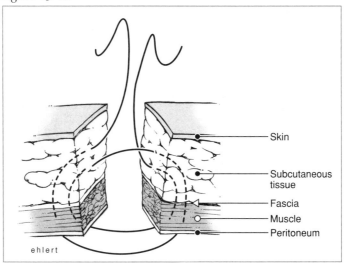

Smead-Jones mass closure. In the Smead-Jones closure, the peritoneum, abdominal wall muscles, and fascia are closed in a single layer, with sutures placed about 1.5 to 2.0 cm apart. The technique is advocated for wounds at high risk of dehiscence.

longitudinal incisions in the presence of morbid obesity or chronic steroid use).

Closure of the subcutaneous tissue is generally not necessary. If the depth of the subcutaneous tissue is greater than 2 cm, however, closure may decrease postoperative wound disruption.

The skin can be closed with staples, subcuticular 4-0 absorbable sutures, or with widely spaced mattress sutures. Pfannenstiel incisions closed with subcuticular sutures result in less postoperative discomfort and are more cosmetically appealing at the 6-week postoperative visit.

Intraoperative Complications

The mortality rate for cesarean delivery is about 6 per 100,000 procedures. Half of these deaths are related to intraoperative complications, while others are related to anesthetic and postoperative complications (Table 19-8). In recent years there has been a shift in the etiology of deaths from hemorrhage and infection to thromboembolic events. The number of deaths from general anesthesia has remained stable over the last 20 years, but regional anesthesia–related deaths have decreased. This has resulted in an increased case-fatality ratio for general anesthesia versus regional anesthesia from 2.3 before 1985 to 16.7 after 1985.

Intraoperative injuries are uncommon, but they can still occur despite careful attention to technique. The operative team is responsible for identifying and repairing injuries or for seeking appropriate assistance to help with repairs. The most common complications are hemorrhage, uterine lacerations, bladder and ureteral injuries, and injuries to the gastrointestinal tract.

HEMORRHAGE

The most common cause of hemorrhage during cesarean delivery is uterine atony. The first management steps are uterine massage and pharmacologic therapy, followed by surgical management. Pharmacologic therapy should proceed in a stepwise fashion from oxytocin 20 to 40 units per liter intravenously to methylergonovine 0.2 mg

Table 19-8

Complications of Cesarean Delivery

Anesthetic complications
  Airway problems
    Aspiration
    Induction/intubation failure
    Inadequate ventilation
    Respiratory failure
  Cardiac arrest
  Local anesthetic toxicity
  High spinal/epidural—hypotension
  Overdosage
  Spinal headache
Intraoperative complications
  Hemorrhage
    Uterine atony
    Placenta previa/accreta
    Lacerations: uterine, broad ligament, vaginal
    Unplanned hysterectomy
  Uterine injury (extension of incision)
  Urinary tract injury
    Cystotomy
    Ureteral
  Gastrointestinal injury
Postoperative complications
  Respiratory
    Atelectasis
    Pneumonia
  Gastrointestinal
    Ileus
    Obstruction
  Infectious
    Urinary tract infection
    Endomyometritis
      Peritonitis, parametrial phlegmon, pelvic
        abscess
      Future subfertility from intrauterine or
        fallopian tube scarring
    Wound infection
      Fascial dehiscence
    Septic thromboembolism
    Septic shock
  Thromboembolism
    Deep venous thrombosis
    Pulmonary embolism
  Uterine
    Repeat cesarean with subsequent deliveries
    Uterine scar disruption: rupture,
      asymptomatic dehiscence
    Placenta accreta
    Unplanned hysterectomy: infertility
  Skin
    Keloid formation

intramuscularly, to 15-methyl prostaglandin F-2-alpha. The initial dose of 15-methyl prostaglandin F-2-alpha is 0.25 mg. That dose can be repeated every 15 minutes for a maximum total dose of 2.0 mg. 15-Methyl prostaglandin F-2-alpha can be administered intramuscularly or directly into the myometrium.

The surgical management of hemorrhage should also proceed in a stepwise fashion, assuming the patient is hemodynamically stable. The first step is bilateral O'Leary sutures of the uterine arteries. These 0 or #1 absorbable sutures are placed in the lateral aspect of the uterus, just superior to the ureters (Fig. 19-13). A second step to decrease uterine bleeding is bilateral ligation of the uterine vessels just medial to the ovaries. The next step, if needed, is to ligate the anterior divisions of the hypogastric arteries just distal to the superior gluteal artery (Fig. 19-14). Finally, if hemorrhage contin-

Figure 19-13

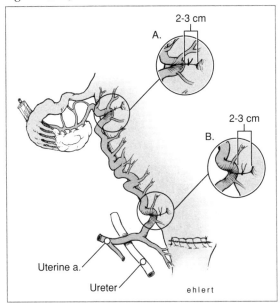

Ligation of the uterine artery. When pharmacologic management fails to stop uterine hemorrhage, the uterine artery arcade can be ligated in two places on the lateral aspect of the uterus. The first is adjacent to the lower segment of the uterus, just superior to the ureter. The second is near the cornu of the uterus, just medial to the ovaries.

ues despite these efforts, or if the patient is hemodynamically unstable, then hysterectomy may be indicated. The surgeon must communicate with the anesthesia staff to ensure adequate patient temperature with the high volume of infused fluids. A central venous catheter may be necessary to follow the patient's volume status.

If the hemorrhage continues in a hemodynamically stable patient, placement of a No. 30 French Foley catheter with a full 30-cc balloon through the cervix into the uterine cavity may tamponade the bleeding. This temporizing measure may allow time for correction of reversible conditions such as coagulopathy or thrombocytopenia. An IV fluid bag can be attached to the catheter as it exits the vagina to provide traction. If these efforts fail, a hysterectomy may be necessary.

Other modalities to stop uterine bleeding include selective arterial embolization for generalized uterine bleeding or oversewing with a 2-0 absorbable suture for areas of localized hemorrhage. When patients require large-volume transfusions, autotransfusion technology may offer advantages for remote hospitals with limited blood-bank resources. It also eliminates the risk of transmitting infectious agents during transfusion.

UTERINE LACERATIONS

Lacerations of the uterus are more common with malpresentations, macrosomia, and a very thin lower uterine segment. If the lower uterine segment is completely attenuated, then the surgeon may place the incision slightly higher than normal to decrease the likelihood of a uterine laceration; in this situation it is important to be cognizant of the altered delivery mechanics.

To achieve a satisfactory repair, the full extent of the laceration must be exposed and visualized. The first suture should be placed just beyond the apex of the laceration. The remaining sutures can be placed in a locking or interrupted fashion.

It may be necessary to visualize ureteral peristalsis throughout its course in the broad ligament to ensure that the uterine repair did not injure the ureter. If necessary, the ureter can be cannulated

Figure 19-14

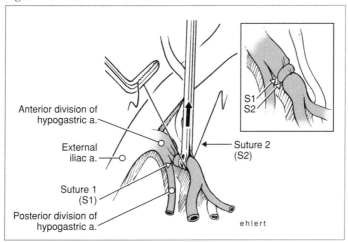

Hypogastric artery ligation. When uterine artery ligation is unsuccessful in stopping uterine hemorrhage, the anterior division of the hypogastric artery can be ligated. The hypogastric artery is a branch of the external iliac artery. It is located over the hypogastric vein, just lateral to the ureter. Grasp the anterior division of the hypogastric artery just distal to the superior gluteal artery with a Babcock clamp. Suture is placed around the artery. Care must be exercised to avoid injuring the ureter or uterine vein.

with a No. 8 French ureteral catheter through a cystotomy in the dome in the bladder. The cystotomy can subsequently be closed with two layers of 00 absorbable suture.

BLADDER INJURY

Bladder injury is more common with a Pfannenstiel incision, repeat cesarean delivery, uterine rupture, and cesarean hysterectomy. It is less common with sharp dissection between the lower uterine segment and bladder than with blunt dissection.

The dome of the bladder can be repaired with two layers of 00 absorbable suture. If the base or trigone of the bladder is involved, then the ureters should be cannulated to facilitate their identification during the repair. A urethral catheter should remain in place for 5 days after cystotomy. Intraoperative consultation with a urologist may be appropriate.

URETERAL INJURY

The ureter is most often injured during efforts to control bleeding from lateral uterine lacerations. Ureteral injury is reported to occur in 0.1% of cesarean deliveries and in 0.2% to 0.5% of cesarean hysterectomies. This injury may go unrecognized, but, if suspected, it is necessary to dissect and observe the length of the ureter to ensure that ureteral peristalsis is present. Ureteral repair usually requires urologic consultation.

GASTROINTESTINAL INJURY

Gastrointestinal injuries occur in 1 of 1300 cesarean deliveries and are more common when patients have adhesions from prior surgical procedures. The risk of bowel injury can be minimized by limiting sharp dissection to transparent peritoneum and, for lysis of adhesions, to sharp dissection with the scissors pointed away from the bowel.

Full-thickness defects of less than 1 cm are repaired in a double-layered fashion that avoids the possibility of bowel lumen narrowing (e.g., transverse closure of a longitudinal laceration). The mucosa is repaired with 3-0 absorbable suture in an interrupted fashion. The muscular and serosal layers are closed with a 3-0 silk suture in an interrupted fashion. Larger or complex lacerations may require consultation and assistance from a general or colorectal surgeon.

If fecal contamination of the operative field occurs, then copious irrigation and broad-spectrum antibiotics with gram-negative aerobic and anaerobic coverage are needed. Appropriate antibiotics include an aminoglycoside or a cephalosporin, plus either metronidazole or clindamycin, or an extended-spectrum penicillin. Prophylactic wound drainage is rarely needed. If an abscess is encountered, then debridement, copious lavage, and closed drainage through a separate site are recommended. Significant contamination may require secondary closure, especially in obese patients.

ANESTHETIC COMPLICATIONS

Despite the advances in anesthesia and the increased use of regional anesthesia, the number of deaths resulting from general anesthesia has not decreased. These deaths are frequently attributed to the inability to intubate or ventilate the patient and are more common when the patient is obese.

Postoperative Care

Cesarean aftercare should aid the mother's transition from the physiologic adaptations of pregnancy to a nonpregnant state with the responsibility of childcare. Cesarean aftercare must balance pain control with the prevention of complications.

Normal Postoperative Course

The amount of bleeding and the tone of the uterus should be continuously monitored. Vital signs and fundal status should be monitored hourly until stable and then every 4 hours. Coughing, deep breathing, and incentive spirometry are recommended to diminish the likelihood of pulmonary atelectasis.

Administer morphine sulfate 5 to 10 mg as needed every 2 hours intravenously or with a patient-controlled analgesia device. An oral analgesic should be started as soon as oral intake is tolerated. Give droperidol 0.5 to 1.0 mg every 4 hours intravenously as needed for nausea.

Early oral intake and ambulation should be encouraged. The IV can be converted to a heparin lock 24 to 36 hours after surgery, and the bladder catheter can be removed in 12 hours or the next morning.

The wound dressing should be removed in 24 hours and the wound monitored daily. The surgical clips can be removed in 3 days and tape strips placed for transverse skin incisions. With vertical incisions, clips are removed and tape strips placed at 5 to 7 days.

Before discharge, the Rh and rubella status should be reviewed and immune globulin and rubella immunizations administered, if appropriate. The postoperative hemoglobin level can be used to determine the need for iron replacement therapy. Discharge can usually be accomplished in 2 to 4 days. The gradual return to full activity is based on patient comfort. Fertility planning should be discussed prior to discharge and at the 6-week visit. The clinician should encourage breast-feeding for all women.

Postoperative Complications—Early

The most common early complications after cesarean delivery are infectious. The rate of infection without prophylactic antibiotic approaches 85%, while the infection rate with prophylactic antibiotics is only about 5%. Hence, routine antibiotic therapy is more than "prophylactic." Life-threatening infections (e.g., septic shock, pelvic abscess, and septic thrombophlebitis) occur in less than 2% of cases. The risk of infection is higher in younger women, lower socioeconomic status, longer labors, longer ruptured membranes, more vaginal examinations, and chorioamnionitis.

ENDOMYOMETRITIS

Endomyometritis presents with uterine or parametrial tenderness, fever (two postoperative temperatures over 38°C beyond 24 hours postdelivery), and leukocytosis. Because the leukocyte count is normally elevated in labor and the early puerperium, averaging 14,000 to 16,000 per mm, the diagnosis of endomyometritis is largely based on the clinical presentation. Furthermore, cultures of the lochia are often misleading, and blood cultures are frequently negative.

Ninety percent of cases will resolve within 72 hours with broad-spectrum intravenous antibiotics. A small percentage of patients will develop septic thrombophlebitis, parametrial phlegmon, pelvic abscess, and peritonitis.

WOUND INFECTION

Wound infection presents with erythema and tenderness, and patients may develop purulence and fever. Wound infection is a clinical diagnosis with laboratory data serving only as an adjunct. The leukocytosis is variable and wound cultures are often misleading. Abdominal wall ultrasound may localize fluid pockets.

Treatment includes broad-spectrum antibiotics and local care. The wound may need to be opened, probed, drained, irrigated, and packed, and the necrotic tissue debrided. The decision about delayed secondary closure versus healing by secondary intention will be influenced by the size of the wound and the logistics of follow-up care.

Fascial dehiscence occurs in approximately 5% of wound infections. Fascial dehiscence presents

with copious discharge followed by protrusion of bowel through the surgical wound. If this occurs, the bowel should be covered with a moist, sterile gauze pad and the wound explored immediately. The wound should be cleansed, debrided, and closed with retention sutures or a mass closure (e.g., Smead-Jones closure) (see Fig. 19-12) using long-term absorbable or nonabsorbable suture. Consultation should be obtained.

URINARY TRACT INFECTION

Urinary tract infections are often associated with the use of an indwelling urethral catheter. Treatment should be initiated with broad-spectrum antibiotics and subsequent antibiotic therapy based on urine culture and sensitivity results.

GASTROINTESTINAL COMPLICATIONS

Ileus presents with abdominal distention, nausea, vomiting, and failure to pass flatus. Physical examination may reveal the absence of bowel sounds. High-pitched bowel sounds and peristaltic rushes suggest a bowel obstruction, rather than ileus. Radiographic studies of patients with ileus show distended loops of small and large bowel, with gas usually present in the colon. In contrast, postoperative obstruction displays single or multiple loops of distended bowel, usually small bowel, with air fluid levels.

Treatment involves withholding oral intake, awaiting the return of bowel function, and providing adequate fluids and electrolytes. The patient may need nasogastric suctioning, or a duodenal or jejunal tube in the case of obstruction. Surgical consultation and possible lysis of adhesions may be needed if an obstruction persists.

THROMBOEMBOLIC COMPLICATIONS

Deep venous thrombosis (DVT) is three to five times more common after cesarean delivery than after vaginal delivery. DVT can progress to pulmonary embolus if untreated. DVT typically presents with leg tenderness, swelling, a palpable cord, Homan's sign, or a positive Lowenberg test. Doppler studies have 90% sensitivity for popliteal, femoral, or iliac thromboses, but only 50% for calf thrombosis. Impedence plethysmography is sensitive in proximal cases, but not in pelvic thrombosis. Venography remains the gold-standard test.

Intravenous heparin therapy is the standard treatment of DVT. If clinical suspicion of DVT is sufficiently high, heparin should be initiated after baseline coagulation studies are obtained, without waiting for the results of vascular studies. Limited research in nonpregnant patients indicates that DVT can be treated with low-molecular-weight (fractionated) heparin. Low-molecular-weight heparin is administered by subcutaneous injection without need to monitor coagulation studies except in obese patients. Outcomes with low-molecular-weight heparin are better than with "standard" unfractionated heparin because resolution of symptoms and rates of pulmonary embolism are the same as with standard intravenous heparin; however, the rate of hemorrhagic complications is lower. No data are available on the use of low-molecular-weight heparin for treating postpartum thromboembolic disease.

Pulmonary embolus presents with tachypnea, dyspnea, pleuritic pain, and apprehension. Findings include rales, friction rub, accentuated second heart sound, and a gallop. Radionuclide ventilation-perfusion lung scan is used for diagnosis, and pulmonary angiography will clarify equivocal findings. If suspicion of pulmonary embolism is high, then oxygen and heparin therapy should be administered before the lung scan results are available. In selected cases with life-threatening pulmonary emboli, injection of thrombolytic agents into the pulmonary artery can be lifesaving.

SEPTIC THROMBOPHLEBITIS

Septic thrombophlebitis is a diagnosis of exclusion. Persistent and unexplained fever is often the only symptom of septic thrombophlebitis, although some patients complain of pelvic pain. Ultrasonography and computerized tomography are frequently negative. Physical examination may reveal unilateral pelvic tenderness and, on rare occasions, ropelike adnexal structures.

Continued nonfocalized fever despite several days of antibiotic therapy suggests septic thrombophlebitis. Defervescence on heparin therapy provides effective treatment and confirms the diagnosis.

Postoperative Complications—Delayed

The delayed complications of cesarean delivery are uterine rupture and/or dehiscence, repeat cesarean delivery, increased likelihood of placenta accreta, and unplanned hysterectomy, as well as adhesion formation and subfertility as consequences of infectious morbidity.

UTERINE SCAR DISRUPTION

Dehiscence and rupture of a uterine scar are uncommon complications that are diagnosed during a subsequent pregnancy. Meta-analysis reveals that patients undergoing VTOL are at no higher risk for dehiscence or rupture in either the antepartum or the intrapartum periods than patients undergoing repeat cesarean delivery.

DEHISCENCE   The term *uterine dehiscence* is commonly applied to asymptomatic scar separation that does not penetrate the serosa and does not produce hemorrhage. Dehiscence occurs following fewer than 1% of pregnancies that follow cesarean delivery. Dehiscence presents as a "serosal window" and is often discovered unexpectedly during a repeat cesarean delivery.

RUPTURE   In contrast to dehiscence, uterine rupture is a through-and-through scar separation that is clinically symptomatic and requires immediate surgical intervention. Uterine rupture occurs in about 1% of women with a prior cesarean delivery. Clinical manifestations include loss of fetal station during labor, abrupt change in fetal heart rate pattern or uterine tone, vaginal bleeding, or hypotension and tachycardia beyond what would be expected for the observed amount of hemorrhage. Uterine or scar tenderness is present in only 25% of cases. Treatment for uterine rupture is dictated by the nature of the defect. In some cases a layered closure of the myometrium with absorbable suture will suffice, although hysterectomy may be necessary.

PLACENTA ACCRETA

One in four patients who undergo repeat cesarean delivery because of placenta previa will require cesarean hysterectomy for hemorrhage caused by placenta accreta. This complication increases with the number of prior uterine incisions, and its incidence has increased concurrently with the rise in cesarean delivery rates. In focal placenta accreta, the placental bed can be oversewn with interrupted sutures placed around the area of hemorrhage. If not successful, then complete hysterectomy is necessary because supracervical hysterectomy may not control the hemorrhage.

REPEAT CESAREAN DELIVERY

A major complication of cesarean delivery is that the patient will likely undergo cesarean delivery with subsequent pregnancies. Nearly two-thirds of repeat cesarean deliveries are performed without VTOL.

CESAREAN HYSTERECTOMY

Indications for cesarean hysterectomy are uterine hemorrhage unresponsive to treatment, placenta accreta, laceration of major pelvic vessels, large myomas, advanced cervical dysplasia or carcinoma, and sterilization. Complications of cesarean hysterectomy are more common during emergent procedures and include increased blood loss and anesthesia time, plus infection, blood transfusion, and unanticipated sterility.

Placement of an umbrella pack may control hemorrhage from the vaginal cuff after a cesarean hysterectomy. An umbrella pack consists of a plastic bag filled with a gauze tape. The bag is placed through the abdominal incision, and the tape protrudes from the bag into the vagina. The bag should occlude the vaginal cuff and be large enough to remain in place when an intravenous infusion bag is attached to the plastic bag. Traction is applied for 24 hours, after which the pack is removed. Removal is accomplished by pulling the tape through the vagina, thereby reducing the size of the bag. The patient should receive prophylactic antibiotics and have an indwelling urinary catheter to prevent urinary obstruction while the pack is in place.

ADHESIONS AND SUBFERTILITY

Adhesion formation can occur with improper handling of devitalized tissue, but more commonly is associated with the presence of infection and inflammation. Subfertility can result from adnexal adhesions, especially following pelvic abscess or phlegmon.

Long-Term Monitoring, Treatment, and Prognosis

The most important issue relating to long-term prognosis following cesarean delivery is the possibility of rupture of a uterine scar during subsequent deliveries. No routine long-term monitoring is necessary for women who have undergone cesarean delivery through a low-transverse uterine incision. The rate of uterine rupture during a subsequent VTOL in these women is 0.5% to 0.8%, which is not significantly higher than the rate in women who undergo repeat cesarean delivery.

Some controversy exists, however, about whether these women should undergo routine uterine scar exploration following VBAC. At present, routine uterine scar exploration is not essential, because even if disruption of a low-transverse uterine scar is found, surgical correction is not necessary unless the disruption is bleeding.

When scar disruption occurs during labor, it may be signaled by a dysfunctional labor pattern during an unsuccessful VTOL. The risk of scar dehiscence or rupture is increased by 2.8 times in failed VTOL versus elective repeat cesarean delivery.

Education

Postoperative Instructions

WOUND CARE

The abdominal wound should be kept dry and is best treated with minimal dressing. The area can be cleansed with warm water and mild soap. After hospital discharge, the patient should notify her clinician if she experiences erythema, drainage, fluctuance, temperature over 100.5°F, or increased warmth at the site.

GENERAL ACTIVITY

The patient can return to general activity based on comfort. She can climb stairs immediately, but should avoid carrying heavy objects on stairs for 2 weeks. Lifting objects that weigh more than 20 pounds and driving can be resumed based on comfort. Kegel, single leg lifts, and pelvic tilt exercises can also resume based on comfort. Coitus can be resumed based on comfort after the lochia subsides. Discuss contraception and infant care prior to discharge and at postpartum visits.

PSYCHOLOGICAL

If the patient has unanswered questions after the cesarean, then an unhurried conversation, when the patient is feeling well, will go a long way toward resolving issues.

UTERINE SCAR INFORMATION

After cesarean delivery, patients should be educated about the risks of vertical uterine incisions versus low-transverse incisions for future pregnancies. In our increasingly mobile society, it is reasonable to provide the patient with a copy of her operative report for presentation to her clinician during a subsequent pregnancy. Patients should be educated that repeat cesarean delivery has more maternal complications than VTOL and is no guarantee of perfect fetal outcome.

Errors

Errors in the management of cesarean delivery relate to decision making about indications for the procedure, technical performance of the procedure, and documentation.

Decision Making About Indications for Cesarean Delivery

Cesarean deliveries are sometimes performed without adequate indication. The most common situations in which this occurs relate to electronic fetal monitoring and breech deliveries. Cesarean deliveries are also performed inappropriately in conjunction with other surgical procedures and to avoid malpractice litigation.

FALSE-POSITIVE ELECTRONIC FETAL MONITORING

The widespread use of electronic fetal monitoring (EFM) has neither decreased acidosis-related newborn morbidity nor decreased the incidence of cerebral palsy. Many subtle EFM findings are indications of preexisting fetal abnormalities not likely to benefit from cesarean delivery. Some self-limited bradycardias can be observed without intervention because the fetus has significant acid-base reserves. This may be the case with uterine hyperstimulation, self-limited eclamptic seizures, or vasovagal episodes.

ROUTINE CESAREAN DELIVERY OF BREECH INFANTS

There is no firm evidence on which to base a recommendation for routine cesarean delivery of infants presenting in a breech position at term that meet standard criteria for vaginal delivery (e.g., frank breech, 1500 to 3500 grams, head flexed). Meta-analysis reveals that long-term morbidity for term infants presenting breech is not decreased by cesarean delivery.

COMBINING CESAREAN DELIVERY WITH OTHER SURGICAL PROCEDURES

The surgeon's primary responsibly is safe operative delivery, even when pathology is found at cesarean delivery. The surgeon should perform the most conservative procedure necessary. Some surgeons choose to perform elective surgical procedures at the time of cesarean delivery. As discussed below, this practice should be discouraged.

REMOVAL OF ABNORMAL ADNEXAE Adnexal pathology is discovered at 1 out of 200 cesarean deliveries; the most common ovarian neoplasm is benign cystic teratoma. The treatment of choice for a teratoma is cystectomy with careful inspection and palpation of the contralateral ovary. Bilateral teratomas are present in 5% to 10% of cases, but biopsy of the contralateral ovary is of little value unless a gross lesion is present, and extensive biopsy or wedge resections may compromise future fertility by producing adhesions. Removal of other adnexal abnormalities such as ovarian and para-ovarian hydatoids and hydrosalpinges should be reserved for obvious malignancy or lesions susceptible to torsion.

Ovarian malignancy, however, is found in only 1 out of 20,000 women who undergo cesarean delivery. Because malignancy is uncommon, and because prognosis in ovarian cancer is related to tumor, grade, and distribution it is inappropriate to attempt definitive surgical procedures for suspected ovarian cancer during cesarean delivery. Incomplete evaluations such as a partial staging procedure without lymph node dissection do not benefit the patient. The surgeon should perform the most conservative procedure possible (e.g., diagnostic biopsy), leaving definitive treatment until after a histologic diagnosis is made.

REMOVAL OF LEIOMYOMAS Most leiomyomas regress after pregnancy and are highly vascular. Removal should not be attempted unless there is an easily accessible pedicle and torsion is anticipated. Such lesions can be removed by cross-clamping and placement of Heaney transfixion ligatures with an absorbable suture.

REMOVAL OF THE APPENDIX A woman's lifetime risk for acute appendicitis is approximately 10% at age 17, but falls to only 3.5% by age 37. Thus, routine elective removal of the appendix at the time of cesarean delivery is not indicated.

Obstruction of the appendix by a fecalith is the primary cause of appendicitis. Therefore, palpation of the appendix during abdominal exploration and expression of fecaliths or other material is appropriate. Removal of the appendix, however, is appropriate only if a fecalith is identified and cannot be easily extruded into the cecum, if signs of appendiceal inflammation are present, or if a mass is noted.

OTHER SURGICAL PROCEDURES Some clinicians choose to perform a cesarean delivery on patients near term if the patient has another indication for surgery, such as a desire for surgical sterilization. Performance of an elective cesarean delivery because of the second surgical procedure should be discouraged because of the increased morbidity and hospital stay. For example, a repeat cesarean delivery plus a tubal ligation may double the length of hospitalization required for a VTOL with a postpartum tubal ligation.

PERFORMING A CESAREAN DELIVERY TO AVOID MALPRACTICE LITIGATION

Many health-care providers incorrectly assume that performing a cesarean delivery helps avoid malpractice claims. Performance of a cesarean offers no protection against allegations of malpractice if a less-than perfect infant is born. The plaintiff's legal team can simply shift the focus to other issues such as the cesarean delivery not being performed sooner and a perceived lack of prenatal care or antenatal testing.

Technical Errors

Common technical errors involve incorrect closure of the uterine incision, malpresentation deliveries, and selection of the surgical procedure.

CLOSING THE UTERINE INCISION

A common error is placement of sutures too far beyond the uterine incision. This may result in increased bleeding from the lateral uterine vessels, and it increases the risk of ureteral injury. Furthermore, an inexperienced operator, or one operating with inadequate exposure, may inadvertently suture incorrect tissue. Therefore, the lateral apices of the uterine incision and any extensions should be carefully identified prior to closure. Poor exposure may result in suturing the upper edge of the uterine incision to a prominent posterior wall of the uterus, instead of the lower uterine incision.

MALPRESENTATION DELIVERIES

Some experienced clinicians consider converting a breech or transverse presentation to a cephalic presentation after opening the abdomen but before the uterine incision. Intraoperative version prior to uterine incision may avoid a traumatic delivery, a classical uterine incision, an inverted "T" incision, or an extension. Adequate exposure and a skilled assistant are critical for atraumatic delivery of a malpresentation.

CHOICE OF PROCEDURE

Randomized, controlled studies have shown that many aspects of the traditional procedure that accompany the Pfannenstiel skin and Kerr uterine incisions are unnecessary. In particular, double-layered uterine closure and closure of vesicouterine and parietal peritoneum do not improve outcomes for patients. The modified Misgav-Ladach cesarean delivery avoids these steps and is associated with less operative time, fewer complications, and a shorter length of stay.

Poor Documentation in Operative Reports

Accurate documentation of the operative procedure can prevent confusion and complications in the future. In particular, the surgeon should take care in describing the uterine incision. For example, "repeat low-transverse cesarean delivery" could mean (1) the prior incision was a classical or low vertical, and the current procedure was a "repeat" cesarean performed via a low-transverse incision; or (2) the previous operation was a low-transverse incision, and the same procedure was used in the current procedure. In the first example the patient should never undergo a VTOL, while the second is a VTOL candidate. A better description of the procedure would be "repeat cesarean delivery, low-transverse uterine incision." It is also important to properly document the extent of active uterine segment involved in a low-vertical incision, the extent of an inverted "T" incision, and the nature of any uterine lacerations.

Controversies

The high rate of cesarean delivery in North America is the subject of controversy. Some causes of the increased cesarean rate are listed in Table 19-1. Four controversies are particularly worthy of discussion: delivery of macrosomic infants by cesarean to avoid shoulder dystocia; safety and success of VBAC; the role of vaginal delivery for breech presentation; and, finally, the role of maternal lifestyle.

Macrosomia

Some clinicians perform cesarean delivery for presumed macrosomia to avoid shoulder dystocia. Cesarean delivery has been recommended variously for fetuses estimated to weigh 4000, 4250,

4500, and 5000 grams, with and without glucose intolerance. Fetal weight is commonly estimated by ultrasound, although ultrasound may be no more predictive than clinical examination.

One outcome of macrosomic birth is brachial plexus injury. Most brachial plexus injuries are self limited, although 5% to 22% result in permanent neurologic injury. Decision analyses indicate that for infants weighing more than 5000 grams of diabetic mothers, it would be necessary to perform only five cesarean deliveries to avoid one brachial plexus injury. At 4500 grams, however, the corresponding figure is 20 cesarean deliveries to prevent one brachial plexus injury. Furthermore, because most brachial plexus injuries resolve spontaneously, researchers have estimated that it would require as many as 3695 cesarean deliveries at an additional cost of $8.7 million to prevent one permanent brachial plexus injury in fetuses over 4500 grams in mothers without diabetes (Table 19-9). The controversy is further complicated by the fact that brachial plexus injuries sometimes occur in fetuses weighing less than 4000 grams born by cesarean delivery.

The controversy regarding cesarean delivery of macrosomic fetuses may be resolved when more accurate and precise antenatal indicators of macrosomia and shoulder dystocia are developed. Some fetal indicators under study are abdominal cutaneous-tissue thickness, humeral soft-tissue thickness, cheek-to-cheek diameter, and femur length ratio, as well as echo-planar imaging.

Vaginal Trial of Labor

Some authors suggest that VBAC and operative vaginal deliveries have inherent risks that are unacceptable compared to the risk of repeat cesarean delivery. Some argue that any specific goal is arbitrary and suggest that VBAC is encouraged simply because vaginal delivery is less costly than cesarean delivery. These arguments ignore data from those countries with cesarean-delivery rates lower than 15%, yet with perinatal mortality rates lower than in the United States. Endorsement of a high cesarean-delivery rate must take into account the many complications associated with cesarean delivery. The number of complications and deaths are likely to increase as the cohort of North American women continues to age and gain weight.

Table 19-9

Cesarean Deliveries to Avoid Brachial Plexus Injury (BPI) in Macrosomic Infants

| | CESAREAN DELIVERIES TO PREVENT | | |
	BIRTH WEIGHT (G)	IMMEDIATE BPI	PERMANENT BPI
All nondiabetic vaginal deliveries	≥ 4000	162	733–3226
	≥ 4500	51	233–1026
	≥ 5000	19	85–373
Operative[a] nondiabetic vaginal deliveries	≥ 4000	74	339–1493
	≥ 4500	38	174–766
	≥ 5000	—	—
All diabetic vaginal deliveries	≥ 4000	48	219–962
	≥ 4500	20	91–400
	≥ 5000	5	23–100

[a]Operative deliveries include forceps and vacuum assisted deliveries.
SOURCE: Reprinted with permission from the American College of Obstetricians and Gynecologists (*Obstet Gynecol*, 1997, 89:643–647).

Breech Vaginal Delivery

About 70% of breech presentations at term can be avoided by appropriate external cephalic version. There is no difference in 10-year outcome measures (i.e., incidence of neurologic deficit, developmental delay, handicap, or psychiatric referral) in children born by vaginal breech delivery versus cesarean delivery.

Maternal Lifestyle

The factors associated with the increased rate of cesarean delivery can be classified as health-care-system–related (Table 19-1) or patient-related. Patient-related factors include those that are easily amenable to change and those that are not. Some maternal factors that are not easily amenable to change include age, short stature, education status, and nulliparity.

Other maternal characteristics, however, are potentially modifiable. These include prepregnancy weight, weight gain during pregnancy, and illicit drug use. Appropriate preconception counseling, along with society-level interventions, to address these modifiable risk factors could decrease the risk of cesarean delivery among patients at risk.

Emerging Concepts

Stapling Devices

Some stapling devices simultaneously cut tissue and hemostatically ligate tissue with an absorbable glyclolide-lactide copolymer. Studies have not replicated the initial decreased operative times or estimated blood loss or the improved operative outcomes previously reported. The use of stapling devices may need further evaluation with the emergence of HIV disease and their use in "bloodless" cesarean delivery.

Bloodless Cesarean Delivery

The procedure of "bloodless" cesarean delivery was developed to decrease the intraoperative transmission of HIV from an infected mother to her infant. The bloodless method does not eliminate maternal blood loss; rather it minimizes exposure of the infant to maternal blood and bodily fluids.

On entry into the peritoneum, all bleeding sites are meticulously cauterized. The operative field is irrigated and draped with fresh sterile towels. The surgeon's gloves are then irrigated with a cleansing solution or changed. Using care not to rupture the amniotic membrane, the uterine cavity is opened. A plane is created between the uterine wall and the amniotic membrane. The uterine wall is elevated with clamps and a disposable stapling device completes the incision. The infant is delivered with the membrane intact, if possible. An assistant continuously irrigates the operative field with sterile saline to lessen exposure to maternal bodily fluids. The infant is bathed with a warm cleansing solution on delivery and is transferred to an attendant who completes the cleansing process.

As the worldwide HIV epidemic continues, bloodless cesarean delivery may be performed more frequently. However, it will be necessary to study the effectiveness of the technique in comparison with treating HIV-infected pregnant women with highly active retroviral therapy.

Perimortem Cesarean Delivery

Historically, cesarean delivery was a perimortem event performed to give birth to an infant whose mother was dead or dying. In recent years perimortem cesarean delivery has reemerged as a procedure to be performed after maternal cardiac arrest. The American Heart Association now recommends that if advanced cardiac life support has not restored effective circulation to a pregnant woman with 4 to 5 minutes of cardiac arrest, then rapid cesarean delivery should be performed. It is not necessary to obtain permission from family members before performing the procedure.

If promptly performed, perimortem cesarean delivery improves infant survival. The best survival

Table 19-10

Steps in Performing a Perimortem Cesarean Delivery

Initiate immediate cardiopulmonary resuscitation and advanced cardiac life support with lateral uterine displacement.

Initiate cesarean delivery after 4 minutes of ineffective maternal circulation.

Attempt procedure if estimated gestational age is greater than 23 weeks (fundal height ≥ 4 cm or ≥ 3 finger-breadth above the umbilicus).

Prepare equipment/personnel for perimortem cesarean delivery and neonatal resuscitation.

Avoid delays for fetal heart tones or waiting for an obstetrician.

The first provider available should initiate the cesarean delivery.

Wear appropriate personal protective equipment to protect health personnel from transmission of infection.

Perform rapid cesarean delivery with the modified Joel-Cohen method or a vertical midline incision, with a vertical uterine incision. Use modified sterile technique, e.g., "splash and slash."

Pack with moist sponges. Continue ACLS throughout. Remove lateral tilt.

If hemodynamically stable, close uterus with a single line of #0 absorbable suture. Obtain hemostasis with interrupted 0 absorbable suture. Depending on available personnel, the wound may be left packed or closed anatomically.

---

rates are obtained when perimortem cesarean is performed within 5 minutes of the onset of ineffective maternal circulation. It is still worthwhile to pursue delivery after 5 minutes, however, because fetal mortality is 100% if no action is taken.

Furthermore, perimortem cesarean delivery increases the chance of maternal survival. Without cesarean delivery, less than 10% of patients suffering in-hospital cardiac arrest will survive to hospital discharge. With cesarean delivery, maternal survival increases because removal of the fetus results in an improvement in maternal circulation during cardiopulmonary resuscitation (CPR). In fact, uterine evacuation during cesarean delivery

at term can raise cardiac output by about 25% by relieving aortocaval compression.

Key considerations in performing perimortem cesarean delivery are shown in Table 19-10. The procedure should not be delayed while attempting to listen for fetal heart tones or perform an ultrasound study to document gestational age. Omission of a perimortem cesarean delivery, or delay in performing the procedure, may lead to the unnecessary loss of two lives. After delivery, the infant should be dried and kept warm because an infant may lose 30% of their available energy reserve within 5 minutes in a room-temperature environment.

All health-care providers should be able to provide this service in or out of the hospital. Equipment desirable for a postmortem cesarean delivery is listed in Table 19-11. If this equipment is not available, then the only necessary equipment is a scalpel and blankets to dry the infant.

Table 19-11

Perimortem Cesarean Delivery Kit

Obstetric supplies
Knife handle, #10 scalpel blade
Bladder blade retractor
Bandage scissors
4 laparotomy sponges
2 medium Richardson retractors
2 Kocher clamps
2 hemostats
2 cord clamps
Bulb syringe
DeLee suction
Needle driver
Finger forceps or pickups
3 each 0 chromic sutures
2 each 1 vicryl sutures
Sterile gloves
Pediatric supplies
3 pediatric blankets
Infant/child self-inflating bag
Resuscitation face masks
Neonate
Infant

References

American College of Obstetricians and Gynecologists: Active management of labor. *ACOG Update,* Vol. 24, No. 9. Port Washington, NY, Medical Information Systems, 1999, p. 5.

Brocklehurst P: Interventions aimed at decreasing the risk of mother-to-child transmission of HIV infection (Cochrane Review), in *The Cochrane Library,* Issue 4. Oxford, Update Software, 1999.

Buchanan TA, Kjos SL, Schaffer, U, et al: Utility of fetal measurements in the management of gestational diabetes mellitus. *Diabetes Care* 21 (suppl 2):B99, 1998.

Centers for Disease Control and Prevention: Rates of cesarean delivery—United States 1993. *MMWR* 44: 303, 1995.

Cetin A, Cetin M: Superficial wound disruption after cesarean delivery: effect of the depth and closure of subcutaneous tissue. *Int J Obstet Gynecol* 57:17, 1997.

Clark SL, Hankins GD, Dudley DA, et al: Amniotic fluid embolism: analysis of the national registry. *Am J Obstet Gynecol* 172:1158, 1995.

Conway DL, Langer O: Elective delivery of infants with macrosomia in diabetic women: reduced shoulder dystocia versus increased cesarean deliveries. *Am J Obstet Gynecol* 178:922, 1998.

Cunningham FG, McDonald PC, Leveno KJ, et al: *Williams Obstetrics,* 20th ed. Stamford, CT, Appleton & Lange, 1997.

Dajani AS, Taubert KA, Wilson W, et al: Prevention of bacterial endocarditis: recommendations of the American Heart Association. *JAMA* 277:1794, 1997.

Depp R: Cesarean delivery, in Gabbe SG, Niebyl JR, Simpson JL (eds): *Obstetrics—Normal & Problem Pregnancies.* New York, Churchill Livingstone, 1996, p. 623.

Ecker JL, Greenberg JA, Norwitz ER, et al: Birth weight as a predictor of brachial plexus injury. *Obstet Gynecol* 89:643, 1997.

Eisinger SH, Koller WS: Malpresentations, malpositions, and multiple gestation, in Kelber MJ, Beasley JW, Damos JR, et al (eds): *Advanced Life Support in Obstetrics Course Syllabus,* 3rd ed. Kansas City, American Academy of Family Physicians, 1996.

Enkin MW, Wilkinson C: Absorbable staples for uterine incision at cesarean section (Cochrane Review), in *The Cochrane Library,* Issue 4. Oxford, Update Software, 1999.

Enkin MW, Wilkinson C: Manual removal of placenta at cesarean section (Cochrane Review), in *The Cochrane Library,* Issue 4. Oxford, Update Software, 1999.

Enkin MW, Wilkinson C: Single versus two layer suturing for closing the uterine incision at cesarean section (Cochrane Review), in *The Cochrane Library,* Issue 4. Oxford, Update Software, 1999.

Enkin MW, Wilkinson C: Uterine exteriorization versus intraperitoneal repair at cesarean section (Cochrane Review), in *The Cochrane Library,* Issue 4. Oxford, Update Software, 1999.

Federici D, Lacelli B, Maggiasca A, et al: Cesarean section using the Misgav Ladach method. *Int J Gynecol Obstet* 57:273, 1997.

Franchi M, Ghezzi F, Balestreri D, et al: Randomized clinical trial of two surgical techniques of cesarean section. *Am J Obstet Gynecol* 178:S31, 1998.

Frishman GN, Schwartz T, Hogan JW: Closure of Pfannenstiel skin incisions: staples vs subcuticular suture. *J Reprod Med* 42:627, 1997.

Gregory KD, Korst LM, Cane P, et al: Vaginal birth after cesarean and uterine rupture in California. *Obstet Gynecol* 94:985, 1999.

Hawkins JL, Koonin LM, Palmer SK: Anesthesia-related deaths during obstetric delivery in the United States, 1979–1990. *Anesthesiology* 86:277, 1997.

Hodnett ED: Caregiver support for women during childbirth (Cochrane Review), in *The Cochrane Library,* Issue 4. Oxford, Update Software, 1999.

Hofmeyr GJ, Hannah ME: Planned cesarean section for term breech delivery (Cochrane Review), in *The Cochrane Library,* Issue 4. Oxford, Update Software, 1999.

Hofmeyr GJ, Kulier R: External cephalic version for breech presentation at term (Cochrane Review), in *The Cochrane Library,* Issue 4. Oxford, Update Software, 1999.

Holmgren G, Sjoholm L: The Misgav Ladach method of cesarean section: evolved by Joel Cohen and Michael Stark in Jerusalem. *Trop Doc* 26:150, 1996.

Hopkins L, Smaill F: Antibiotic prophylaxis regimens and drugs for cesarean section (Cochrane Review), in *The Cochrane Library,* Issue 4. Oxford, Update Software, 1999.

Howell CJ: Epidural versus non-epidural analgesia for pain relief in labour (Cochrane Review), in *The Cochrane Library,* Issue 4. Oxford, Update Software, 1999.

Johnstone FD, Prescott RJ, Steel JM, et al: Clinical and ultrasound prediction of macrosomia in diabetic pregnancy. *Br J Obstet Gynecol* 103:747, 1996.

Katz VL, Dotters DJ, Droegemueller W: Perimortem cesarean delivery. *Obstet Gynecol* 68:571, 1986.

Lopez-Zeno JA, Peaceman AM, Adashek JA, et al: A controlled trial of a program for the active management of labor. *N Engl J Med* 326:450, 1992.

Lurie S, Zalel Y, Hagay ZJ: The evaluation of accelerated fetal growth. *Curr Opin Obstet Gynecol* 7:477, 1995.

Marcovici I, Scoccia B: Postpartum hemorrhage and intrauterine balloon tamponade: a report of three cases. *J Reprod Med* 44:122, 1999.

National Center for Health Statistics: Cesarean delivery in the United States, 1990. *Vital and Health Statistics,* Series 21, No. 51, Data on Natality, Marriage and Divorce. DHHS Publication No. (PHS) 94-1929, Hyattsville, MD, 1994.

National Center for Health Statistics: Rates of cesarean birth and vaginal birth after previous cesarean, 1991–1995. *Monthly Vital Statistics Report,* Vol. 45, No. 11(suppl 3) Hyattsville, MD, 1997.

Nozton FC: International differences in use of obstetric interventions. *JAMA* 263:3288, 1990.

Rebarber A, Lonser R, Jackson S, et al: The safety of intraoperative autologous blood collection and autotransfusion during cesarean section. *Am J Obstet Gynecol* 179:715, 1998.

Rouse DJ, Owen J, Goldenberg RL, et al: The effectiveness and cost of elective cesarean delivery for fetal macrosomia diagnosed by ultrasound. *JAMA* 276:1480, 1996.

Sachs BP, Castro MA: The risks of lowering the cesarean delivery rate. *N Engl J Med* 340:54, 1999.

Sewell JE: *Cesarean Section—A Brief History.* Washington, DC, American College of Obstetricians and Gynecologists, 1993.

Smaill F, Hofmeyr GJ: Antibiotic prophylaxis for Cesarean section (Cochrane Review), in *The Cochrane Library,* Issue 4. Oxford, Update Software, 1999.

Thacker SB, Stroup DF: Continuous electronic heart rate monitoring versus intermittent auscultation for assessment during labor (Cochrane Review), in *The Cochrane Library,* Issue 4. Oxford, Update Software, 1999.

Thorp JA: Epidural anesthesia for labor: effect on the cesarean birth rate. *Clin Obstet Gynecol* 41:449, 1998.

Towers CV, Deveikis A, Asrat T, et al: The bloodless cesarean section and perinatal transmission of the human immunodeficiency virus. *Am J Obstet Gynecol* 179:708, 1998.

U.S. Department of Health and Human Services: *Healthy People 2000. National Health Promotion and Disease Prevention Objectives.* DHHS Publication No. (PHS) 91-50212. Washington, DC, Public Health Service, 1990.

Wilkinson CS, Enkin MW: Peritoneal non-closure at cesarean section (Cochrane Review), in *The Cochrane Library,* Issue 4. Oxford, Update Software, 1999.

Vanessa B. Peyton

Episiotomy and Obstetric Lacerations

Introduction

Episiotomy is a surgical incision of the perineum that transects the vaginal mucosa and the underlying fascia and perineal musculature. Episiotomy was introduced in 1742 by Ould as an adjunct to vaginal deliveries. Historically the intent of an episiotomy was to prevent severe obstetric lacerations, including third-degree lacerations (involvement of the rectal sphincter) and fourth-degree lacerations (involvement of the rectal mucosa). However, recent studies have demonstrated that episiotomies actually lead to a higher incidence of third- and fourth-degree lacerations. Effectively treating obstetrical lacerations that occur during a delivery depends on properly classifying lacerations, and identifying and restoring anatomic landmarks.

Pathophysiology

As the fetal head descends during the later parts of the second stage of labor, the muscular and soft-tissue support of the pelvic floor stretch to make room for the descending fetus. With rapid descent and stretching, however, the pelvic muscle and soft tissues may be unable to fully accommodate the fetus, and as a result the pelvic tissues can tear, causing obstetric lacerations.

Obstetric lacerations are first categorized by their location. These include cervical, vaginal, periurethral, and perineal lacerations. Perineal lacerations are further categorized by depth and by the structures injured. A first-degree perineal laceration involves only the vaginal mucosa. Second-degree lacerations involve not only the vaginal mucosa, but also the underlying perineal body, the bulbocavernosus muscles (which are muscles that converge to form the perineal body), and the hymeneal ring. Third-degree lacerations extend through the rectal sphincter, and fourth-degree lacerations extend through the rectal mucosa.

An episiotomy is a surgically created, second-degree perineal laceration. There are two basic types of episiotomy. The first is a midline, or median, episiotomy, which is an incision of the perineum, usually 2 to 3 cm in length, from the 6 o'clock position of the introitus directed toward the rectal sphincter. The second type is a mediolateral episiotomy, which begins at the 6 o'clock position of the introitus and is directed posteriorlaterally, either to the left or the right, at a 45° angle.

Epidemiology

Incidence of Episiotomy

There is substantial geographic variation in the rate of episiotomy, with the procedure being uncommon in some areas and nearly routine in others.

In the United States, episiotomy rates have decreased over the past 2 decades from more than 85% to about 10% of deliveries. The decline in routine use of episiotomies has been caused in part by studies demonstrating that routine episiotomy results in an increased incidence of third- and fourth-degree lacerations, a longer recovery time after delivery, and higher rates of chronic perineal discomfort and dyspareunia.

Benefits and Risks of Episiotomy

Table 20-1 lists the known risks and benefits of episiotomy. Periurethral tears are less common when episiotomy is performed. Also, there is benefit to performing an episiotomy in operative vaginal delivery and when delivering twins, breech infants, and shoulder dystocia.

However, while some proponents of episiotomy argue that the procedure reduces the risk of subsequent pelvic relaxation (cystocele, rectocele) and vesiculovaginal fistulas, there are no data to support these contentions. In fact, there is evidence that outcomes in regard to pelvic muscle function, sexual function, and postpartum pain are superior when no episiotomy is performed, even if a spontaneous second-degree laceration occurs. There is also no difference in the incidence of infections, fetal intracranial trauma, and neonatal acidosis when an episiotomy is performed.

The risk of death following episiotomy and spontaneous lacerations is extremely small. When deaths occur, they are most commonly associated with anesthetic complications (e.g., maternal or neonatal lidocaine toxicity) or infection (maternal necrotizing fasciitis). Serious consequences can be avoided by exercising care to avoid fetal injury, identifying complications through careful examination, and promptly intervening when a problem is identified.

Risk Factors for Obstetric Lacerations

Risk factors (Table 20-2) for sustaining perineal laceration include nulliparity, fetal weight over 4000 g, operative vaginal delivery, and Asian or African-American ethnicity. The risk of perineal lacerations in these situations can often be minimized if the delivering clinician provides adequate perineal protection or support during delivery of the fetal head.

Cervical lacerations most often occur when the patient pushes against an incompletely dilated cervix, or when attempts are made to manually dilate the cervix. Other risk factors for cervical lacerations include rapid progression of the first- and second-stage of labor, delivery of macrosmic infants, the presence of cervical scars from prior surgeries or lacerations, and instrumented deliveries. Vaginal wall tears can occur in compound presentations (e.g., nuchal hand, hand presenta-

Table 20-1

Episiotomy: Risks and Benefits

RISKS	BENEFITS
↑ Incidence of third-degree and fourth-degree lacerations	Easier to repair than spontaneous lacerations
↑ Blood loss	↓ Incidence of periurethral tears
Chronic perineal discomfort	Shortens second stage of labor
Dyspareunia	Facilitates delivery of shoulder dystocia
Longer recovery time after delivery	Facilitates operative vaginal delivery
Fetal lacerations	Facilitates breech delivery
Altered body image	

Table 20-2

Risk Factors for Obstetric Lacerations

TYPE OF LACERATION	RISK FACTORS
Perineal (second degree)	Nulliparity
	Fetal weight >4 kg
	Instrumented delivery
	Asian or African-American ethnicity
Third and fourth degree	Nulliparity
	Fetal weight >4 kg
	Instrumented delivery
	Short perineum
	Routine episiotomy
Vaginal	Compound presentation
	Rapid progression of stage II of labor
	Instrumented delivery
Cervical	Incomplete cervical dilation at onset of pushing
	Rapid progression of labor
	Instrumented delivery
	Fetal macrosomia
	Cervical scars

tion, etc.), rapid progression of the second stage of labor, and instrumented deliveries.

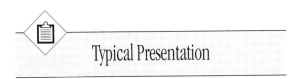

Typical Presentation

Clinicians most commonly perform an episiotomy in primiparous women who, because of maternal fatigue or fetal bradycardia, require an instrumented delivery. Spontaneous lacerations most often occur in primiparous women who experience either (1) a rapid second stage of labor with no time for distention and relaxation of the pelvic floor, or (2) a prolonged second stage of labor with significant perineal edema. Most of these lacerations are second-degree midline or periurethral lacerations. Third- and fourth-degree lacerations are most commonly seen with instrumented deliveries.

Cervical lacerations typically present as vaginal bleeding with the onset of pushing or as persis-

tent bleeding during or after the third stage of labor. Vaginal sidewall lacerations are most often seen following forceps deliveries.

Some obstetric lacerations are uncommon. For example, a rectal mucosal tear may occur without concomitant injury to the rectal sphincter. Rarely, a vaginal or cervical laceration may extend into the peritoneal cavity, broad ligament, or lower uterine segment, in which case repair of the laceration (frequently by laparotomy) by an experienced surgeon is required.

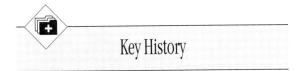

Key History

Detecting Contraindications

Prior to delivery, history should be directed at detecting contraindications to episiotomy. These include inflammatory bowel disease (because of the possibility of developing rectovaginal or rectocutaneous fistulas), large venereal warts (which may bleed with incision), and a patient's refusal to undergo the procedure.

Detecting Indications

The delivering clinician should be alert for development of intrapartum conditions for which episiotomy might be indicated. These include instrumented delivery, malpresentations, shoulder dystocia, and extremely small perineal size. Marked perineal edema, particularly in association with a prolonged second stage of labor, may also be an indication for performing an episiotomy.

Once the decision to perform an episiotomy has been made, the delivering clinician must determine if a median or mediolateral episiotomy should be performed. In the United States, midline episiotomies are performed far more frequently than mediolateral episiotomies because midline incisions are easier to anesthetize with local anesthesia, easier to repair, and they cause less bleeding, postpartum pain, and dyspareunia. Mediolateral episiotomy is indicated when patients are at very high risk for third- and fourth-degree lacerations because of a markedly shortened perineum.

Key Physical Examination

Routine Examination

Virtually all clinicians examine the perineal and periurethral areas after every delivery to detect lacerations that may have occurred. Many clinicians also recommend that all deliveries be followed by a routine rectal examination and inspection of the cervix and vaginal walls, although others perform these examinations only in special situations such as (1) after instrumented deliveries, (2) when there is unexplained bleeding, (3) if there are risk factors for a cervical lacera-

tion (i.e., pushing prior to complete cervical dilation), or (4) if the delivery was not otherwise straightforward. There is no research evidence with which to determine which of these approaches leads to superior outcomes for patients.

Cervical Examination

The cervix is examined to detect lacerations. The standard method for examining the cervix involves opening the vagina by having the examiner place three or four fingers of the nondominant hand into the vagina and exert downward pressure on the pelvic floor. Then, a ring forceps is used to "walk" around the cervix and visualize it through its entire circumference. If a cervical laceration is detected, repair is required if the laceration is bleeding or if it is greater than 1.5 cm in length.

Cervical visualization, especially of the posterior aspect of the cervix, can be difficult, particularly when there is heavy vaginal bleeding and before delivery of the placenta. It may be necessary to use retractors to help visualize the cervix. Common instruments for retraction include a "sponge stick" (4″ × 4″ gauze, folded and clamped into the end of a ring forceps), Sims' retractors, or the blade end of nonfenestrated obstetric forceps (Fig. 20-1).

Rectal Examination

The purpose of the rectal examination is to detect defects in the rectal mucosa, rectal sphincter, or rectovaginal septum. The best technique involves inserting one finger into the rectum while visualizing the vaginal mucosa of the rectovaginal septum, the rectal sphincter, and the perineum. The rectal mucosa and sphincter are carefully inspected and palpated for defects. If the rectal sphincter is torn, it will often be asymmetric, with one half of the muscle retracting back within the muscle's capsule, while the other half protrudes into the wound. Careful observation and identification of anatomic landmarks will facilitate repair of any defects that are detected.

Figure 20-1

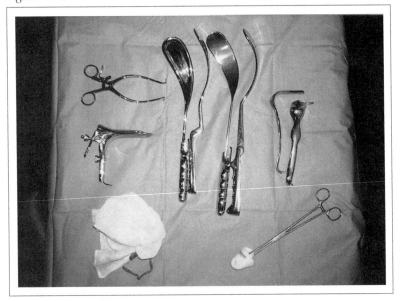

Retraction devices. A variety of devices and instruments can be used to retract tissues to facilitate visualization of the cervix and vagina. These include, starting clockwise at the lower left: vaginal packing, sterile speculum, Gelpi retractor, obstetric forceps with nonfenestrated blades (two sets shown), Sims' retractors, and sponge stick.

Ancillary Tests

Ancillary tests are rarely needed when dealing with episiotomies and obstetric lacerations. If there is suspicion that a laceration has extended into the peritoneal cavity, but the extension cannot be visualized on physical examination, an upright abdominal x-ray can be obtained. The x-ray will demonstrate free air under the diaphragm if an extended laceration is present.

Algorithm

Figure 20-2 is an algorithm displaying the decision-making process involved in determining if an epi-

siotomy should be performed. The algorithm in Figure 20-3 outlines the general approach to patients with a suspected obstetric laceration.

Treatment

Anesthesia for Episiotomy and Repair of Lacerations

Performing an episiotomy and repairing a laceration requires anesthesia to prevent maternal pain. For some women, epidural or intrathecal anesthesia used for pain control during labor may provide adequate anesthesia for episiotomy or laceration repair. For others, however, these anesthetic techniques may not provide sufficient pain control, and additional anesthesia will be needed. For such patients, and for those who have not received epidural or intrathecal anesthesia, options for pain control include local perineal infiltration and pudendal nerve blocks.

LOCAL INFILTRATION

Local perineal infiltration is usually accomplished by injecting up to 10 to 15 cc of 1% lidocaine (without epinephrine) into the perineum through a fine needle (e.g., 22-gauge). The goal is infiltration of the tissues of the perineum and vaginal vault surrounding the area of the laceration or of the tissues to be cut during episiotomy. When infiltrating a laceration, the needle should be inserted through the open wound of the laceration, rather than through intact skin or mucosa, as

Figure 20-2

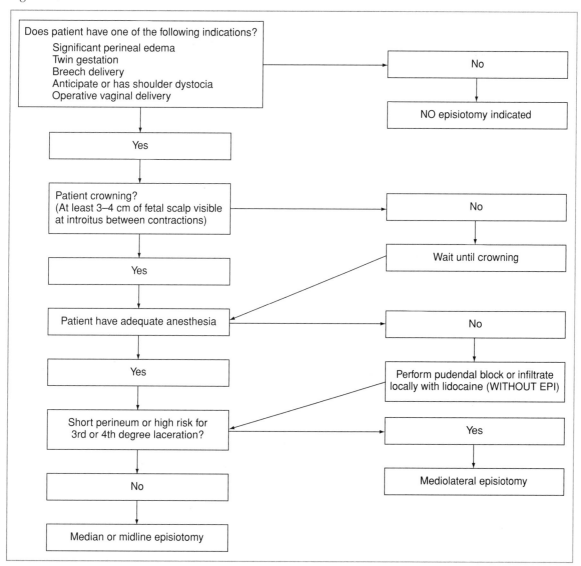

Algorithm for determining the need for an episiotomy.

Figure 20-3

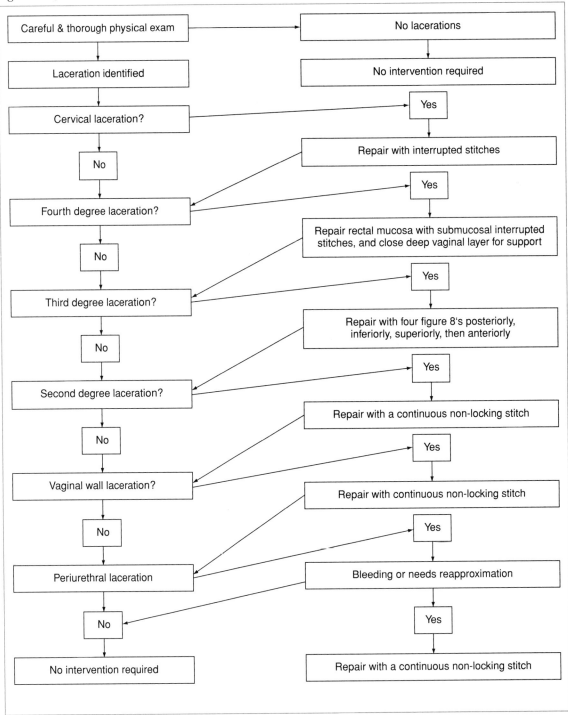

Algorithm for evaluation and management of obstetric lacerations.

injection through the wound will cause less discomfort for the patient.

To avoid complications, the clinician should aspirate the syringe before injecting lidocaine to be certain the tip of the needle is not in a maternal blood vessel. Lidocaine is then injected while withdrawing the needle from the injection site. If lidocaine is being infiltrated in anticipation of an episiotomy, care must be taken to not inject the fetal scalp, as lidocaine injected into the fetus can cause neonatal seizures and cardiac arrhythmias.

PUDENDAL BLOCK

A pudendal block is often difficult to perform once the fetal head has descended to 3 to 5 cm below the ischial spines, and it may take 5 to 10 minutes for the anesthetic effect to become apparent. Furthermore, pudendal nerve blocks do not provide adequate anesthesia for repairing cervical lacerations. Thus, the technique has limited utility.

Pudendal block may, however, be useful for repairing extensive vaginal lacerations, thereby avoiding the injection of large quantities of lidocaine. Pudendal anesthesia is also useful in anticipation of episiotomy when an instrumented (forceps) delivery is expected.

The first step in performing a pudendal nerve block is to palpate the ischial spines. This is accomplished with the nondominant hand. It is important to emphasize that pudendal nerve block cannot be performed if the ischial spines cannot be identified.

The injection for pudendal nerve block is then made with the dominant hand, using a needle positioned through a plastic inserter. The inserter is introduced into the vagina with the needle tip retracted and is placed at the injection sites adjacent to the ischial spine (Fig. 20-4). Once the appropriate adjacent sites have been identified, the needle is advanced through the tip of the inserter. If injecting prior to delivery, it is important to protect the fetal head with the fingers of the nondominant hand. It is also important to aspirate from the syringe prior to injection to ensure that the needle tip is not in a maternal blood vessel.

Figure 20-4

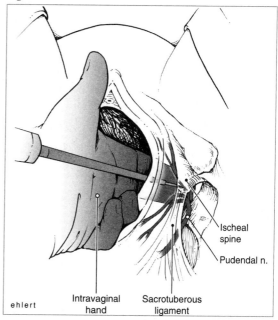

Pudendal nerve block. As described in the text, pudendal anesthesia is administered by injecting just posterior and inferiomedially to the ischial spine. Two fingers of the intravaginal hand are used to identify the ischial spine and to control the location of the needle tip, while the other hand manipulates the syringe.

The first injection site is just posterior to the tip of the ischial spine. Between 2.5 and 5.0 cc of 1% lidocaine (without epinephrine) is injected at this site. The second injection site is slightly medial and inferior to the ischial spine (into the sacrospinous ligament), where a similar volume of lidocaine is injected. Anesthesia will take effect within 10 minutes and will last for 20 to 60 minutes.

Performing an Episiotomy

To perform an episiotomy, the delivering clinician should wait until 3 to 4 cm of the fetal scalp is visible at the introitus between contractions. At this point, the perineum will begin to blanch because of pressure on the perineum from the fetal head, which decreases blood flow to the perineum. An incision made at that time will result in less bleeding than episiotomies performed before the fetal head tamponades the perineum.

For midline episiotomies, an incision is made using Mayo scissors, beginning the incision at the 6 o'clock position and extending it toward the rectal sphincter for approximately 2 to 3 cm (Fig. 20-5). The incision should stop at least 1 to 2 cm above the sphincter. For mediolateral episiotomies, the incision begins at the 6 o'clock position of the introitus and extends 2 to 3 cm at a 45° angle.

Figure 20-5

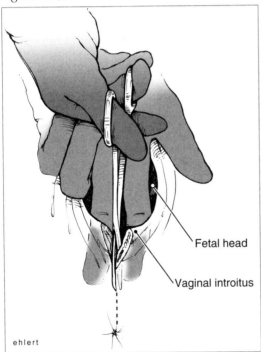

Fetal head

Vaginal introitus

ehlert

Cutting a midline episiotomy. With Mayo scissors, an incision is begun at the 6 o'clock position of the vaginal introitus and extended along the midline toward the rectum. The incision should stop well short of the rectum and rectal sphincter. Note how the operator inserts fingers into the vagina to create a space into which the scissors can be inserted, thereby avoiding injury to the fetal head.

Repair of Episiotomy and Lacerations

There are multiple ways to repair episiotomies and obstetric lacerations, and each approach has purported advantages and disadvantages. Limited research, however, has evaluated outcomes using these different approaches, and, with the exception of Flemming's work demonstrating different outcomes with different methods of repairing second-degree lacerations (see below), no studies are available to compare the relative benefits of the various repair techniques.

On completion of any repair, it is vital to perform a careful examination not only of the repair sites but also of the rectum to ensure that sutures have not inadvertently been passed through the rectal mucosa, as this may occur even with repair of simple episiotomies and second-degree lacerations. Thus, a digital rectal examination should be performed to palpate for sutures in the rectum, and any palpable stitch must be removed to minimize the risk of infection and fistula formation. If a third- or fourth-degree repair was performed, examination to ensure that the rectal sphincter is intact can be accomplished by having the patient squeeze while one of the examiner's fingers is inserted into the rectum.

SUTURE TECHNIQUES AND MATERIALS

The suture technique used for repair affects healing and postpartum pain. Flemming demonstrated that when repairing an episiotomy or a second-degree laceration, a locking stitch and a "snug" repair cause more postpartum pain than a continuous running stitch with a loose closure. A locking stitch should be reserved for situations in which bleeding is profuse and a hemostatic stitch is required.

Grant demonstrated that the choice of suture material not only affects postpartum pain, but also influences the rate of subsequent dyspareunia. This research showed that polyglycolic acid suture (Vicryl or Dexon) causes less postpartum pain and dyspareunia than chromic catgut. The recommended suture materials and stitching techniques are summarized in Table 20-3.

Table 20-3

Suture Material and Technique for Episiotomy and Laceration Repairs

REPAIR	SUTURE TYPE	SUTURE SIZE	NEEDLE TYPE	NEEDLE SIZE	STITCH
Second degree	Vicryl or Dexon	3-0 or 2-0	Taper	Large (CTX, CT, or CT-1)	Running continuous
Third degree	Vicryl[a]	2-0 or 1-0	Taper	Medium (CT-1)	Interrupted figure 8s
Fourth degree	Chromic[b]	4-0 or 3-0	Taper	Small (SH-1)	Interrupted
Vaginal wall	Vicryl or Dexon	3-0 or 2-0	Taper	Large (CTX, CT, or CT-1)	Running continuous
Cervical	Chromic or Vicryl	3-0 or 2-0	Taper	Medium (CT-1)	Interrupted
Periurethral	Vicryl or Dexon	4-0 or 3-0	Taper	Small (SH-1)	Running continuous

[a] Vicryl suture is preferred for repair of third-degree lacerations (i.e., rectal sphincter repair) because its absorption time is greater, thus providing more strength to the repaired rectal sphincter muscle.

[b] Chromic suture is preferred for repair of fourth-degree lacerations (i.e., rectal mucosa repair) because it is absorbed more quickly, thereby reducing the likelihood of developing a rectovaginal fistula.

REPAIR OF EPISIOTOMY AND SECOND-DEGREE LACERATIONS

SUPPLIES   Supplies required for repairing a simple episiotomy or second-degree laceration include nontraumatic tissue forceps, needle holder, suture scissors, 2-0 or 3-0 delayed absorbable suture on a taper needle (2-0 Vicryl or Dexon on a CT-1 needle), vaginal packing, and retractors for deep vaginal extensions.

REPAIRING THE VAGINAL COMPONENT   The repair begins with the vaginal component of the laceration/episiotomy, placing the first stitch above the distal apex of the wound (Fig. 20-6A). With a running continuous stitch, the vaginal laceration is repaired and dead space closed by taking deep "bites" of tissue (Fig. 20-6A), taking care not to stitch through into the rectum. The individual stitches should be placed approximately 1 cm apart.

REPAIRING THE HYMENEAL RING   The second part of the repair involves reapproximation of the hymeneal ring (Fig. 20-6A, inset A₁). This is achieved by reapproximating the ring by having the same suture used for the vaginal repair entering on the vaginal aspect of one half of the hymeneal ring and exiting on the vaginal aspect of the other half of the ring. Once the vaginal laceration has been repaired and

hymeneal ring reapproximated, the direction of suturing changes to begin the perineal repair. The suture is inserted near the midline, inside the hymeneal ring, and exits in the superiomedial aspect of the perineal laceration (Fig. 20-6A, inset A₂).

REPAIRING THE PERINEUM   The goal of perineal repair is not to have a "seam-tight" closure but rather to reapproximate the tissues. The approach is first to close the deep tissues, followed by closure of the dermis, using the same suture that was used to repair the vagina and which was brought under the hymeneal ring.

The deep tissues are closed by first approximating deep muscular tissue with interrupted sutures (Fig. 20-6B₁). Then, closure of the perineal tissues is achieved with a continuous running stitch, using the same suture that was brought under the hymeneal ring. The suture should be inserted superiorly to inferiorly, taking deep bites of tissue, and should exit subcutaneously (Fig. 20-6B₂). This suture continues until it reaches the inferior apex of the wound.

The final step is subcutaneous closure of the skin, again performed using the same suture, in a continuous running subcuticular fashion, moving upward from the apex to the vaginal opening (Fig. 20-6C). While skin closure is standard practice, it is of note that a recent study by Gordon et al

Figure 20-6

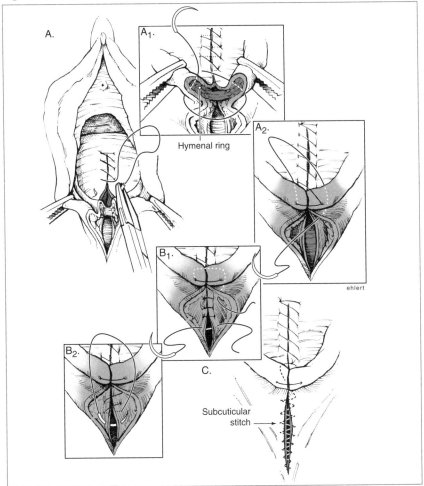

Repair of episiotomy or second-degree laceration. **A.** Vaginal mucosa. Repair of the vaginal mucosa is accomplished by placing the first stitch above the apex of the wound and then closing the vaginal mucosa with a single, continuous, running suture. The continuous suture continues to, and then exits under, the hymeneal ring *(inset A_1)*. The suture is not cut or tied at this point, but, instead, remains available for closing the perineal dermis *(inset A_2)*. **B.** Closing the perineal tissues. The deep, perineal, muscular tissues are closed with running or interrupted sutures *(B_1)*, after which the more superficial tissues are closed using the same suture that was used for the vagina. This latter suture continues as a running suture that closes the perineal dermis, moving from the hymeneal ring toward the rectum *(B_2)*. To achieve good closure, it is important that the needle enters and exits the wound as close as possible to the skin surface. **C.** Closing the skin. A subcuticular stitch is used to close the skin. The stitching begins at the apex near the rectum and then moves upward to the hymeneal ring. The needle is then passed back up under the hymeneal ring into the vagina, where a final tie-down stitch is made.

found that leaving the skin unsutured and permitting it to heal spontaneously results in less pain and dyspareunia at 3 months postpartum, with no apparent disadvantages and no increased risk of wound breakdown.

If a subcutaneous closure is performed, the last step is a tie-down stitch. This tie-down stitch should be within the vaginal vault, rather than in or adjacent to the perineal skin, to reduce postpartum pain.

REPAIR OF THIRD-DEGREE LACERATIONS

SUPPLIES Supplies required to repair a third-degree laceration include nontraumatic tissue forceps, nee-

dle holder, suture scissors, 2-0 or 1-0 delayed absorbable suture (Vicryl or Dexon) on a taper needle (e.g., CTX, CT, CT-1), two Allis clamps, and vaginal packing. Retractors may also be needed.

REPAIR TECHNIQUE Most clinicians recommend cleansing third-degree lacerations with a povidine iodine solution prior to repair, with the intention of reducing the incidence of infection. Following this iodine cleansing, the operator should grasp each end of the torn rectal sphincter, along with its respective capsule, using an Allis clamp (Fig. 20-7). Inclusion of both the capsule and the muscle

Figure 20-7

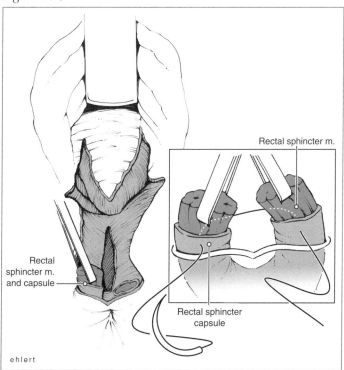

Rectal sphincter m.

Rectal sphincter m. and capsule

Rectal sphincter capsule

ehlert

Repairing third-degree and fourth-degree tears. This figure shows a layer of suture, seen from within the perineal wound, that has closed the defect in the rectal mucosa (i.e., the fourth-degree tear). To repair the rectal sphincter (third-degree tear), Allis clamps are used to grasp each end of the rectal sphincter muscle and to pull them into the surgical field (*inset*). The muscle capsule should be included in the grasp of the clamp, rather than excluded as shown in the inset. Figure-of-eight stitches are then placed into the rectal sphincter muscle, as described in the text.

is essential to ensure that the repair is strong and to prevent the muscle from retracting back into the capsule.

Four, interrupted, figure-of-eight stitches are then placed through both the capsule and the muscle itself (Fig. 20-7, inset). The first of the four sutures is placed posteriorly, followed by sutures in the inferior, superior, and anterior (P-I-S-A) positions. Placing the stitches in a different order makes it difficult to complete the repair properly.

After completion of the repair, it is important to carefully examine both the sphincter and the rectal mucosa to make certain the repair is intact and that there is no suture palpable in the rectum. Any sutures palpable in the rectum must be removed to avoid development of a rectovaginal fistula.

REPAIR OF FOURTH-DEGREE LACERATIONS

SUPPLIES Supplies required to repair a fourth-degree laceration include nontraumatic forceps (such as Russian forceps); needle holder; suture scissors; 4-0 or 3-0 delayed absorbable suture (chromic) on a small, noncutting, tapered (e.g., SH) needle; vaginal packing; and retractors.

REPAIR TECHNIQUE Adequate visualization is essential for proper repair. This is achieved with retractors (a Gelpi self-retaining retractor is helpful) and a vaginal pack. Use of vaginal packing will prevent the repair site from being obscured by blood. In addition, it is often useful to have an assistant present to help maintain retraction and the visual field.

Repair begins by identifying the distal apex of the rectal laceration and by placing the first stitch above the distal apex to prevent further extension of the wound. Interrupted submucosal stitches are then placed approximately 0.5 cm apart, from the apex to the base of the laceration.

It is essential to ensure that sutures are not placed within the rectal lumen, as this can lead to infection and formation of rectovaginal fistulas. Therefore, it is necessary to perform frequent rectal examinations during the repair; some clinicians even maintain a finger within the rectum while

placing sutures. After each rectal examination sterile gloves must be replaced to avoid contaminating the wound with fecal material.

After completing the mucosal repair, a careful rectal examination is again performed to ensure that the mucosa is intact and that no sutures are palpable in the rectal lumen. If a suture is palpable in the lumen, the stitch must be removed. Most clinicians then insert a second layer of support by placing a continuous running stitch in the deep vaginal fascial/muscular layers. At this point, the laceration has been converted to a third-degree wound, and repair proceeds as described earlier.

REPAIR OF CERVICAL LACERATIONS

SUPPLIES The following supplies are needed to repair a cervical laceration: nontraumatic tissue forceps, needle holder, suture scissors, 3-0 or 2-0 delayed absorbable suture (e.g., Chromic catgut, Vicryl, or Dexon) on tapered (noncutting) needle (e.g., CT-1), and two ring forceps. Because visualization is a key factor in successful repair of cervical lacerations, it is also necessary to have several devices available for retraction. Commonly used retraction devices include Sim's retractors, Gelpi self-sustaining retractors, and sponge sticks. As noted earlier, the blades of nonfenestrated obstetric forceps can also be used for retraction.

REPAIR TECHNIQUE Each side of the cervical laceration is grasped with a ring forceps. If possible, repair should begin with the first stitch above the apex of the laceration (Fig. 20-8). However, difficulty visualizing the entire laceration may preclude beginning the repair at the apex. In this situation, the repair begins at the edge of the laceration that is most easily visualized, which is usually the proximal/medial edge.

Individual interrupted sutures are placed. As each stitch is placed, placement of subsequent stitches will be facilitated by having an assistant maintain traction on the sutures. If repair did not begin at the apex, placement of sutures continues until the distal apex is in view, placing the final stitch above the distal apex. After completing the

Figure 20-8

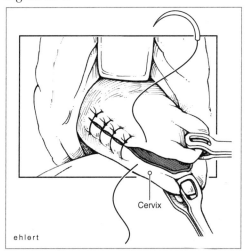

ehlert

Repair of a cervical laceration. To repair a cervical laceration, the cut ends of the laceration are first grasped with a ring forceps. The laceration is then repaired with interrupted stitches, approximately 0.5 cm apart. Placing traction on the tied sutures will help maintain visualization of the apex of the cervical laceration. Note the need for excellent exposure, provided with the aid of multiple retractors and an assistant.

repair, the cervix should be reexamined to ensure that hemostasis has been achieved and that no additional lacerations are present.

REPAIR OF VAGINAL WALL LACERATIONS

SUPPLIES Supplies required to repair a vaginal wall laceration include nontraumatic tissue forceps, a needle holder, suture scissors, 2-0 or 3-0 delayed absorbable suture (Vicryl or Dexon) on a taper needle, and retractors to facilitate visualization of both the apex and the base of the laceration.

REPAIR TECHNIQUE Excellent visualization is vital, as extensions of vaginal lacerations into the peritoneal cavity, into the lower uterine segment, or involving the ureter must be identified because they require repair by an experienced surgeon. Repair usually begins by placement of an anchoring stitch above the distal apex. Closure of the wound is then achieved with a continuous running stitch. Each stitch should be 1 cm deep, and they should be spaced 1 cm apart.

REPAIR OF PERIURETHRAL LACERATION

SUPPLIES Supplies required for repairing a periurethral laceration include nontraumatic tissue forceps, a needle holder, 3-0 or 4-0 delayed absorbable suture (Vicryl or Dexon with a SH needle), and a Foley or red-rubber urethral catheter.

REPAIR TECHNIQUE Repair of periurethral lacerations has two goals. The first is to repair the wound, in which the objective is reapproximation of the tissues, not strength. The second goal is to avoid injuring the urethra during the repair process.

To repair the laceration the clinician should place a running stitch, beginning at the apex of the upper end of the wound and working inferiorly. Each stitch should incorporate approximately 0.5 cm of tissue, and they should be spaced approximately 0.5 to 1.0 cm apart.

To avoid urethral injury, a urethral (Foley) catheter is inserted into the bladder and remains in place until the laceration is repaired. The catheter facilitates identification of the urethra and aids in preventing urethral needle punctures while repairing the laceration. If a suture is inadvertently inserted into the urethra, it must be removed. There are thought to be no long-term consequences from a stitch into the urethra if the stitch is promptly removed.

Postoperative Care

NORMAL POSTOPERATIVE COURSE

The majority of patients who have had an episiotomy or laceration repair experience substantial improvement of perineal discomfort within the first week after delivery. By 5 to 7 days postpartum, suture that is completely embedded within tissue begins to be absorbed; absorption times may be longer for suture material exposed to the air. As suture material is absorbed, patients may notice pieces of suture material when wiping, this is normal.

By 6 weeks postpartum, if the laceration or episiotomy is healing normally, a physical examination of the perineum will be normal. A scar may not even be evident. There is generally no pain at this time, and most patients are able to resume sexual intercourse.

Postoperative care for patients who have had an episiotomy or laceration repair involves pain control, good perineal hygiene, and avoiding trauma from hard stools. Table 20-4 provides a summary of instructions for patients who have had an episiotomy or laceration repair.

PAIN CONTROL

Pain control in the days following delivery is usually accomplished with acetaminophen or ibuprofen, although occasional patients may require narcotic analgesics (e.g., codeine). However, narcotics should be avoided when possible because they can cause constipation with passage of hard stool; this may result in disruption of sutures after repair of third-degree and fourth-degree lacerations.

PERINEAL HYGIENE

Patients who practice good perineal hygiene heal and become pain-free more quickly. Standard recommendations for perineal hygiene involve "periwash" and sitz baths. Periwash is a flushing of the perineal area with warm tap water using a squirt bottle. Sitz baths, another technique for washing the perineal area, is described in the chapter on hemorrhoids. Typically, periwash is performed after each void and sitz baths are administered three times a day.

AVOIDING TRAUMA

Patients with fourth- and third-degree lacerations must avoid constipation and diarrhea, as constipation can result in rectal trauma through stretching and wound dehiscence, and the liquid stool of diarrhea may penetrate the wound and lead to infection. The incidence of constipation and diarrhea can be reduced by using stool softeners and a low-residue diet (Table 20-5), which

Table 20-4
Summary of Postpartum Instructions for Wound Care

TYPE OF LACERATION	INSTRUCTIONS
All perineal lacerations	Wound cleansing after each toiletting
	Sitz baths TID
	Avoid perfumed toilet paper, perfume, or powder in genital area
	Pelvic rest (no intercourse, no douching, no tampons)
	Return for increasing pain or pain persisting for >1 week
	Return for increased bleeding
Third- and fourth-degree lacerations	Avoid constipation
	Avoid narcotics
	Avoid bulking agents (e.g., Metamucil)
	Avoid laxatives and suppositories
	Low fiber, low residue diet (see Table 20-5)
	Stool softeners (e.g., docusate 100 mg BID)
Periurethral lacerations	Call if difficulty urinating

Table 20-5

Low-Residue, Low-Fiber Diet

FOOD GROUP	FOODS THAT ARE LOW IN FIBER	FOODS TO AVOID
Breads, cereals, grains	Breads, rolls, muffins, bagels made from white flour and without nuts or seeds Pancakes (except buckwheat) Graham crackers, saltines Pasta Ready-to-eat cereals made from corn, rice, or white flour Hot cereals: Cream of Wheat or grits Broth and noodle or rice soups (e.g., chicken noodle soup)	Breads, muffins, bagels made from whole wheat, bran, rye, pumpernickel, oat, nut, or fruit Whole wheat or rye crackers Brown rice, barley, bulgar Ready-to-eat cereals made from granola, whole wheat, oat, or bran Hot cereals: oatmeal, wheat, or whole grains Popcorn
Fruits, vegetables	Canned or peeled fruit Cooked vegetables (except those listed under foods to avoid) Fruit and vegetable juices Mushrooms Iceberg lettuce Vegetable soups (except those listed under foods to avoid)	Fresh oranges, berries Dried fruit Raw vegetables Broccoli, corn, succotash, peas (green or black-eyed), mixed vegetables, potato skin, beans (except green or wax), cooked or raw Soups: bean, pea, lentil, minestrone
Meats, fish, poultry, eggs	Any	None
Dairy	Any	None

together promote the formation of nonbulky soft stools. Patients should not use any suppositories or laxatives, as they can cause diarrhea.

Postoperative Complications

Both short- and long-term complications can occur following episiotomy and laceration repairs. The most important short-term complications are hematoma and infection. The most important long-term complications are fecal incontinence and persistent perineal pain.

HEMATOMA

PRESENTATION   Patients with hematomas have often had a forceps delivery, and typically present with pain or rectal pressure out of proportion to what would be expected from the repair performed. They may also have urinary retention. On rare occasions, if blood loss into the hematoma has been considerable, the patient may present with hypovolemic shock. Physical examination reveals unilateral perineal or vaginal swelling and a palpable mass on bimanual examination.

DIAGNOSIS   Perineal hematomas are usually obvious to the examiner. Patients have unilateral marked swelling with discoloration, pain, urinary obstruction, and a palpable tender mass at the site of the hematoma. Vaginal hematomas, on the other hand, are often missed because there may be no findings apparent on casual inspection of the perineum. Therefore, patients who complain of vaginal pain or rectal pressure should undergo a bimanual examination to permit identification of a tender unilateral mass within the vagina. For both vaginal and perineal hematomas, it is important to carefully note the size of the lesion as a reference for subsequent examinations, to permit detection of an enlarging hematoma.

TREATMENT   General measures should be instituted to provide circulatory support, including intravenous fluids and blood transfusions if needed. Hemoglobin and hematocrit levels should be monitored, and a Foley catheter should be inserted to provide relief of urinary obstruction, as well as to monitor urine output. Consultation with an experienced surgeon should be considered on identification of a hematoma, so that surgical intervention (i.e., evacuation of the hematoma), if needed, will not be delayed.

Management of perineal hematomas involves application of ice packs to the perineum and evacuation of enlarging hematomas with closure of the dead space after evacuation. A compression dressing should be applied, regardless of whether the hematoma required evacuation.

Vaginal hematomas can be managed with vaginal compression packing to tamponade the hematoma. Packing is usually left in place for 12 to 24 hours and then slowly removed (removing a small part of the packing every 20 to 30 minutes). If the hematoma expands despite vaginal packing, it will require evacuation.

INFECTION

PRESENTATION   The majority of women with an infected episiotomy or laceration will complain of pain and foul-smelling discharge. They may also be febrile. However, it is often difficult to distinguish normal postpartum pain from the pain associated with an infection, making physical examination essential if infection is suspected.

DIAGNOSIS   When examining a patient with a suspected infection of an episiotomy or laceration, it is important to keep in mind that the perineum will normally show some inflammatory changes (i.e., erythema and tenderness) during the first few postpartum days. Infections are distinguished from the normal postepisiotomy inflammation by the degree of inflammation and the presence of foul-smelling purulent discharge and/or necrotic tissue.

Other tests such as white blood cell counts and cultures usually are not helpful in making the diagnosis of infection, because white blood cell counts are usually elevated in all laboring and postpartum women, and cultures taken from the infection site usually grow multiple organisms. However, white blood cell counts may be helpful when following the trend in leukocytosis when patients have an active infection, and cultures that grow group A beta-hemolytic streptococci may indicate the presence or development of necrotizing fasciitis.

TREATMENT   Infections of the perineum require prompt surgical intervention. Surgical intervention may be as simple as opening the wound or as complicated as an extensive resection of necrotic tissue when patients have necrotizing fasciitis. For patients with necrotizing fasciitis, the earlier the intervention the better the outcome.

Antibiotics should be started at time of diagnosis. Broad-spectrum coverage, to include gram-positive, gram-negative, and anaerobic organisms, is usually required.

FECAL INCONTINENCE

PRESENTATION   Fecal incontinence will develop in as many as 10% of women following repair of third- and fourth-degree lacerations, even if repair techniques were appropriate. Incontinence may develop immediately postpartum, or its presentation may be delayed for days or weeks. Delayed presentation most commonly results from wound dehiscence and/or infection. The incontinence may occur on performance of a Valsalva maneuver (stress fecal incontinence), or it may present as urgency or as fecal soiling.

DIAGNOSIS AND TREATMENT   Physical examination may reveal a rectovaginal fistula or decreased or absent rectal sphincter tone. In some cases, an overt defect in the anal sphincter ring may be seen. Fecal incontinence following third- or fourth-degree perineal lacerations requires referral to a colorectal surgeon for evaluation and treatment.

PERSISTENT PERINEAL PAIN AND DYSPAREUNIA

PRESENTATION   By 6 weeks postpartum, perineal pain normally has resolved. Some women, however, complain of persistent pain. The pain may be sharp or dull, worse with certain activities or positions, and may or may not be relieved with acetaminophen or ibuprofen. Other women will report pain with intercourse (usually on entry).

DIAGNOSIS   Physical examination may reveal a cause for the pain. The most common identifiable causes are wound dehiscence or scar formation in the vagina or hymeneal ring. Sometimes, there will be an overtly palpable perineal scar.

TREATMENT   For wound dehiscence, treatment consists of allowing time to permit healing of the wound by secondary intention. A minor dehiscence will usually heal by 3 months postpartum, but larger defects may take up to 6 months.

Pain caused by scarring may be relieved by massaging the site with a lubricant to stretch the scar. The patient can perform massage with her fingers or with a vaginal dilator. When dyspareunia occurs, the usual approach is to have the patient gently introduce one finger, then two or more fingers, into the vagina, gradually increasing the number of fingers until intercourse is possible. The process usually occurs over several weeks, and a lubricant such as KY Jelly or Astroglide should always be used.

Long-Term Monitoring, Treatment, and Prognosis

The majority of patients with episiotomies or lacerations have an extremely good outcome, with resolution of pain after 6 weeks postpartum and minimal scarring. In the absence of complications, no long-term monitoring or treatment is required.

Education

Important issues about which patients should be educated include the need for episiotomy as well as self-management and expected outcomes following episiotomy or lacerations.

The Need for Episiotomy

Many women will inquire during their prenatal visits about whether they will require an episiotomy. These inquiries often stem from a concern that a successful delivery means no episiotomy and that performance of an episiotomy often creates an air of "failure."

During prenatal visits, therefore, it is important to briefly explain the indications for episiotomy (perineal edema, breech delivery, twin delivery, instrumented delivery, shoulder dystocia) and the benefits of performing an episiotomy when these indications are present. Similarly, an explanation of the female anatomy and birth process will provide the patient with an understanding of why lacerations sometimes occur.

When obtaining the patient's signature on informed consent forms at the time of delivery, the reasons for episiotomy should again be reviewed, but patients should also understand the potential complications of the procedure. Complications that should be mentioned include bleeding, infection, extension into the rectal sphincter and mucosa, and need for repair. Some patients will refuse an episiotomy, even in the presence of legitimate indications, and their refusals should be respected. However, most patients refuse an episiotomy out of fear, and such refusals may be avoided with adequate prenatal counseling.

Self-Management and Expected Outcomes

Postpartum instructions for patients are provided in Table 20-4. Patients should be informed that majority of patients recover from episiotomy and lacerations without consequence. Pain usually resolves by 4 to 6 weeks, at which time sexual intercourse may be resumed.

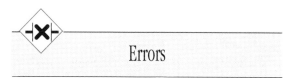

Errors

Four errors related to episiotomy and lacerations are worthy of discussion. The first is performing episiotomy without indication. Other errors include performing indicated episiotomy too soon, failure to diagnose lacerations, and errors in compliance with postpartum instructions.

Performing an Episiotomy without Indication

Because of past teachings about the purported benefits of episiotomy, many clinicians continue to perform episiotomy as a routine procedure. This practice should be discouraged because of recent research demonstrating that routine episiotomy leads to higher rates of third- and fourth-degree lacerations, sexual dysfunction, and incontinence.

Performing an Episiotomy Too Soon

If an episiotomy is to be performed, many clinicians make the error of performing it too early in the second stage of labor. The primary consequence of early episiotomy is bleeding, which can often be reduced by application of pressure to sites of bleeding, although this may be difficult if the delivering clinician is involved in performing a forceps or vacuum delivery. Early episiotomy most often occurs when there is marked fetal caput, with apparent crowning of the presenting part representing caput rather than fetal skull. Early episiotomy is also common during instrumented delivery, when clinicians make the episiotomy incision before the fetal head has dilated the introitus to 3 to 4 cm. When possible, the episiotomy incision should be delayed until there is a sufficient degree of pressure on and stretching of the perineum.

Failure to Diagnose a Laceration

A variety of complications may occur when obstetric lacerations are not identified and repaired. These include short-term complications such as postpartum bleeding and longer recovery times and longer-term complications such as chronic pain, rectovaginal fistulas, and fecal incontinence. The most common cause of failure to diagnose a laceration is failure to perform a careful and thorough examination of the perineum, vagina, and cervix—an entirely avoidable error.

Patient Noncompliance with Postpartum Instructions

New mothers often have little time for sleep, let alone time to follow a clinician's instructions regarding wound care. Prior to hospital discharge, therefore, it is essential that patients, and their families if appropriate, receive education about the importance of self-care to promote wound healing and recovery. Phone or office follow-up, before the routine 6-week postpartum visit, is appropriate for patients with severe lacerations, to reinforce instructions and to ensure that the patient has no complications.

Controversies and Emerging Concepts

The developing trend of "evidence-based medicine" is leading to reexamination of many long-standing medical practices and controversies. The value of many practices related to episiotomy and lacerations has never been studied, such as whether there is measurable benefit to sitz baths and stool softeners, and the preferred type of sutures for episiotomy repair. Similarly, many clinicians debate the relative advantages of midline versus mediolateral episiotomy, and whether episiotomy is of any benefit for preventing pelvic relaxation (rectocele, cystocele) and urinary incontinence. It is likely that future research will be directed at resolving these controversies.

Another future direction for research involves the role of newer, wound-closure techniques such as cyanoacrylate adhesives in repair of episiotomy and lacerations. These techniques have the potential to speed healing and reduce postpartum pain, but there has been no research to study these potential benefits.

References

Bansal RK, Tan WM, Ecker JL, et al: Is there a benefit to episiotomy at spontaneous vaginal delivery? A natural experiment. *Am J Obstet Gynecol* 175:4, 1996.

Belizan JM, Carroli G: Routine episiotomy should be abandoned. *BMJ* 317:1389, 1998.

Cunningham FG, MacDonald PC, Gant NF, et al: *Williams Obstetrics,* 20th ed. Norwalk, CT, Appleton & Lange, 1997.

Ecker JL, Ta WM, Bansal RK, et al: Is there a benefit to episiotomy at operative vaginal delivery? Observations over ten years in a stable population. *Am J Obstet Gynecol* 176:2, 1997.

Flemming N: Can suturing method make a difference in postpartum perineal pain? *J Nurse Midwifery* 35:19, 1990.

Goldaber KG, Wendel PJ, McIntire DD, et al: Postpartum perineal morbidity after fourth-degree perineal repair. *Am J Obstet Gynecol* 168:2, 1993.

Grant A: The choice of suture materials and techniques for repair of perineal trauma: an overview of evidence from controlled trials. *Br J Obstet Gynaecol* 96:1281, 1989.

Helwig JT, Thorp JM, Bowes WA: Does midline episiotomy increase the risk of third- and fourth-degree lacerations in operative vaginal deliveries? *Obstet Gynecol* 82:2, 1993.

Klein MC, Gauthier RJ, Kaczorowski J, et al: Relationship of episiotomy to perineal trauma and morbidity, sexual dysfunction, and pelvic floor relation. *Am J Obstet Gynecol* 171:591, 1994.

Klein MC, Janssen PA, MacWilliam L, et al: Determinants of vaginal-perineal integrity and pelvic floor functioning in childbirth. *Am J Obstet Gynecol* 176:403, 1997.

Labrecque M, Baillargeon L, Dallaire M, et al: Association between median episiotomy and severe perineal lacerations in primiparous women. *Can Med Assoc J* 156:6, 1997.

Lede RL, Belizan JM, Carroli G, et al: Is routine use of episiotomy justified? *Am J Obstet Gynecol* 174:5, 1996.

Mackrodt C, Gordon B, Fern E, et al: The Ipswich Childbirth Study. I. A randomised evaluation of two-stage postpartum perineal repair leaving the skin unsutured. *Br J Obstet Gynaecol* 105:435, 1998.

Mackrodt C, Gordon B, Fern E, et al: The Ipswich Childbirth Study. II. A randomised comparison of polyglactin 910 with chromic catgut for postpartum perineal repair. *Br J Obstet Gynaecol* 105:441, 1998.

May JL: Modified median episiotomy. *Obstet Gynecol* 83:1, 1994.

Renfrew MJ, Hannah W, Albers L, Floyd E: Practices that minimize trauma to the genital tract in childbirth: a systematic review of the literature. *Birth* 25:143, 1998.

Signorello LB, Harlow BL, Chekos AK, et al: Midline episiotomy and anal incontinence retrospective cohort study. *BMJ* 320:86, 2000.

Thacker SB, Banta HD: Benefits and risks of episiotomy: an interpretative review of the English language literature, 1860–1980. *Obstet Gynecol Surv* 38:6, 1983.

Way S: Episiotomy and body image. *Modern Midwife* 6:18, 1996.

Williams FL, du V Florey C, Mires GJ, Ogston SA: Episiotomy and perineal tears in a low-risk UK primigravidas. *J Public Health Med* 20:422, 1998.

Wood J, Amos L, Rieger N: Third-degree anal sphincter tears: risk factors and outcomes. *Aust N Z J Obstet Gynecol* 38:414, 1998.

Wooley RJ: Benefits and risks of episiotomy: a review of the English-language literature since 1980. Part I. *Obstet Gynecol Surv* 50:11, 1995.

Wooley RJ: Benefits and risks of episiotomy: a review of the English-language literature since 1980. Part II. *Obstet Gynecol Surv* 50:11, 1995.

Index

Page numbers followed by f indicate figure; those followed by t indicate table.